APHASIA AND
ASSOCIATED DISORDERS
TAXONOMY, LOCALIZATION, AND RECOVERY

APHASIA AND ASSOCIATED DISORDERS
TAXONOMY, LOCALIZATION, AND RECOVERY

Andrew Kertesz, M.D., F.R.C.P. (C)

Associate Professor, Department of Clinical Neurological Sciences and the Department of Medicine, University of Western Ontario, London, Ontario

Head, Department of Clinical Neurological Sciences, St. Joseph's Hospital, London, Ontario

Honorary Lecturer, Communicative Disorders Programme, University of Western Ontario, London, Ontario

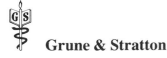

Grune & Stratton

A Subsidiary of Harcourt Brace Jovanovich, Publishers

New York   London   Toronto   Sydney   San Francisco

Grune & Stratton, Inc.
111 Fifth Avenue
New York, New York 10003

Distributed in the United Kingdom by
Academic Press, Inc. (London) Ltd.
24/48 Oval Road, London NW 1

Library of Congress Catalog Card Number 79-17013
International Standard Book Number 0-8089-1193-7

Printed in the United States of America

To My Teachers in Neurology and Aphasiology

TABLE OF CONTENTS

FOREWORD

In the English speaking countries of North America there are probably about 200,000 new cases of stroke a year among which there are, by a reasonable guess, over 50,000 patients suffering from a disabling degree of aphasia. Many of these patients, indeed probably the majority, remain severely disabled by this deficit for many years. In the face of frequency of this problem in everyday clinical practice and in the face of the many years of chronic disability caused by this disorder, it is remarkable that aphasia has been so neglected by physicians—not only by the medical profession at large but also by specialists in neurology and neurosurgery. In my medical school days the word aphasia could almost never be found, except in passing in the medical journals. Although an interest in aphasia was one of the main reasons for my taking up neurological training, I was amazed to discover that many neurologists regarded the study of disorders of language as an esoteric field suitable only for those with an excessively philosophical bent and void of either practical interest or of relevance to research on the nervous system. There was, in fact, a common idea, often explicitly put into words, that an interest in aphasia was the first sign of dementia in a neurologist!

These rather curious and, in fact, bizarre attitudes have not wholly disappeared. Yet aphasia is not rare; it is a major cause of disability, and, since it involves a function whose development in the human brain far outstrips that in any other species, it represents a problem of major theoretical importance. The doctor who is ignorant in this area is capable of making major errors, both in diagnosis and prognosis. Even today there are probably still patients with the fluently aphasic types of disorders and without elementary motor or sensory findings who are misdiagnosed as psychotic. Furthermore, while it is true that the prognosis of most persistent aphasias is poor, it is unfortunate that patients with those syndromes, who often have excellent recovery, are given unduly poor prognoses.

The reader of this book, even the casual reader, will certainly not make such elementary errors. The careful reader of the book who refers to it repeatedly will have expert knowledge. The book repeatedly stresses the practical aspect of the syndromes of aphasia. The elegant testing procedures can be used readily for diagnosis and prognosis. The discussions of techniques of localization and particularly the use of computerized tomography will be extremely valuable to anyone who has to assess patients and to decide on etiology. Finally, the particularly difficult problem of recovery from aphasia, both spontaneous and in relation to therapy, is very well discussed and is an excellent practical guide for the clinician dealing with the patient and the family.

It is a particular pleasure for me to write the foreword to this book, not only because of its inherent value, but also because Dr. Kertesz is an old and close associate. He was one of the early fellows to serve on the Aphasia Ward of the Boston Veterans Administration Hospital during my stay at the institution. Since his return to Canada he has become one of the authorities in this field. I have no doubt that he will be in the forefront of many of the changes that will occur in the next few years, and the reader of his book will equally be prepared for those changes. The therapy of aphasia will probably undergo radical changes. One is already observing the development of ingenious new retraining approaches that combine both recent knowledge of hemispheric specialization with advances in technology. The widespread availability of computers in the home will probably open a new era in aphasia therapy, while the rapid advance of biological knowledge concerning the connections in pharmacology in the brain will probably lead to a new period of medical therapies. It will continue to be essential to have simple and powerful methods for evaluating the effects of new forms of therapy. Andy Kertesz and his readers will be prepared for these changes.

Norman Geschwind, M.D.
James Jackson Putnam Professor of Neurology
Harvard Medical School

Director, Neurological Unit
Beth Israel Hospital
Boston, Massachusetts

PREFACE

Much of this book is related to more than ten years of experience in our aphasia laboratory with more than 500 patients, most of them aphasics with infarcts. The uniqueness of our laboratory is its setting in an acute hospital, allowing us to see patients early and localize their lesions, as well as follow them at regular intervals. A major goal of this book was the synthesis of information from the literature to complement the individual experience from the laboratory, thereby creating a dual purpose text:
1. to summarize up-to-date knowledge in a form that is not available elsewhere, and
2. to present new data with a novel approach and technique.

The crucial issues of classification, testing, localization, and recovery are covered, as well as the relationship of aphasia to intelligence, apraxia, alexia, and agraphia. Many linguistic and neuropsychological issues, although greatly relevant to aphasia, were not included, of course, since other recent reviews have done an excellent job of covering these.

The technical information is sufficiently referenced and built up gradually so as to make it intelligible to those who are getting acquainted with the topic; the new data are presented in depth for those already involved in the field. The statistics cited in this book are used only as a tool and not as an end in themselves. Those not mathematically inclined can easily leave out the details of the taxonomic method and the statistical tables of various chapters. The introductory sections of all chapters, and specifically Chapters 1 through 3, 8, 11 through 16, can be perused as a textbook of aphasiology. Chapter 4 deals with the standardization of our text and the population on which the data in this book are based. Many chapters contain new data to support the theoretical framework.

Although it is impossible to describe accurately all the contributions and input received, I am greatly indebted to the Boston School of Neurologists, Psychologists, and Aphasiologists for their important ideas and inspiration. I am grateful to Dr. C. Shewan for her contribution to the statistics and reliability studies and for her editorial advice with Chapters 2 through 4, 15, and 16, and to Dr. J. Phipps for the actual performance of the computations of taxonomic steps and numerous discussions on numerical taxonomy. A great deal of credit is due to my associates of long duration, Betty Poole and Patricia McCabe, for their endurance and skill in testing so many patients. Wil Harlock and Patricia McCabe contributed substantially to the actual collection, analysis, and organization of data in the book. Some data collection and analysis were done by Bob Kormos, Shel Krakofsky, Greg Hasen, Jonathan Lomas, Jeanette McGlone, and Mitch Roelfe. The speech pathologists collaborating in the reliability studies were Donna Bandur, Jane Brenneman, Janice Elliott, Sue Lockie, and Dr. C. Shewan. Radiologists Robert Coates, Tom Brown, and David Lesk traced the lesions on the scans. Sally Beech and Chris Sloma provided the secretarial work, and most of the illustrations were the art of Trudy Vandenberg and the photography of Ruth Cooper. Dr. J. Gilbert helped with the clinicopathological correlation in Chapter 8.

While the data were collected and the book was written, I was the recipient of Ontario Health Research Grants PR 721 and DM 324, and an operating grant to our laboratory from the University of Western Ontario. Finally, without the encouragement of Ryo Arai, this work would not have been possible.

1

Classification of Aphasia

*There is only one aphasia . . . – . . . anarthria, . . . anarthria with aphasia, . . .
temporal aphasia, . . . angular gyrus aphasia . . . global aphasia . . .*

Pierre Marie (1906–1917)

INTRODUCTION

Most clinicians will agree that although aphasic disability is complex, many patients are clinically similar and will fall into recurring identifiable groups. This is a basic thesis of this book. There are many classifications, indicating that none is altogether satisfactory, but also that this effort is useful and even necessary to diagnose and treat aphasics or to understand the phenomena. The bewildering proliferation of the nomenclature deters most but the truly devoted to master classification. With clinical experience comes the realization that:

1. Indeed there is a need for classification.
2. The patients and their symptomatology are complex yet similar enough to the experience of others.
3. Many of the classifiers describe the same phenomena from a different angle, and in fact, complement rathe. than contradict each other.

1

The opponents of classification point out the numerous disagreements among observers, the many exceptions that cannot be fitted into categories, and the frequent evolution of certain types into others. They also object to the oversimplification involved in any practical, descriptive system.

The controversy can be reduced to a few issues. Is aphasia a unitary disturbance or are there several kinds of aphasias? The answer, of course, is yes to both. There is something qualitatively different about aphasic language disturbance which sets it apart from dysarthria, mutism, confusion, psychotic speech, just to mention the main problem areas in differential diagnosis. What makes aphasic disturbance so palpably different is difficult to define to everyone's satisfaction, but a multidisciplinary approach may be acceptable to most: *aphasia is a neurologically central disturbance of language characterized by paraphasias, word finding difficulty, and variably impaired comprehension,* associated with disturbance of reading and writing, at times with dysarthria, nonverbal constructional, and problem-solving difficulty and impairment of gesture.

Ever since Broca described "aphemia," and Wernicke sensory aphasia, many clinicians have tried to record their experience and improve the results of classification, and the voluminous literature seems to indicate a need for this. In order to ease the shock and confusion initially experienced when reading about the subject, a table was constructed to summarize the various classifications and to show that these, in fact, cover the same phenomena (Table 1-1). In this table the various terms describing the same disturbance appear underneath each other. Four columns appear to represent the entities, that almost invariably, everybody identifies.

BROCA'S APHASIA

What Broca (1861) described as aphemia, Wernicke (1874) called motor aphasia. Marie (1906) did not consider Broca's aphemia true aphasia. Pick (1913) labeled it "expressive aphasia with agrammatism," and Weisenburg and McBride (1935) popularized "expressive aphasia," which still enjoys favor among many. The problem with the term "expressive" is, of course, that all aphasics have some "expressive" difficulties. Then came the "innovators," such as Henry Head (1926), whose distaste for his predecessors' diagrams resulted in a unique psycholinguistic classification which is difficult to apply to clinical cases. Broca's aphasia thus became "verbal aphasia." After Head, only Wepman (1951) used similar terminology extensively in the literature. Luria's (1964) physiological concepts led to "efferent motor" aphasia. Jacobson's (1964) linguistic approach used "contiguity" or "combination" disorders for this phenomenon, and Osgood (1963) called it "encoding" disturbance. Schuell's (1964) classification is highly individualistic and difficult to correlate with others. Her Group 3, "severe reduction of language" with "sensorimotor" disturbance, corresponds best to Broca's aphasia. Bay (1964), like Marie (1906), considered "aphemia" different from aphasia and gave it the term "cortical dysarthria," a theoretical deviation from the consensus which considers these patients aphasic. "Anarthria," the term used by Marie for the same phenomenon, is used by modern neurologists to describe the most severe dysarthria, due to bulbar or "pseudobulbar" paralysis (Critchley, 1970). Recently, interest in aphemia or cortical dysarthria has been renewed by Darley (1964) and other speech pathologists, who have popularized the term "apraxia of speech" or "verbal apraxia" to identify a purely motor speech disorder, distinct from dysarthria and often seen in association with aphasia. Darley (1964) and Johns and Lapointe (1976) emphasize the necessity to separate this entity from the rest of the aphasias, from the point of view of therapy. The relationship of Broca's aphasia to apraxia of speech remains controversial. Geschwind (1965), DeRenzi et al. (1966), and Heilman (1973) suggest that Broca's aphasia and facial apraxia may vary independently. Many cases of marked "verbal apraxia" have comprehension deficit, and the articulatory disorder is similar to the phonemic paraphasias seen in other aphasics. Yet there are some patients in whom the articulatory disorder is distinctive enough to justify nosologic separation.

More recent clinically and linguistically oriented classifications place an emphasis on the fluency – nonfluency dichotomy in aphasia. Goodglass and Kaplan (1972) and many others have recognized the clinical relevance of measuring fluency. They also advocate the retention of the classic eponym "Broca's aphasia," rather than using "motor" or "expressive" aphasia, in order to avoid suggesting that speech output is normal in other forms of aphasia. The agrammatism of Broca's aphasia is characterized by the relative preservation of substantive words in contrast to the syntactical modifiers. Short nouns are more likely to remain than verbs (telegraphic speech). Only short propositional phrases or automatic sentences appear. The linguistic analysis of comprehension in Broca's aphasia suggested that this parallels the expressive difficulties. These patients have more difficulty comprehending grammatical modifiers than substantive words; a similarly specific deficit for reading exists also.

Much of the controversy about Broca's aphasia centers around the existence of comprehension deficit. These patients are characterized by relatively well-preserved comprehension and their major disability is in language output. However, if comprehension is examined extensively, it is found to be impaired to a certain extent, almost without exception. This prompted many investigators to emphasize that comprehension deficit is an all-pervasive feature of aphasia, and that the variable amount of motor difficulty, at times labeled "cortical dysarthria," superimposed on aphasia results in the variation of the clinical picture called "Broca's aphasia." Mohr (1978) makes the point that persisting Broca's aphasia, with severely reduced speech output and agrammatisms, is the result of a large infarct extending beyond Broca's area, and Broca's area involvement results in mild, usually transient, motor speech disturbance. He usefully splits the

Table 1–1

Classification of Aphasias

AUTHORS		1	2		
Broca	1861	Aphemia	Verbal Amnesia		
Wernicke	1874 and 1886	Motor / Subcortical Motor	Sensory / Subcortical Sensory	Conduction	
Marie	1906 and 1917	Anarthria Anarthria + Aphasia	Temporal Aphasia		
Pick	1913 and 1931	Expressive (Frontal)	Impressive (Temporal)	Agrammatism	
Head	1926	Verbal	Syntactic		
Kleist	1934	Word Muteness	Word Deafness		
Weisenburg and McBride	1935	Expressive	Receptive	Mixed	
Goldstein	1948	Peripheral Motor Cortical Motor	Cortical Sensory	Central	
Wepman	1961	Syntactic (Verbal)	Pragmatic Jargon		
Schuell	1964	III (Sensorimotor)	I + II + III	IV (?)	
Nielsen	1946	Apractic	Auditory Verbal Agnosia Formulation		
Brain	1961	Pure Word Dumbness Broca's	Pure Word Deafness	Central	
Bay	1962	Cortical Dysarthria	Sensory		
Luria	1964	Efferent Motor	Sensory	Afferent Motor Acoustic Amnestic	
Osgood	1963	Encoding	Decoding		
Jacobson	1964	Contiguity (Combination)	Similarity (Selection)		
Howes and Geschwind	1965	Type A (Nonfluent)	Type B (Fluent)		
Benson and Geschwind	1971	Aphemia Broca's	Pure Word Deafness Wernicke's	Conduction	
Leischner	1972	Motor Motor Amnestic	Sensory Mixed Sensory Amnestic Central		
Goodglass and Kaplan	1972	Broca's	Wernicke's	Conduction	
Taxonomic	1977	Broca's	Wernicke's	Efferent Conduction Afferent Conduction	

The authors of the left-sided column originated or popularized the terminologies. The columns labeled 1–4 are

3	4			
		Transcortical Motor	Transcortical Sensory	
Angular Gyrus Aphasia	Global			
Pseudoagrammatism		Adynamic		
Semantic Nominal				
Paragrammatism		Transcortical		
Amnesic	Mixed			
Amnesic	Global	Transcortical Motor	Transcortical Sensory	Mixed Echolalic
Semantic	Global			
I (Simple)	V (Severe)			
Semantic (Formulation) Object				
Nominal	Mixed Total			
Amnesic		Echolalic		
Semantic Amnestic	Global	Dynamic		
Semantic Paradigmatic				
Anomic	Global	Transcortical Motor	Transcortical Sensory	Isolation
Semantic Amnestic	Total			
Anomic	Global	Transcortical Motor	Transcortical Sensory	
Semantic Anomic	Global	Transcortical Motor	Transcortical Sensory	Isolation

the most frequently described entities and are described in detail in the text.

traditional entity of Broca's aphasia on the basis of persistence, and lesion size and location.

Most clinicians agree, however, that motor aphasia, primarily expressive aphasia or Broca's aphasia, is an identifiable, common, aphasic syndrome with scant, hesitant, effortful and paraphasic, spontaneous speech, at times, slightly better repetition, and relatively good comprehension. Besides the restriction of vocabulary and grammar, there is, often, impaired articulation. They read aloud poorly, but reading comprehension is often good. Writing is affected similarly to speech. The variability of features and severity led to splitting and redefinition of the syndrome by some authors, although it continues as a real entity in the clinic and in research.

WERNICKE'S APHASIA

Sensory aphasia, as described by Wernicke (1874) in his famous paper "Der aphasische symptomenkomplex" is recognized by everyone, with the notable exception of Hughlings Jackson. Jackson's (1879) hierarchial view of language dissolution included "jargon" as a disturbance of expression, but these recurrent utterances were more stereotypic than the profuse phonemic or semantic jargon of sensory aphasia. Marie (1906) claimed that sensory aphasia was the only true aphasia and this is still championed by Bay (1964). Schuell (1964) was also impressed by the auditory disturbance as the *sine qua non* of aphasia. Curiously, her classification does not have a single group which could be identified unequivocally with sensory or Wernicke's aphasia. Head (1926), like Wepman and Schuell after him, in order to avoid the input−output dichotomy and the notion of pure language defects, created novel classifications, deviating from the clinically obvious, and confusing generations of readers for many years. His syntactic aphasia is not the same as Wepman's, who called sensory aphasia "pragmatic," and the motor, "syntactic." Jacobson's (1964) "similarity" or "selection" disorder encompasses a range of clinical disturbances, such as "sensory," "semantic," and "acoustic amnestic" aphasia, as he used Luria's (1964) terminology. According to Jacobson, sensory aphasia is characterized linguistically by preserved syntactic units, and phonemic combinations, although certain phonemic distinctions are lost. Osgood's (1963) decoding disturbance is in this category also.

Jargon aphasia is at times identified as a separate entity, although most writers will classify it with Wernicke's or sensory aphasia. The fluent, profusely paraphasic speech may be usefully subdivided into semantic and neologistic jargon (Kertesz and Benson, 1970), depending on the degree of phonemic distortions or neologisms [the paraphasic and asemantic jargon of Alajouanine (1956)]. These patients are often curiously unaware of their faulty communication and this is described as "anosognosia" for speech. Their speech is often under pressure, "logorrheic." The variability of language production in Wernicke's aphasia induced some to split the symptom complex further. Huber et al. (1975), for instance, differentiate four varieties, such as with (1) predominantly semantic paraphasias, (2) semantic jargon, (3) phonemic paraphasias, and (4) phonemic jargon, although a qualitative basis for the discrimination is not provided.

Wernicke's aphasia, as described by Goodglass and Kaplan (1972), features impaired comprehension and fluently articulated, but paraphasic, speech. Nouns are most often substituted by paraphasias and other substantive, informative elements of speech are missing, in spite of the fluent use of grammatical connecting words, complex verb tenses, and embedded subordinate clauses. The syntax and prosody of language is retained to a greater extent. Their speech is paragrammatic rather than agrammatic, as in Broca's aphasia. Augmentation and pressure of speech is, at times, associated with phonemic or semantic jargon. Impaired recognition, naming or word-finding difficulty, and impaired reading and writing are always present. At times, the fluent paraphasic writing with repetitious phrases resembles spoken jargon (see a sample of this "graphorrhea" in Chapter 12). Since various degrees of impairment are seen and the fringes of the entity are often ill-defined and controversial, retention of the eponym seems useful to describe this clinically valid and common aphasic impairment.

ANOMIC APHASIA

Probably the largest group of aphasics, which is variously called anomic or amnesic aphasia, have relatively little expressive or receptive difficulty. Their speech is fluent, although at times very circumlocutory or empty, occasionally paraphasic, and shows obvious word-finding difficulty. Their verbal paraphasias are semantic substitutions, rather than phonemic (literal) distortions. They have near normal comprehension and repetition, but their naming is most often impaired. However, at times, naming on a confrontation test is surprisingly good and word-finding difficulty is only evidenced in spontaneous speech or prolonged testing with low frequency items. Other times, spontaneous speech is nearly normal and the main deficit is in naming. This syndrome often appears *de novo* or it may be the end result of recovering from other syndromes, such as Wernicke's, conduction, or the transcortical aphasias. Some aphasiologists object to classifying the recovered group as anomic aphasics even though they are very difficult to distinguish from the primary syndrome objectively.

Although Broca himself spoke about "verbal amnesia," this entity was not defined until Goldstein (1924) described amnesic aphasia as an impairment of "abstract attitude." An argument against this "categorical defect" is that often the circumlocutions by the patients are excellent abstractions. Henry Head (1926) described nominal aphasia as a difficulty in naming, but included impaired understanding of names as part of the disturbance, which is contrary to what clinicians usually find in this picture.

Luria (1977) described three different forms of amnestic aphasia. The first is a disturbance of the "optical" basis of naming, close to optic agnosia. The second is a disturbance of perception and retention of the phonemic structure, resulting in literal paraphasias. This is also characterized as a sensory disturbance in word finding, seen in temporal lesions. The third variety is a selection of disturbance with semantic paraphasias and good response to prompting. This primary or "pure" amnesic aphasia is seen with parietal lesions.

GLOBAL APHASIA

Another common aphasic group is universally called global or total aphasia, because of the severity of involvement of both expressive and receptive functions. The patient does not communicate, and what is said is only a stereotypic repetitive utterance, at times, an expletive without semantic value. Occasionally these utterances are used quite fluently, with inflection and associated emotional expression conveying some meaning. Comprehension seems almost entirely absent and even when one has the impression that the patient "looks comprehending," the expressive outlets are so limited that it cannot be tested. Similarly, repetition and naming are very poor. Recent studies of recovery indicate that quite a few global patients regain enough comprehension to be considered Broca's aphasics. (Kertesz and McCabe, 1977; Mohr et al., 1978). There is as yet no reliable feature initially to distinguish these patients who will recover comprehension from those who will not, except that those who will recover are often more attentive and alert. In our computerized tomography (C.T.) study (Chapter 10), the lesion size of these patients appears to be an early predictor of clinical recovery; those patients who are reclassified at 3−6 months as Broca's aphasics do not have as much temporo-parietal tissue destruction as those who remain global. Blumstein et al. (1977) used the term "mixed anterior" aphasia for this group of nonfluent aphasics with significant comprehension impairment. This group is seen with some recovery from global aphasia. At times, some of its members are designated as persistent severe Broca's aphasia. These patients appear to occupy a distinct enough place between global and Broca's aphasia on the nosological continuum that in the future they may be treated as separate by most investigators.

There are a few patients, often elderly, with severe aphasia who have fluent but mumbling speech, which may be mistaken for jargon, but the utterances are stereotypic, lacking the phonemic variability of neologistic jargon aphasia. These patients may be misclassified as Wernicke's aphasia. When repetition is not tested, the occasional patient with isolation syndrome (see below) may be considered to have global aphasia.

CONDUCTION APHASIA

There are aphasics who are less universally classified. A group of relatively fluent patients having good comprehension but poor repetition, and a great deal of phonemic paraphasias, was called *conduction aphasia* (Leitungsaphasie) by Wernicke (1874), on the basis of the theoretical consideration that conduction of sensory impulses to motor patterns is impaired. Lichtheim (1885) specified the disturbance of repetition as a feature of conduction aphasia, and Wernicke incorporated this idea in his 1908 paper. Kleist (1916) viewed conduction aphasia as word deafness associated with speech apraxia and partially compensated for by the right hemisphere. Many clinicians doubted the justification of separating this group from others with sensory and motor impairment. Weisenburg and McBride (1935) claimed that they have not seen a case which would clearly show the picture of conduction aphasia, in contrast to Goldstein's (1948) description of "central" aphasia, and those of Isserlin (1936), Konorski (1961), Geschwind (1965), Benson (1973), Green and Howes (1977), and many others who considered it an independent form. Delineation is possible on the basis of disturbed repetition, which is out of proportion to the relatively fluent, spontaneous, or responsive speech and good comprehension.

The fluency in conduction aphasics is variable. At times it is restricted to brief bursts of speech. At other times some of these patients have a great deal of struggling to approximate the target phonemes (conduit d'approche). Some of these patients resemble Broca's aphasics and it is difficult to separate them with certainty. Luria called this group of patients afferent motor aphasics (1964). Dubois et al. (1964) considered conduction aphasia a form of expressive aphasia, although the pattern of impairment appeared distinct from motor aphasia. They called it a disorganized execution of the encoding program, related to disturbed "auditory feedback." The patient's awareness of his own mistakes and his efforts to correct them were emphasized. The repetitition deficit in conduction aphasia has also been viewed as a disturbance in short term verbal memory (Warrington and Shallice, 1969), an ordering deficiency (Tzortzis and Albert, 1974), and a disorder of reproduction (Shallice and Warrington, 1977). The unity of conduction aphasia has also been questioned (Benson et al., 1973). Our numerical taxonomic studies (Kertesz and Phipps, 1977), in fact, showed the bimodal distribution of conduction aphasics. There is also evidence from studies of localization of defects in conduction aphasia confirming the existence of a less fluent group with more anterior lesions, along with a more fluent group with more posterior lesions (Kertesz et al., 1977). We took the liberty of calling the first group "efferent conduction aphasia," and the second, "afferent conduction aphasia" in a cautious attempt to update the terminology.

TRANSCORTICAL APHASIAS

The clinical picture opposite to conduction aphasia is called echolalic or *transcortical aphasia,* when repetition is preserved out of proportion compared to the other language functions. These patients were subdivided by Wernicke (1908) and Goldstein (1948) into *transcortical motor* (TCM), showing poor output but good comprehension and repetition; *transcortical sensory* (TCS), characterized by poor comprehension but fluent speech and good repetition; and *mixed echolalic,* featuring poor comprehension, poor output but good repetition, similar but qualitatively different from nonaphasic echolalia. The identity of these syndromes is defined by repetition and one has to test for it specifically. However, one only has to see a few TCM cases to recognize the patient who says practically nothing spontaneously, but comprehends everything and repeats amazingly well. Pick (1905) described "Adynamie der Schprache." Kleist (1934) subsequently wrote about adynamic and Luria about dynamic aphasia (1964), which seems to be the same entity as transcortical motor aphasia. Luria and Tsvetkova (1968), however, insisted that dynamic aphasia was distinct, representing a disturbance of the predicative function of speech or "inner speech." The localization of lesions producing transcortical motor aphasia has been known to be related to the "supplementary speech area" of Penfield (see Chapter 8); recent isotope studies (Rubens, 1975; Kertesz, 1977) confirmed this feature. At times, the same or similar syndrome seems to be produced by smaller lesions, right under or in Broca's area. The uniformly rapid recovery and good prognosis underline the importance of this clinically distinct entity.

Isolation of the speech area was described by Goldstein (1948) as the mechanism for mixed transcortical aphasia where repetition is spared but spontaneous speech and comprehension are lost. He thought that the speech mechanism had to be intact but isolated from the rest of the conceptual processes in the brain. One such patient was observed to sing along with a radio and complete and repeat sentences without comprehension or spontaneous speech, and on autopsy was found to have lesions due to carbon monoxide poisoning surrounding but not directly involving the parasylvian speech area (Geschwind et al., 1968). A detailed linguistic analysis of the dissociation of voluntary and automatic aspects of language was done in an echolalic demented patient by Whitaker (1976). Automatic aspects of grammar and linguistically restricted comprehension appeared to be spared. Nonaphasic echolalia is considered a common, nonspecific feature in dementia. Some authors do not consider these syndromes aphasic. Partial isolation syndrome has been seen in strokes and trauma in our clinic (see Chapters 9 and 10).

Transcortical (echolalic) sensory aphasia is characterized by fluent but often irrelevant speech, good repetition, and poor comprehension. It is most often seen in posttraumatic cases and is often transient. At times, it is lumped together with the isolation syndrome. Investigators in rehabilitation units do not see these patients as often as those in general hospitals, and TCS does not seem to occur with strokes as frequently. Many classifications will acknowledge the existence of only those aphasic defects which tend to persist in time. This way, some very interesting and theoretically important language disturbances remain unrecognized.

SEMANTIC APHASIA

Semantic aphasia was described originally by Head, and meant impaired word–meaning relationships and difficulty in formulating the goals of the speaker. The linguistic classification of Jacobson and Luria continued to use the term. Although discussed in detail by Jason Brown (1972), there is no succinct definition. Semantic paraphasias differ from those in anomic aphasia, in that they tend to be less related to the target word, and they tend to condition further discourse. The patient is unaware of the errors, unlike in anomic aphasia. Luria (1964) conceived semantic aphasia as the deficit of simultaneous synthesis. Complex comparative constructions, interrelated subordination of words, and prepositional relations appear to be impaired most in the 30 cases described by Luria (1977). Interestingly, in our mathematical taxonomy, there is a group which is close but distinct from anomic aphasia, with more paraphasias and comprehension difficulty, which is not severely enough affected to group it with Wernicke's (or sensory) aphasia. It may be realistic to preserve the distinction between semantic and anomic aphasia, reserving the term anomic for the purer disturbance of word-finding and naming, and semantic for mild impairment of comprehension, associated with verbal, semantic paraphasias. Undoubtedly, others would classify some of these patients as having mild Wernicke's aphasia.

MODALITY SPECIFIC APHASIAS

Modality specific aphasias are rare and seldom if ever "pure." Isolated output processing disorder, *"pure word dumbness," "aphemia," "anarthria," "verbal apraxia"* (also discussed under Broca's aphasia) is rarely without some associated disturbance of comprehension, provided the appropriately difficult tests are used; therefore, it should be considered aphasia rather than dysarthria. Liepmann (1900) used the term *articulatory apraxia,* and even before him, Broca described a "disordered faculty of coordinating the movements necessary for articulate language." *Aphemia* was Broca's term for what we now consider severe, persistent Broca's aphasia, but Bastian (1898) and more recently Geschwind (1965) used the term for the pure motor disturbance. Marie called this *anarthria,* a term which is now infrequently used; to some people, it means severe dysarthria, in which writing is intact. *Subcortical motor aphasia* was Wernicke's (1874) term for pure motor aphasia (Dejerine, 1914), but it is rarely if ever used now. Alajouanine et al. (1939) called it phonetic disintegration of language and tried to show that it was due to paresis, apraxia or dystonia of the speech musculature. Hecaen (1972) thought that phonematic aphasia was accompanied by agraphia most of the time, in contrast to most other authors. None of these terms, including *apraxia of speech,* are entirely satisfactory or acceptable to the majority of aphasiologists, even though most acknowledge the existence of a purer and milder motor disturbance in which the articulatory and prosodic difficulties are outstanding. It appears different from Broca's aphasia, which has more agrammatism and comprehension difficulty.

Pure Word Deafness (P.W.D.), a term originating with Kussmaul (1877), is rarely if ever "pure." Lichtheim (1885) called it *isolated speech deafness* and *subcortical sensory aphasia.* Most descriptions acknowledge the additional presence of word finding or naming difficulty and/or paraphasias, and variable amounts of hearing deficit to pure tones or other acoustic stimuli. Reading comprehension, writing, spontaneous speech and hearing noises are preserved, but the comprehension and repetition of speech are very poor. It is usually found in the course of evolution of Wernicke's aphasia (Klein and Harper, 1956; Gazzaniga et al., 1973). Although P.W.D. is usually associated with auditory agnosia for meaningful nonverbal sounds (impaired identification of noises like barking, typewriter, train, etc.), according to Vignolo (1969), their dissociation has been reported also (Spreen et al., 1965; Albert and Bear, 1974). Albert and Bear (1974) postulated that the improved comprehension of slower than normal rates of speech indicated right hemisphere linguistic processing in their left temporal lobe damaged patients with word deafness.

Modality specific anomia is controversial; an often recognized example is the difficulty naming fingers and discriminating right from left in the Gerstmann (1927) syndrome. Although Benton (1961) pointed out that this cluster of symptoms, including agraphia and acalculia, is rarely pure and the components are often disturbed in aphasics, this does not detract from its usefulness in calling attention to the dominant parietal lobe (see Chapter 12).

Pure alexia is a well recognized entity and it will be discussed further in Chapter 11. It is often associated, however, with hemianopia and color-naming defect, just like "pure agraphia" is associated with apraxia or a mild anomia as a rule.

A CRITIQUE

This review of classifications did not intend to be complete. Some systems, although quite extensive, were not included because they are difficult to compare to others. Some authors, such as Nielsen (1946), have overclassified on theoretical grounds to such an extent that it is difficult to justify or relate to clinical facts. Such nomenclature, of course, never becomes widespread. Many authors, fortunately, exercise restraint in devising new terms and try to do research within the framework of existing terminology. There are some aphasiologists who consider the complexity of aphasic phenomenon an unsurmountable barrier to classification. Critchley (1970), in his erudite essay on aphasiological nomenclature, suggested that the logical classification of aphasics was still impractical. In contrast to this, the "diagram makers" such as Lichtheim (1885) attempted to organize the existing clinical experience into a simplified logical system, based on the sensory-motor dichotomy and the associationist theoretical framework. The Lichtheim-Wernicke classification (first row in Table 1-1) withstood the test of time in contrast to the abstract theoretical psycholinguistic system of its chief critic—Henry Head. The "Procrustean beds" have different names, but we cannot avoid them if we are to differentiate among aphasic types. An alternate approach is to take the typical cases only under a certain category and call the rest "mixed aphasics" (Leischner, 1972; Prins, 1978).

The results of classification will be modified to a great extent by the tests used to measure language deficit (see Chapter 2) and to some extent, by the etiology of aphasia. Neoplasms produce different (atypical) syndromes from infarcts and trauma. Unfortunately, this principle is not remembered often enough. We deal with this issue in the chapters on taxonomy, localization and recovery.

The problem of latent, mild, or ingravescent aphasia has concerned most clinicians. Anyone interested in clinical diagnosis or research has come to grips with certain criteria as to where aphasia ends and nonaphasic disturbances or normal language begins. Our chapters on test standardization and recovery address this problem. The disorders of tone and prosody deserve a separate mention in the classification of articulatory or motor disorders of speech. Broadbent (1872) observed an increase in foreign accent in aphasia, and Pick (1913) recognized the importance of modulation as an expression. Monrad-Krohn (1947) described and established firmly the entity of dysprosody as distinct, although at times, associated with aphasia. Schizophasia and the language of psychotics rarely represents a problem in differential diagnosis. Reviews of psychotic language were done by Critchley (1964) and Benson (1973), schizophasia by Chaika (1974) and Lecours (1976), and mania by Durbin and Martin (1977).

Few aphasiologists emphasize the frequency of change from one variety of aphasia to another in the course of recovery, although Leischner (1972) called this instability of categories "Syndromenwandel." In our taxonomic, localizing and recovery studies, careful attention is paid to this important feature.

There is no classification yet which has gained universal acceptance; adoption of a standard one has not been attempted by such interdisciplinary bodies as the American Academy of Aphasia. Perhaps there is fear that a standard classification, even though acceptable or practical, would inhibit fresh approaches or innovative thinking. It is much more likely that any adopted system of nomenclature would quickly become obsolete as new information is acquired. Some classifications are not easily adaptable from one discipline to another. A linguistic typology may not be of much use to a neurologist who wants a reliable system for the localization of lesions.

The contentious issue of mixing anatomical and psychological terms can hardly be avoided in the classification of aphasias. Hughlings Jackson warned against it sternly, yet distinguished neurolinguists such as Pick, Goodglass and Kaplan, etc., continue to make use of the relevant anatomical terms in association with psychological and linguistic ones. Purists (often without anatomical training) object to anatomoclinical classifications. Preconceived and speculative anatomical terminology and classification is not justifiable on the available evidence. On the other hand, designating patients as anterior and posterior aphasics on the basis of their linguistic features alone is not very satisfactory either. Psychological phenomena do not exist in a vacuum, however, and a terminology that reflects our growing knowledge of brain—behavior relationships using anatomical and linguistic concepts is acceptable. As some of the evidence presented further on in this book indicates, there is a discernible relationship between the location of lesions and the clinical syndromes caused by them.

Even though aphasics often need to be classified for diagnosis, therapy, or research, aphasiologists are reluctant to define aphasic types according to measurable parameters. Most investigators are satisfied with impressions of unmeasured performance or established criteria on the basis of one or two parameters, such as the severity or fluency-nonfluency scale. Often, aphasic profiles are constructed according to the performance on various subtests, but the limits or cutoff scores for each symptom complex are not determined. Some authors, like Goodglass and Kaplan (1972), compare individual scores to the z scores of their aphasic population, define the range of scores, and illustrate each syndrome with a typical example. Unless further exclusive limits are defined, this will not allow every patient to be classified unequivocally. This point is made by Goodglass and Kaplan, with the example that mild Wernicke's or Broca's aphasics cannot be distinguished reliably from anomics, at the severity levels of 4 or 5 on the Boston Diagnostic Aphasia Examination. Recently, attempts were made to define clinically recognizable aphasic groups, according to numerical limits of scores obtained in certain tests (Vignolo, 1964 and Kertesz and Poole, 1974). Beyond these intuitive classifications (taxonomies), a mathematical approach to classification became available to biologists and clinicians. Numerical taxonomy, as it is called, can provide objective clusters of aphasics on the basis of test scores, free from the constraints of previous classifications. We published the first classification based on numerical taxonomy (Kertesz and Phipps, 1977). The groups derived from this study have been designated with the traditional terminology and listed in the last line of Table 1-1.

SUMMARY

A brief but comprehensive survey of classifying aphasia reveals that most investigators describe at least four major groups, conveniently labeled Broca's, Wernicke's, anomic, and global aphasia. Conduction and transcortical aphasias are less generally described and modality specific syndromes rarely, if ever, exist purely. The lumpers and splitters have not had their final say in aphasiology, but objective numerical taxonomy may solve some of the problems of classification.

2

Aphasia Tests: Description, Comparison and Evaluation

Round and round like a stage army moves the procession: the clinical appearances are identical, but each fresh group of observers views them with new eyes and with different preconceptions.

Henry Head (1926)

INTRODUCTION

Aphasia testing has been carried out for a long time, though at the earlier stages of descriptive aphasiology, it often consisted of asking the patient questions. From time to time, other items were added to this. Broca, for instance, besides asking Lelong, his second patient, conversational questions, also described his gestures and tested his tongue movements, writing, and arithmetic. Hughlings Jackson tested sign making, writing, comprehension, repetition, reading, and tongue movements, regularly, in addition to spontaneous speech. Pierre Marie felt that comprehension deficit underlies all aphasia and it is only a matter of using difficult enough tests to detect it. He also emphasized that nonverbal intellectual functions were also disturbed. He described the now famous three-paper test of comprehension in which the patient is asked to do various things with three pieces of paper, in sequence. Moutier (1908), Pierre Marie's pupil, published a monograph with a rather complete set of systematic tests for aphasia. In this chapter, an attempt will be made to describe, compare, and evaluate the major clinical tests for aphasia in the English language. Table 3-1 compares the items between subtests of the WAB and other tests.

HENRY HEAD'S TEST

Henry Head (1926) published the first detailed account of a systematic aphasia examination in English. Although his test was not standardized and did not gain popularity as a whole, many parts of it have been reproduced or subsequently modified, and many of his ideas of testing have been adopted. This is a summary to illustrate the careful detail he used to explore all potentially disturbed aspects of language.

Naming and Recognition of Common Objects

Head chose six objects—a pencil, a key, a penny, a matchbox, scissors, and a knife—and asked the patient to point to the object which was presented to him visually, tactually (nonverbal matching), then orally. Next, Head asked the patient to name each object. Following that, he gave the patient cards which bore the names of the objects. The patient was asked to write the name of each object and then, to match the object to its printed name. A similar series of tests were also performed with colors.

The Man, Cat, and Dog Tests

These tests investigated mainly reading and writing, in their most elementary form. The patient was asked to read three word sentences and then form these sentences from pictures only. He was then asked to write them down, and finally, to copy them from print into cursive handwriting.

The Clock Tests

These tests consisted of setting a clock to a sample, then to oral and printed commands. Finally, the clock was set by the examiner and the patient would tell the time aloud or write it down.

The Coin−Bowl Test

This test consisted of placing a coin in one of the bowls, following printed and oral commands. (''Put the second coin into the fourth bowl.'') Henry Head made the statement that no normal person failed to carry out this test correctly, but that in cases of aphasia, it caused considerable difficulty. These sequential commands were similar to those in the Token Test of DeRenzi and Vignolo (1962).

The Hand−Eye−Ear Test

This test was a similar but more complicated version of a sequential comprehension test in the coin−bowl test. The patient was seated opposite the observer and attempted to imitate a series of movements, consisting of touching an eye or an ear with one or the other hand, first on the same side, then crossing the body. Then the patient was placed in front of a large mirror and was asked to imitate the reflected movements of the observer. The patient was then given cards, each of which represented a human figure carrying out one of the target movements. This was the most difficult of all the serial tests and, according to Head, the answers of a normal person might also be defective. The initial commands required a single act only, and then a combination of these orders added up to the complexities of the full Hand−Eye−Ear Test. It was also a test of R (right) and L (left) orientation and, to some extent, praxis.

There were many other tests Henry Head employed more sporadically: writing down the alphabet, the days of the week, or the months of the year; understanding a paragraph from the newspaper; describing a picture; counting, taking arithmetical tests of various complexity; naming coins; drawing objects from a model and from memory; and sketching a ground plan of a familiar room. Visual imagery, spatial orientation, finding the way along some familiar route, playing games, such as dominoes, chess, cards, or billiards, and completing jigsaw puzzles, were often used.

Henry Head considered his testing incomplete and capable of improvement. He thought that testing should be adapted to the capacity of the patient and that it should not be applied in a routine manner, even though he described in some detail the way the tests should be applied.

WEISENBURG AND McBRIDE'S BATTERY

Weisenburg and McBride's detailed testing procedure was characterized by the adaptation of psychological tests standardized for normals, in addition to modified tests for aphasics.

1. Recording the patient's spontaneous speech or reactive speech.
2. Automatic word series of counting and days of the week, months of the year, and the alphabet, reciting a prayer or nursery rhyme.

3. Naming objects and colors, as by Henry Head (see above).
4. Repeating single words containing all English sounds and a series of short, familiar phrases, and easy sentences.
5. Testing comprehension. Weisenburg and McBride recognized that a satisfactory test for understanding the spoken language was difficult to construct, mainly because the patient's comprehension had to be judged by his response, and that this might not be satisfactory, due to disturbances of expression. Following directions could be impaired as well, making the performance unreliable. They used the Gates Word, Phrase, and Sentence Reading Test, covering the printed material and asking the patient to select the correct one out of four pictures to match the word, phrase, or sentence spoken by the examiner. They then asked the patient to perform the test with the printed stimuli, testing comprehension of written material. In the ''Test of Following Directions,'' commands of increasing complexity were included, such as requesting that the patient put the back of his hand on the top of his head (undoubtedly a test of apraxia, as well). They used complicated commands, with three or four directions, such as putting a key on a chair, shutting the door, and bringing in a box, which is part of the Stanford−Binet Scale and also, Marie's Three-Paper Test. Tests involved comprehension of spatial terms and relationships, such as tests of right and left, from the Stanford−Binet scale comprehension test, from the Binet−Simon scale, Henry Head's Hand−Ear−Eye test and Abelson's geometrical figures, with instructions such as ''point inside the circle and the triangle but not in the square'' (reminding one very much of the recently popular ''Token Test'').
6. Testing reading by the ''Gates Graded Word Pronunciation Test,'' and the ''Gray Oral Reading Paragraphs.'' For reading comprehension, the ''Gates Word Recognition and Word Phrase and Sentence Test,'' were used.
7. Testing writing by using samples of spontaneous writing of the patient's name and by having the patient compose letters and reports. They also had the patient write to dictation and used formal dictation tests such as the ''Morrison−McCall Spelling Scale'' and the new ''Stanford Achievement Dictation Test.'' They tested oral spelling by using the ''Gates List of 36 Words of Graded Difficulty.'' For copying, they used a random assortment of single letters, as well as the patient's own name and a long paragraph from the ''Thorndike−McCall Reading Scale.''
8. They tested arithmetical ability with arithmetic tests from the ''Stanford Achievement Arithmetic Examination,'' including computation and reasoning.

Less frequently used tests were those of language intelligence, such as oral opposites, part−whole tests, oral analogies [horn is to blow as bell is to *(ring)*], the printed analogies test, sentence completion test, and oral absurdities test, such as: the judge said to the prisoner: ''you are to be hanged, and I hope this will be a warning to you!'' They used tests to assess recognition of printed absurdities and gave reading tests from the "Stanford—Binet Scale" and the "Thorndike Current Test of Word Knowledge." Immediate memory for digits, letters and disconnected words, and reproduction of a short story of the "Auditory Verbal Memory Test" were also tested occasionally.

Nonlanguage tests from various performance scales of intelligence tests, and drawing tests, from a model and from memory, were extensively used. Among the supplementary tests, an interesting experiment was conducted to see if the patient had difficulty recognizing nonspeech sounds. Various objects were assembled in front of the patient, such as a comb, a nickel, a rubber band, etc., and noises were made behind a screen—dropping a nickel, snapping a rubber band, and running a finger along a comb. Interestingly, the patient was asked to reproduce the sound, with the objects on the table, instead of just pointing to them (which should have been easier for aphasics with apraxia).

They constructed shorter batteries, one for use in "severe" disorders, with a probable time of 2—3 hours, and one for "slighter" disorders, for the same duration. Definitions of severity were not given and standardization was not attempted.

EISENSON'S EXAMINATION FOR APHASIA

Eisenson's Examination for Aphasia (1954) was devised as a clinical instrument, with informal instructions for administration, expecting experience with aphasics from the tester. The material is graded to estimate various levels of ability in each language function and the tests are supposed to be easy for a grammar school-educated adult. The entire examination takes 30—90 minutes, depending on the severity of the impairment.

1. Receptive disturbances are examined in the first part. Recognition of common objects is tested by either naming, pointing, or selecting choices given by the examiner. Similarly, colors, forms, reduced size pictures, numbers, letters, printed words, and printed sentences are examined for recognition. Auditory verbal comprehension of sentences followed by a series of questions, allows the patient the choice of four in the response. Oral paragraphs are followed by similar questions, with four choices. Reading comprehension is composed of paragraphs adopted from other reading tests.
2. Expressive disturbances are also examined, including apraxia, by carrying out actions with the body, with objects, and, also, to pretend actions. On the verbal apraxia test, the patient is asked to repeat numbers, words, and sentences. Automatic speech, writing, spelling, naming, word finding, calculation, clock setting, and oral reading are all tested and impairment on each subtest is summarized on a five point scale, as complete, severe, moderate, little, or none.

Eisenson, like Henry Head, considered a formal scoring system inapplicable to aphasia, in which inconsistency of response is a major feature. The test has not been standardized for an aphasic population, but it was widely used by clinicians as a guide for treatment.

THE LANGUAGE MODALITIES TEST FOR APHASIA (LMTA)

This test by Wepman and Jones (1961) provides a psycholinguistic analysis by a standardized procedure. There is a four-way organization of the presentation of stimuli and responses. The visual stimuli are presented on film strips and the auditory stimuli by the examiner. Oral and graphic responses are scored for both kinds of stimuli. The stimulus material includes pictures of common objects, such as a tree or dog, simple words, numbers, and sentences of three, four, or five words. Responses are speaking, writing, or matching. The LMTA tests the comprehension of language symbols, as well as the ability to imitate them when presented both visually and auditorily. Form recognition, arithmetic, spelling, and articulation are scored as well. It also includes four pictures about which the subject is asked to tell a story. The standardized samples of spontaneous speech thus obtained allow examination of the use of syntax and vocabulary. The scoring scale for all oral and graphic responses consists of: (1) the correct response, (2) phonemic or graphic errors, (3) syntactic errors, (4) semantic errors, (5) jargon or illegible response, (6) no response. There are two equivalent forms available for retesting. The procedure takes about an hour. The scoring system is to differentiate between defective symbol processing and input or output problems and to indicate the therapy needs of the patient.

On the basis of oral responses to the LMTA, five classes of aphasic patients can be identified.

1. Syntactic patients whose difficulties are largely with syntactic words such as "of," "with," "in," singulars, plurals and verb endings.
2. Semantic patients who have semantic or word-finding problems.
3. Pragmatic patients whose comprehension is usually poor and whose speech conveys little meaning. They often use neologisms and inappropriate substantive words.
4. Jargon patients who, unlike pragmatic patients, use few, if any, meaningful words but unintelligible jargon words instead.
5. Global patients who often have no speech at all except for a few automatic phrases, such as "I don't know" or meaningless combinations of sound.

THE MINNESOTA TEST FOR DIFFERENTIAL DIAGNOSIS OF APHASIA (MTDDA)

This test by Schuell and her co-workers (1964), consists of 69 tests, with more than 595 test items. The main six sections are:

1. Tests for auditory disturbances (10)
2. Tests for visual and reading disturbances (11)
3. Tests for speech and language disturbances (20)
4. Tests for visuomotor and writing disturbances (14)
5. Tests for numerical relations and arithmetic processes (8)
6. Tests for body image (6)

Scores consist of numbers of errors. One hundred and fifty-seven aphasics and 50 normal patients were used for a factor analysis which was interpreted to show five major factors:

1. Language behavior
2. Visual discrimination, recognition, and recall
3. Visuospatial behavior
4. Gross movements of the speech musculature
5. Recognition of stimulus equivalents

Test−retest data were available for 75 subjects, with an interval from 1−13 months.

SCHUELL'S SHORT EXAMINATION FOR APHASIA

This test by Schuell (1957) consists of the tests from the MTDDA with the highest diagnostic and prognostic value.

Section A, *Auditory Disturbances,* includes *auditory recognition,* tested by the subject pointing to objects and pictures of objects, after the examiner speaks only the single word, and after a pause, repeats it. *Auditory retention span* consists of pointing to objects called out serially by the examiner, and also, by a *repetition task,* where the patient repeats increasingly complex words and sentences. *Auditory comprehension* is also tested by following directions, again with increasing complexity, including several sequences of relational words between stimuli. Finally, comprehension of a paragraph is tested by the examiner reading a story and asking "yes" and "no" questions about it.

Section B, *Reading Disturbances,* are tested at the word level, when the stimulus is a printed word and the patient has to select a picture from an array. Auditory *recognition of words* consists of an auditory stimulus with a pointing response to a choice of printed words. *Reading comprehension* is tested by reading sentences and a paragraph, and asking "yes" and "no" questions.

Section C includes the *examination of cranial nerve involvement.* Initiating and sustaining phonation, deviation of the tongue, inequality of lateral movements and deviation of the uvula, and movements of the soft palate or difficulty swallowing are included. *Sensorimotor involvement* is tested by repetition tasks and mispronunciations are scored as errors. A naming task is also included here, utilizing line drawings of simple items. *Functional speech* consists of a vocabulary test, in which the patient has to explain the meaning of words and proverbs.

Section D includes tests of *visual and writing* disturbances, such as *drawing* a man, reproducing letters, spelling, writing words and sentences on dictation, and spontaneous writing, tested by writing a paragraph about a picture.

THE FUNCTIONAL COMMUNICATION PROFILE (FCP)

This test by ML Taylor (1965) consists of 45 items considered common language functions. Ratings of each behavior are made on a continuum along a nine-point scale, on the basis of informal interaction with the patient, in a conversational situation, without cues or assistance. "Good," "fair," and "poor" are to be defined with an estimate of the specific subject's "normal" performance. Ratings take into account speed, accuracy, consistency, "voluntary control without external cues," and compensatory function. Each rating is converted into percentages in each of the five modalities: movement, speaking, understanding, reading, and a miscellaneous category which includes writing and calculation. An overall score is a single measure of an individual's communication effectiveness in everyday life. The profile visually differentiates among types of verbal impairment.

THE NEUROSENSORY CENTER COMPREHENSIVE
EXAMINATION OF APHASIA (NCCEA)

This test by Spreen and Benton (1968) consists of 20 language tests and four control tests of visual and tactile functions. The subtests of the NCCEA include:

1. Visual naming of common objects
2. Description of use of the same objects
3 & 4. Tactile naming, with right and left hand
5. Sentence repetition of tape recorded sentences
6. Digit repetition
7. Digit reversal
8. Word fluency, using three one-minute trials for all the words recalled, beginning with a specific letter
9. Sentence construction from five sets of up to three words
10. Object identification by name (auditory recognition task), where the patient points to objects named by the examiner
11. Identification by sentence, using a shortened version (36 items only) of the Token Test (Spreen and Spellacy, 1969)
12. Oral reading of names of objects presented before
13. Oral reading of the 12 command sentences in test 11
14. Silent reading of names, which involves matching the written name of an object to a display of objects

15. Reading sentences for meaning. The patient is instructed to execute 12 of the written commands used in test 11

16. Visuographic naming requests the patient to write the names of ten objects presented visually

17. Writing names, which scores test 16 for correctness of spelling. If the naming portion is not performed, then the patient is dictated a name and asked to write it

18. Writing on dictation of two sentences

19. Copying sentences

20. Articulation, (which is also a test of repetition) of 30 meaningful and eight nonsense words, presented from a tape recording

Careful instructions for administering and scoring ensure a basis for comparison. Scores are entered on profile sheets and can be compared with norms for normal adults and for an aphasic population as percentiles. Corrections for age and educational level are applied for some tests. It has been standardized for 81 patients.

THE PORCH INDEX OF COMMUNICATIVE ABILITIES (PICA)

This test is by Porch (1971). The index is made up of 18 subtests, four in verbal, eight in gestural, and six in graphic response modalities, using ten common objects as stimuli. The first verbal test requires a description of what to do with each object, the second is a gestural task requiring the patient to demonstrate the use of the object, the third is also a gestural response, with the object being handed to the patient, the fourth is a naming task, the fifth is matching printed sentences, describing the use of the objects, with the actual objects and is primarily a test of reading ability, the sixth is a test of sentence comprehension (the patient is only scored for pointing), the seventh is a test of reading aloud, the eighth is matching pictures with objects, the ninth is sentence completion, the tenth is pointing to an object, after auditory stimulus, the eleventh matches objects with objects, and the twelfth is repetition after a tape recorded voice.

Graphic Test A is a written description of objects and B is writing the names of these; C is to write the name on dictation, D is to write the name after spelling; and E is to copy the name. Finally, Test F is the copying of geometric forms.

The scoring is described in detail for each subtest, in categories from 1 to 16. The responses are differentiated along the dimensions of accuracy, responsiveness, completeness, promptness, and efficiency and these are incorporated into the scoring system. An overall score serves as a single index of the patient's communicative ability. Response levels for modalities and for subtests can be plotted and a ranked response summary is achieved by arranging the subtests in order of difficulty. When the patient's overall response level exceeds 10, adequate communication is usually achieved. Once basic profiles have been established, modalities which fall in a lower percentile are expected to improve to a greater degree. *Three* common types of aphasia are differentiated, such as the patient with

1. Severe verbal formulation difficulty
2. Severe dysarthria
3. Inadequate verbal monitoring

Bilateral damage and aberrant patterns have different profiles.

Percentiles of response levels were determined on 280 left-hemisphere damaged patients. The mean overall score was 10.02; the fiftieth percentile score was 10.64. It is suggested that these scores should be plotted into this population percentile, as the patient recovers, to achieve recovery curves. There is a great deal of manipulation of data, considering the restricted number of test items and the relative simplicity of the tests. The test has been criticized for not including assessment of conversational speech. The detailed scoring categories were considered critically by Martin (1977). Despite the criticisms, the test achieved popularity in recent years among some speech pathologists.

THE APPRAISAL OF LANGUAGE DISTURBANCES (ALD)

This test by L Emeric (1971) is systematized according to the modalities of stimulation and response, incorporating in each subtest various items. The *Oral to Oral* subtests include automatic speech, repetition, supplying opposites to words, sentence completion, definitions, and disparities (word finding). The *Oral to Visual* group of tests include pointing to objects, pictures and words, comprehension, and reading. The *Oral to Gesture* subtests are partly tests of praxis, such as shaking the head, coughing, whistling, humming, pointing to body parts, and demonstrating actions. The *Oral to Graphic* subtest is writing on auditory stimuli; the subtests are similar to the Oral to Oral tests, except the patient responds in writing. The *Gestural to Visual* subtest assesses comprehension of gestures, with multiple choice objects, pictures, and words. The *Visual to Gesture* subtest examines praxis, with actual objects. The *Visual to Oral* subtest contains reading and naming tasks; the *Visual to Graphic* subtest includes copying, writing the names of objects, and writing about a picture.

Central language comprehension is said to be examined by matching of silhouettes to line drawings, pictures to each other, and pictures to written words; the Peabody Picture Vocabulary Test; sorting and arranging tasks, such as object assembly, color sorting, and sorting by shape; a special test of demanding or asking; arithmetic; and the examination of tongue, lip and jaw movement, and phonation.

Test−retest reliability was measured on 76 aphasics, with variable interval between tests and the correlation was 0.74. Not all patients were neurologically stable in this sample. When only 3 months post-onset patients were included in the calculation ($n = 39$), then an r of 0.80 was obtained. Interscore reliability between 2 trained clinicians was 0.86.

THE BOSTON DIAGNOSTIC APHASIA EXAMINATION (BDAE)

This test (Goodglass and Kaplan, 1972) was intended to provide test scores corresponding to the common aphasic syndromes, as recognized by clinicians. Like the PICA, it has become a widely used test since its' publication.

1. The examination of *conversational* or expository *speech* is of great importance. Six features of speech production, *melodic line, phrase length, articulatory agility, grammatical form* or variety of grammatical constructions, *paraphasia in running speech,* and *word finding,* are rated subjectively, by the examiner, on a $1-7$ scale. Auditory comprehension, which is also measured by objective test scores, is included in the rating scale profile. These profiles of speech characteristics rated by three judges were found to be highly correlated, except for ratings of paraphasias and word finding. The severity rating estimates the overall efficiency of oral communication from zero (no communication) to five (no perceptible handicap).
2. *Auditory comprehension* is measured by
    a. *Word discrimination,* which is a multiple choice auditory word recognition test, sampling six semantic categories, such as objects, geometric forms, letters, actions, numbers, and colors
    b. *Body parts and finger identification* are separately scored, but correlate well with word discrimination
    c. *Commands* of increasing complexity requiring some praxis
    d. *Complex ideational material,* requiring only "yes" and "no" responses to matched questions. Both questions for each item must be answered correctly to be rated.
3. *Oral expression* comprises a variety of subtests.
    a. *Oral agility* is divided into:
        (1) *Nonverbal agility,* alternating movement of the tongue and lips, which are tests of dysarthria and have a poor correlation with the remainder of the subtests
        (2) *Verbal agility,* rapid repetition of words, correlating well with automatized sequences
    b. *Automatized sequences* of days, months, numbers and the alphabet
    c. *Recitation* of nursery rhymes, singing and tapping rhythms, which have a low correlation with language skills and are scored on a three step scale
    d. *Repetition* of words, including letters, numbers and a tongue twister

e. *Repetition of phrases* and sentences, divided into high probability and low probability items. Paraphasic items are not given credit.

f. *Word reading* is correlated best with oral sentence reading and visual confrontation naming. Bonus is given for the speed of response.

g. *Responsive naming* correlates best with visual confrontation naming; scoring depends on the estimation of delay of the response.

h. *Visual confrontation naming* is tested in various categories, using the same items as for the word discrimination test. Credit is given for shorter reaction time. No credit is given for cueing or assistance.

i. *Body part naming* is an experimental item.

j. Animal naming, measuring *fluency in controlled association,* shows the highest correlation with confrontation naming, but has a negative correlation with phrase length rating (fluency of spontaneous speech), as aphasics with the highest fluency in connected speech may be poor in word finding. The score consists of the number of different words named in the 60 most productive seconds.

k. *Oral sentence reading* is scored all or nothing and credit is given for a correct performance only.

4. Understanding written language is measured without any need for output, other than pointing to multiple choice items. *Word recognition* involves the selection, from a multiple choice of five written words, of the one which has been spoken by the examiner. This may reveal the phenomenon of responding to the connotative meaning of a written word, without appreciating its phonetic value. This is also a test of *phonetic association. Comprehension of oral spelling* uses auditory stimuli. A purely visual recognition task is the multiple choice matching of letters and short words across different styles of writing, called *symbol and word discrimination.* The comprehension of written words is tested with *word–picture matching,* as well as *reading sentences* and *paragraphs.* The test of *reading comprehension* is accomplished by pointing to a multiple choice of words, completing the test sentence or paragraph.

5. *Writing* is tested by instructing the patient to write his *name* and *address* and then, *copy a printed sentence.* The "mechanics of writing" is scored on a $0-3$ scale. The recall of written symbols is accomplished by *serial writing* of the alphabet and numbers and *dictation* of individual numbers, letters, and words, at a primary level. *Spelling* to dictation and *written* confrontation *naming,* with a range of words of average difficulty, is also used. Finally, *written formulation* is tested by getting the patient to write connected sentences about a picture, with the patient being scored on a five point scale, from $0-4$. Sentences about the picture are also dictated. Substitutions and insertions of irrelevant words and paragraphia are scored on a three point scale.

Supplementary language tests explore psycholinguistic factors in comprehension, expression, and screen for hemispheric disconnection symptoms. Auditory comprehension is explored with special reference to the preposition of location, timing, and direction, passive subject—object discrimination, and comprehension of possessive relationship. Repetition and sentence manipulation tasks are used to explore linguistic competence with forms which may not occur in free conversation. Contrast among indicative, interrogative, and conditional construction is examined. Sentence completion tests are used to determine whether the patient can adjust the verb tense to past and future to follow the semantic demands of the sentence. The patient is then asked to formulate questions with an initial unstressed auxiliary verb, such as "do," "can," or "may," or with interrogative pronouns or adverbs, such as "who," "where," "how," "what," and "why." Repetition of difficult words, grammatical words, numbers, and number—word combinations are further expanded to test conduction aphasics. Dissociation of modalities in naming can be found when naming is tested by touch, in either hand, with the subject's eyes shut. Agraphia of the minor hand is tested for corpus callosum disconnexion.

Supplementary nonlanguage tests include drawing on command and copying, reproduction of stick figures and three-dimensional block designs, finger comprehension, finger naming, visual finger matching, right—left test, arithmetic test, clock setting, finger identification, and matching two-finger positions.

Aphasics were assigned to six clinically defined severity levels and two scores were computed on each level. Clusters on an intercorrelation matrix of 111 patients were considered an artifact of patient populations and the test. When pairs of subtests correlated, this was considered the result of either a common psychological factor or anatomical contiguity of areas producing the deficit. The Kuder—Richardson method of subtest reliability indicated good internal consistency within subtests, with respect to what the items were measuring.

THE SKLAR APHASIA SCALE (SAS)

In this test, Sklar (1973) quantifies language disturbances into four major language skills:

1. *Auditory decoding* uses identifying body parts, understanding simple questions, identifying words and objects in the environment, identifying useful objects, and recalling the object's name (memory span).
2. *Visual decoding* is tested by matching printed words, matching words with pictures, sentence completion, arithmetic, and silent reading with pointing to correct answers.
3. *Oral encoding* scores functional speech, repeating spoken words, naming

objects, reading an article aloud and telling about five items remembered, and describing actions of people in a picture incident.

4. *Graphic encoding* requires the patient to write his name and address, copy words from a model, write names of pictured objects, sentences from dictation, and describe a picture.

Each item is scored correct (0), retarded (1), assisted (2), distorted (3), or erased or no response (4). A total impairment score is determined by adding the four subtest scores and dividing the sum by four. The patients are classified into categories of minimal impairment $0-10$, mild impairment $11-20$, moderate impairment $21-60$, severe impairment $61-90$, and total or global impairment $91-100$, and these categories are also described in terms of functional communication. Recommended supplementary testing is also described. A verbal behavior check list is provided for jargon, automatism, perseveration, dysarthria, oral apraxia, agrammatism, omissions, substitutions, distortions, retardation, word hunting, unintelligible responses, self-monitoring impairment, and dysphonia. When the SAS was administered to 20 normal adults, the language items were within the ability of an average adult with an eighth grade education. Twelve chronic aphasics who had the SAS were examined on Eisenson's test, the Halstead–Wepman Aphasia Screening test, and on Schuell's Short Examination for Aphasia. Mean scores and standard deviations were similar for the four tests and correlation coefficients indicated that all four tests measure similar types of language behavior. The SAS was also compared with the Wechsler–Bellevue Intelligence Scale, the Bender Visual Motor Gestalt test, the Goldstein–Scheerer Cube test, and the Rorschach test. With the exception of the Rorschach, significant correlations were obtained indicating that language intelligence, visual motor perception, and the ability to abstract all deteriorate in a similar fashion. A factor analysis of the SAS scores of 108 patients produced four factors: (1) visual decoding, (2) auditory decoding, (3) oral encoding, and (4) graphic encoding. No factorial representation appeared for speech comprehension and reading comprehension.

A German version of the SAS discriminated aphasics from schizophrenic, brain damaged, and normal controls with a high level of confidence (91.8 percent). It did not discriminate between fluent and nonfluent aphasics (Cohen et al., 1977). A factor analysis showed a main loading represented the severity of language disorders. The second loading appeared to be a memory factor, and the third a sensory–motor or fluency–nonfluency dimension.

THE APHASIA LANGUAGE PERFORMANCE SCALES (ALPS)

This test by J. Keenan and E. Brassell (1975), contains four ten-item scales, one for each of the commonly recognized language modalities. Each scale contains items which sample performance in one modality only and requires linguistic performance ranging from nearly normal to minimal.

1. Listening consists of ten commands of increasing complexity.
2. Talking includes imitation of vowels, counting, naming, responding to questions, describing actions of the examiner, and spontaneous conversational speech.
3. Reading consists of pointing to named numbers, nouns, and verbs, following short instructions, and matching pictures to short and long descriptions in a multiple choice task.
4. Writing includes copying, writing numbers, letters, nouns, phrases, and increasingly complex sentences on dictation.

Emphasis is placed on informal conversational approach, and the examiner is allowed to omit tests if they are judged too difficult or too easy for that patient, and the items may be scored assuming the predicted performance or failure. This shortens the time required for the test (30 minutes). Some complicated test responses receive all or nothing scoring, just like the simple items, and "prompting" is incorporated. Test—retest reliability on 22 patients' split half reliability and internal consistency was measured on about 90 tests. Comparison between PICA and ALPS on 50 aphasics was carried out, among other standardization procedures.

The next two tests of comprehension are described as examples of the many special tests designed to sample one aspect of aphasic behavior in depth. The Token test is widely used in research as it provides a sensitive instrument of comprehension. The Auditory Comprehension Test for Sentences examines some linguistic principles which were thought to be useful in addition to the WAB, and the test was added to our protocol to examine aphasic recovery and therapy.

THE TOKEN TEST

This is a special test of comprehension, designed by DeRenzi and Vignolo (1962) for mild sensory disturbances, or to detect such in expressive syndromes. It consists of 61 commands of graded length and complexity. The patient has to point, touch, or pick up tokens of five different colors, two shapes, and two sizes. The fifth part of the test uses prepositions, conjunctions, or adverbs to vary the linguistic complexity of the commands. The commands are elementary conceptually; they were not considered to load the memory capacity of the patient. Redundancy and clues given by the nature of the objects are eliminated. Initially, the test was given to 19 patients, who did not have difficulty in understanding conversation; they were recovered sensory aphasics or "pure motor aphasics." They all made errors as the difficulty level of the test progressed.

Subsequently, the test was used to study various populations in many countries. The extensive literature on the token test has been reviewed recently by Boller et al. (1978). It is generally considered too difficult for many aphasics but a sensitive test for mild or latent comprehension disturbance. Nonaphasic left and right hemisphere lesioned patients had a relatively high "false positive" rate. Quite different types of aphasics obtain similar scores. Although it is an excellent research tool, clinicians find its applicability to the assessment of aphasia limited. A shortened version has been incorporated in the N.C.C.E.A. (16 items). A 36 item short version has been recently recommended by DeRenzi (1978). See the section on comprehension in the next chapter for further discussion.

THE AUDITORY COMPREHENSION TEST FOR
SENTENCES (ACTS)

This test described by Shewan and Canter (1971), contains 42 sentences, which vary systematically in the parameters of length, vocabulary difficulty, and syntactic complexity. The patient responds by pointing to the correct picture from an array of four corresponding to the sentence presented orally by the examiner. There are seven types of sentences with six examples of each type, created by increasing the difficulty of the three parameters independently, to a moderate and high degree. Scoring uses a weighted system with prompt (0–3 sec), correct (4–10 sec), and delayed (11–30 sec) responses. Incorrect, perseverative categories are scored as zero. The time estimated to administer the test is 20–30 minutes. The clinician administering the test is exhorted to scrutinize additional response parameters, such as time lag and degree of self-correction, but no quantitation is attempted in this respect. This test has been revised and standardized on a group of 150 aphasics and a smaller group of normal adults of comparable age and education (Klor, Freedman, and Shewan, 1976). The test demonstrates an internal reliability coefficient of 0.82 and a test–retest coefficient of 0.87. All parameters contribute equally to the total score and are independent of one another. The difficulty levels differentiate from one another at a significant level. External validity was established by a high correlation (0.80), between a functional comprehension scale and total test score. Error data were analyzed qualitatively for position and type (Shewan, 1976).

DISCUSSION

The proliferation of aphasia tests is similar to that of classifications, though not quite to the same extent because of the efforts involved in test construction and standardization. The variety of needs and approaches is reflected in the methods of presentation, the stimuli, the number of items, and the scoring. Many tests show some relationship to previous tests either in the similarity of the items or the modalities explored. The early aphasia tests, in turn, borrowed generously from intelligence measures. In fact, comprehensive aphasia batteries resemble intelligence tests by exploring not only verbal behavior but also incorporating nonverbal performance variables. Most aphasia tests are too long and fatiguing to the patient and examiner; therefore, often only selected items are used for diagnostic evaluation. It is difficult to advocate any one test, and the particular test chosen is a reflection of one's training and locale. The exact usage is difficult to determine, but the Schuell, PICA, and BDAE are probably the most widespread. The NCCEA formed the basis for an international cooperative effort to establish a worldwide standardized test (Benton, 1967). A table comparing these tests with the Western Aphasia Battery is constructed in Chapter 3.

Common defects of aphasia assessment were cited by Benton (1967): lack of explicit instructions for administration and criteria for scoring, poor scaling of items with respect to level of difficulty, inadequate normative information, and excessive length. Unusual selection of tests based upon various idiosyncratic concepts of aphasia leads to artifactual diagnostic categories not shared by other clinicians. On the other hand, a mechanical exploration of the endless combinations of input and output modalities, regardless of clinical emphasis, results in meaningless categories and impractically long test batteries. Obviously, there is no test that satisfies everyone, but the balance between selectivity and comprehensiveness is probably the key to the value ot each test, provided other criteria concerning standardization, grading, and validity are satisfied. The ease of administration and scoring will contribute to the popularity of a test, but too short an examination may not fulfill some requirements of research or even clinical diagnosis.

SUMMARY

This chapter provides a descriptive summary of the major aphasia examinations in English. None are entirely satisfactory to everyone. Many offer special features, different approaches, but the basic language parameters of speech output, comprehension, reading, and writing are measured by most. Variable emphasis is placed on various language parameters, and the length, scoring, and the extent of standardization differs, depending on the purpose of testing. Many tests are unnecessarily long and therefore not practical. Most clinicians end up selectively using certain items which are suitable for their aim. The need for a practical yet sophisticated, relevant, and reliable measure of aphasia is evident!

3

The Rationale of the Western Aphasia Battery (WAB)

The purposes of aphasia testing: (1) diagnosis of presence and type of aphasic syndrome, leading to inferences concerning cerebral localization; (2) measurement of the level of performance over a wide range, for both initial determination and detection of change over time; (3) comprehensive assessment of the assets and liabilities of the patient in all language areas as a guide to therapy.

> Goodglass H, Kaplan E: Assessment of Aphasia and Related Disorders.
> Philadelphia, Lea & Feberger, 1972

INTRODUCTION

Aphasia testing has proven to be complex and difficult to standardize. Requirements of clinicians and research vary greatly, and it is likely that old tests will continue to be modified and new tests will appear, claiming this or that advantage. Specialized testing procedures for a certain aspect of language or behavior will continue to grow in number, alongside the fewer and more standardized diagnostic batteries designed for the practicing clinician. Even fewer will attempt to be comprehensive enough for research, yet manageable enough for practice. It is this ideal combination which stimulated our efforts to produce a test which will satisfy the requirements of taxonomic analysis by being comprehensive, yet will allow us to examine a reasonable number of patients in the clinic.

A consensus has emerged from clinical experience and the literature that an ideal aphasia test should do the following:

1. Explore all potentially disturbed modalities.
2. Employ subtests that discriminate among various clinically meaningful types of aphasia.
3. Include graded test items so that a representative range of severity can be examined.
4. Contain enough items to eliminate most of the day to day, and test to test, variability.
5. Be practical enough in length to administer it, preferably, in one sitting.
6. Minimize the effects of intelligence and education to measure language performance as purely as possible.
7. Be standardized as to scoring and administration, so that various examiners achieve the same results.
8. Discriminate between normals and aphasics, dementia and aphasia.
9. Have internal consistency and comparability of scores.
10. Have face and content validity.

Most clinically useful aphasia tests will explore these language parameters:

1. Description of spontaneous or conversational speech
2. A measure of information value
3. A measure of fluency
4. Auditory comprehension
5. Naming
6. Repetition
7. Reading comprehension
8. Writing
9. Arithmetic
10. Gestural expression (praxis)

Various other items can be added, in endless combinations, and these major areas can be subdivided through different modalities of stimulation and response. Porch (1971) indicated the desirability to sample, in a consistent manner, the input modality used in receiving the instructions, the input modality while the task is performed, and the output modality of the response. On the other hand, the attention paid to the details of sampling, administration, and scoring of the tests should not obscure the goals of testing. Brookshire (1975) pointed out the need for a test to provide information for prognosis and the method of possible treatment.

At the time when we began to use the first version of our aphasia battery, incorporating some of the material from the yet unpublished test of Goodglass and Kaplan, Benton (1967) had the following comments about aphasia tests: . . . None have been generally adopted. . . None of them have been published in usable form. . .None of them present exact criteria for scoring or offer detailed guides for the interpretation of performance. . .None of them present convincing evidence that the battery possesses a degree of clinical utility which is significantly greater than any other series of aphasia tests which might be assembled. Since these critical words were written, significant advances were made in clinical aphasia testing (reviewed in Chapter 2), especially the publications of the Porch Index of Communicative Ability (PICA) (Porch 1971), and the Boston Diagnostic Aphasia Examination (BDAE) by Goodglass and Kaplan (1972). We continued to use our modification of the "Boston psycholinguistic approach" and published our first standardized version of the test and our experience with 150 patients and 59 controls in 1974 (Kertesz and Poole).

The Western Aphasia Battery (WAB) is designed for research and clinical use. The language subtests can be administered in an hour to most ambulant patients, although two such sessions are often required for the full battery. Severely affected patients may take less time. The tests are selected for all grades of severity, but present no difficulty to a patient with intact language, as attested by the score of 59, age-matched controls. The standardization of the test will subsequently be described in detail. In this chapter, the main features and their rationale will be described and compared to other tests. In Table 3-1, the WAB subtests are lined up with their equivalents on the most commonly used aphasia examinations.

The oral language subtests—(A), spontaneous speech, (B) comprehension, (C) repetition, and (D) naming—are used to assess the severity and the type of aphasia. The summary of their scaled scores provides the Aphasia Quotient (AQ) (Kertesz and Poole 1974). When reading, writing, praxis, drawing, block design, calculation, and Raven's Progressive Matrices scores are added, the Performance Quotient (PQ) is obtained, and the AQ and PQ combined provide the Cortical Quotient (or CQ), a summary of the cognitive function, as tested in our laboratory, for diagnosis and research. Not all patients will have the full battery, although an effort is made to test every aphasic or nondominant hemisphere damaged patient as fully as possible.

SPONTANEOUS SPEECH

Examination of spontaneous or conversational speech is universally acknowledged to be important for diagnosis and classification, for purposes of prognosis as well as considerations of localization and psycholinguistic research.

Table 3–1
Comparison of the Subtests of Major Aphasia Batteries with the WAB

Western Aphasia Battery	Neurosensory Center Comprehensive Examination for Aphasia	Porch Index of Communicative Ability	Boston Diagnostic Aphasia Examination	Schuell's Short Examination for Aphasia
Spontaneous Speech			*Conversational Speech*	*Functional Speech*
Fluency	Description of use	Description of use	Melodic line, phrase length, articulatory agility, grammatical form, paraphasias in running speech, word finding	Definition
Information Content				Proverbs
Comprehension				*Auditory Disturbances*
"Yes–no" questions	Object identification by name	Pointing to objects	Complex ideational material	Following a paragraph
Auditory word recognition			Word discrimination	Auditory recognition
Sequential commands	Identification by sentence	Sentence comprehension	Commands	Auditory retention span
				Following directions
Repetition				
Numbers	Repetition of digits		Repetition of words	Repetition of words
Words		Repetition of words	Repetition of phrases	Repetition of sentences
Sentences	Sentence repetition		Oral agility	Articulation (cranial nerves)
	Articulation			
Naming				
Object naming	Visual naming	Naming	Confrontation naming	Naming
Word fluency	Word fluency		Fluency in controlled association	
Sentence completion	Sentence construction	Sentence completion	Sentence completion	
Responsive speech			Responsive naming	

Reading

Reading comprehension of sentences	Reading sentences for meaning	Matching written sentences to objects	Reading sentences and paragraphs	Reading comprehension of sentences and paragraphs
Reading commands aloud, performing commands	Oral reading (sentences)		Word reading	
	Oral reading (names)			
Written word stimulus–object choice matching				
Picture stimulus–written word choice matching	Reading names for meaning (pointing)	Matching shorter sentences to objects		
Word stimulus–picture choice matching			Word–picture matching	Word–picture matching
Phonetic association			Word recognition	Word recognition
Letter discrimination			Symbol and word discrimination	
			Comprehension of oral spelling	
Spelled word recognition				

Spelling

Spelling			Spelling dictation	Oral spelling

Writing

Writing on request	Writing names		Mechanics of writing	
Written output		Written description	Narrative writing	Spontaneous writing
Writing on dictation	Writing to dictation	Dictation	Sentences written to dictation	Sentence on dictation
Writing of dictated or visually presented words	Visual–graphic naming	Writing names of objects	Spelling to dictation	Written spelling
Recall of written symbols			Recall of written symbols	
Writing of dictated letters or numbers		Writing names of objects after spelling	Primer-level dictation	

Copy

Copy	Writing from copy	Copying	Copy	Copy letters

Table 3–1 (continued)

Western Aphasia Battery	Neurosensory Center Comprehensive Examination for Aphasia	Porch Index of Communicative Ability	Boston Diagnostic Aphasia Examination	Schuell's Short Examination for Aphasia
Praxis				
Upper limb			Intransitive limb	
Buccofacial			Buccofacial	
Instrumental		Object use	Transitive limb	
Complex		Demonstrate use	Serial actions	
Drawing		*Copying of Forms*	*Drawing to Command*	*Revisualization*
Calculation	Reversal of digits	Match pictures to objects	*Arithmetic*	
	Tactile naming	Match objects to objects	Automatic sequences	
			Recitation, singing	

40

Among the tests compared, only the PICA (Porch, 1971) lacks this feature, and although one of the verbal tests requires a description of what to do with each object, this is probably insufficient. The difficulty of scoring conversational or spontaneous speech meaningfully has been acknowledged universally. Goodglass and Kaplan, in the BDAE, have developed a complicated and sophisticated method of scoring spontaneous speech. An important feature is to ask the patients conversational questions, and to standardize them by using the same or equivalent questions with all patients, so that responses can be compared. Picture description provides some constraint on vocabulary and tests the word-finding ability of the patients as well. Goodglass and Kaplan (1972) noted that the quality of the speech often changes from conversational questions to picture description, because some patients with empty speech can use available, overlearned expressions to circumlocute and avoid words with which they may have trouble.

Fluency

Fluency appears to be one of the most important factors differentiating various aphasics, even though there is some variation in how fluency is defined (Howes and Geschwind, 1964; Benson, 1967; Kerschensteiner et al., 1972; Goodglass and Kaplan, 1972; Wagenaar et al., 1975). Goodglass et al. (1964) pointed out that the most significant difference between the major groups of patients is in the character of their speech production and not, as commonly assumed, in the opposition between the function of language intake and output. Our "fluency" rating incorporates phrase length and variety of grammatical construction, as well as the presence of jargon, word-finding difficulty, and circumlocution. Rather than dissect spontaneous speech into component attributes, we try to integrate them into clinically meaningful categories.

We rated fluency according to set criteria applied to the "spontaneous speech," elicited by recording the responses to standardized questions, and by asking the patient to describe a picture (a simple drawing of a house, a pond, people, and animals, used by Schuell). The examiner is to categorize the spontaneous speech of the patient according to one of the following definitions. Each category is assigned a score, and scores span a range of 0−10.

    0 = No response or short, meaningless utterances
    1 = Recurrent utterances used in a meaningful way, with varied intonation
    2 = Single words, mostly inappropriately used
    3 = Fluent, stereotypic utterances or mumbling, very low volume jargon
    4 = Predominantly single words, often appropriate, with occasional verbs or prepositional phrases. Automatic sentences only: "Oh, I don't know."
    5 = Predominantly telegraphic, halting speech, but some grammatical organization. Paraphasias may be prominent. Few propositional sentences.

6 = More complete propositional sentences. Normal rhythmic patterning may be present within phrases.

7 = Phonemic jargon with semblance to English syntax and rhythm, with varied phonemes and neologisms

8 = Circumlocutory, fluent speech. Marked word finding difficulty. Semantic jargon. Often complete sentences.

9 = Mostly complete sentences; hesitation over parts of speech, auxilliary verbs, or word endings; some paraphasias; some word-finding difficulty

10 = Sentences of normal length and complexity, without perceptible word-finding difficulty

We agreed to these categories after several sessions with experienced speech pathologists, watching videotaped conversations of aphasics, and choosing various categories best describing their speech. We think that selection by the examining clinician from these categories is the most practical way to standardize the description of the important fluency dimension of spontaneous speech. These ten categories do not form a smooth continuum, in all respects, but the most important feature, fluency, which is the title of this rating scale, was the basis for ranking them. Other features were incorporated as well. For example, the placing of frequent stereotypic and relatively fluent, low volume mumbling at a low level of fluency rating, and the grade of variable jargon speech at a high level, is based on the consideration of the variability of phonemic pattern. Only rarely will the differentiation of the two represent a problem. Similarly, the first four ''nonfluent'' categories include automatic expressions, with normal melodic line extending to three or four words, such as ''I don't know.'' It is the distinction between barely fluent (5) and mildly nonfluent (4) speech which requires some experience. In order to standardize the ratings of fluency and information content of spontaneous speech, we have tried to make the description of each category comprehensive, from the linguistic point of view, yet concise and recognizable, clinically.

The variability of grammatical complexity in spontaneous speech of normals casts some doubt on the validity of rating grammatical forms. Nevertheless, this is an important concept, provided premorbid linguistic habits and competence are considered. Unfortunately, this can only be estimated in some cases and cannot be assessed at all in others. The melodic line incorporates disturbances of prosody and dysarthria, which may not be aphasic features in all cases. Other aspects of melodic line overlap phrase length, to a great extent, and one questions the necessity or advantage of placing a separate score on it. Rating melodic line, phrase length, and variety of grammatical construction separately did not seem to have any special clinical advantage, even though these are important theoretical linguistic considerations. It is difficult for the clinician to assign ratings on some of these scales on the BDAE since only the extremes and the middle are defined to any extent.

There is a great deal to be said for rating paraphasia; this is one of the major contributions of the psycholinguistic approach of Goodglass and Kaplan (1972). In addition to assessing it in running speech, they also count paraphasias on examining oral expression. Rating of paraphasias, particularly the incidence of literal paraphasia, contributes to their diagnostic classification. One has the impression, however, that the paraphasia rating is overly generous, such as placing one per minute of conversation in the middle of the range, suggesting a milder group of aphasics than one generally encounters. This is borne out by looking at the z scores of paraphasias on more structured tests, indicating a high occurrence of these in the majority of patients. No z scores are available for spontaneous speech. This shift of the z scores much above zero decreases the specificity of paraphasia ratings, somewhat. In a phonological analysis of spontaneous speech, Blumstein (1973) showed that most literal paraphasias consist of sound substitutions, obeying certain linguistic rules, and to a lesser degree, omissions and augmentations. They are most prominent in the speech of Broca's conduction and Wernicke's aphasia. Paraphasia rating alone will not distinguish between various types of aphasics, therefore, we integrated it with fluency in our scoring of spontaneous speech.

The rating of word finding in the BDAE has the peculiarity that the most normal speech is in the middle of the rating, called information proportional to fluency. The high rating (7) is given for speech consisting exclusively of content words or agrammatical or telegraphic speech. The lowest rating is given for fluent speech without information. Although this rating is of theoretical interest, it seems to deviate from the direction of the other items.

Information Content

Information content is assessed in a separate rating scale which correlates well with the severity of aphasia (the aphasia quotient). This is often called the communication value or the functional value of speech. We extended the rating scale $0-10$, with accurate definitions, considering the levels of information conveyed by the patient in conversation.

(10) Correct responses to all six questions, sentences of normal length and complexity, integrating people and action in the picture, and referring to at least three of the principal activities. There is no perceptible circumlocution or word-finding difficulty.

(9) Correct responses to all six questions. Some sentences or longer phrases used in integrating people and actions of the picture; at least ten important people, objects, or actions should be named. Circumlocution may be present.

(8) Correct responses to five of the first six questions; incomplete description of the picture.

(7) Correct responses to four of the first six questions and mention of at least

      six of the key nouns or verbs in the picture with some meaningful grouping
      of words into phrases.

(6)   Correct responses to any four of the first six questions plus some response
      to description of the picture.

(5)   Correct responses to any three of the first six questions plus some response
      to description of the picture.

(4)   Correct responses to any three questions.

(3)   Correct responses to any two questions.

(2)   Correct response to any one question.

(1)   Incomplete responses only, e.g., first name or last name only.

(0)   No information.

      The functional value of speech is a popular concept; some clinicians such as
Sarno (1969) and Holland (1977) feel that aphasic disability can be best assessed
by judging how well the patient functions in everyday situations. The Functional
Communication Profile by Sarno (1971) uses conversational rather than structured questions; the scores are estimates of the patient's capacity. Our information content scale approximates the assessment of functional communication,
because it only scores the amount of information actually communicated in
response to everyday, conversational questions and to descriptions of a picture
(as close as one can come to eliciting "spontaneous speech").

COMPREHENSION

      Comprehension is one of the most important but also the most difficult
feature of language to measure. Patient performance is often complicated by
difficulties of verbal expression and apraxia. Intellectual function is closely
linked and, at times, difficult to separate from comprehension testing. Comprehension tests of graded complexity have become the cornerstone of every
aphasia battery. Our comprehension task attempts to cover various aspects of this
feature, by using "yes−no" questions, a pointing task of auditory recognition,
and a series of sequential commands. The curious "on and off" nature of
comprehension and the variability of responses compels aphasia testers to provide a large number and variety of items to eliminate some of the variation in an
individual's performance.

"Yes−No" Questions

      The patient is asked to reply or nod "yes" or "no" only to 20 questions. If
one uses commands only to test comprehension, patients with apraxia or impairment of gestural output may have difficulties which are added to any problems in
comprehension. There is no easy way to overcome this, since even a "yes" and
"no" task requires the appropriate choice of these words, which is commonly

impaired in severely affected aphasics and some degree of "yes" and "no" confusion may be seen even in more moderate impairments. It is essential, however, to use a "yes" and "no" task which requires less motor activity. We constructed "yes" and "no" questions that were relevant to the patient's own person and environment, as there seems to be a clear dichotomy in some patients who can respond to these questions quite adequately, but have a great deal of difficulty with more abstract questions or items, requiring comprehension of various grammatical and linguistic forms. We also have items incorporating these features, such as "Is a lion larger than a dog?," to examine the comprehension of grammatical relationships ("larger than"), and others, such as "Will a stone sink in water?" to assess the comprehension of semantic relationships. Half of the questions require "yes" and half "no" answers and gestural responses, even eye blinks, are accepted and encouraged. The use of "yes" and "no" responses avoids the pointing difficulty or apraxia the patient may have in carrying out an auditory sequencing task. Time is taken to have the patient understand the task, and attempts are made, before and during the task, to remain with the "set" of answering "yes" and "no" only. The patient is gently reminded to comply with this, even though this seems to be difficult for some aphasics. The phenomenon of yes—no confusion often interferes with the accurate assessment of comprehension. Behavioral clues indicate that the patient comprehends, even though the wrong answer is given. The patient shakes his head sideways while saying "yes" (the oriental "yes"). This response is often spontaneous and not in response to the examiner's inadvertent disapproval. It is also frequently wrong, that is, the patient may be frustrated with the correct answer! In some cases, eye closure may be substituted, with improvement of the score. Self-correction is accepted, but if two equivocal answers are obtained (a head shake closely followed by nodding), zero score is given. The examiner takes care not to provide cues as to the correctness of the answer. We have deliberately stayed away from complex ideational material, with a possible intellectual factor, as used in the BDAE. Even though the length and complexity of the questions are restricted, a detailed yet practical sampling of language comprehension is obtained, without entering the issue of verbal intelligence. Using only auditory stimuli, and accepting any brief indication of comprehension (verbal or gestural), a reasonably pure test of comprehension of language is achieved.

Auditory Word Recognition

The patient is asked to point to an item, spoken by the examiner, from an array in the same category; a choice of six or more, in the case of furniture or body parts. In the pointing task, we used six objects, six line drawings of objects, six letters, six numbers, six geometric forms, six colors, six items of furniture in the room, six body parts of the patient, five items of finger recognition, and seven of right and left orientation. There are patients who do much better in pointing to items in front of them than to their own body parts and there are those for whom the reverse is true; there is also a dichotomy between pointing to items close at hand and in the surrounding environment, as well as between line drawings and real objects (more transmodality perceptual cues). To achieve uniformity, instructions are provided for administration and scoring. One repetition of each command is allowed if no response is obtained or if the patient asks. The common occurrence of the patient pointing to more than one item is dealt with by giving the patient credit if he recognizes his mistake and chooses one item, firmly, eventually. No time limit is set, but it is our custom to wait about 5 seconds before repeating the command or passing on to new items.

Sequential Commands

Our task of sequential commands is patterned after Goodglass and Kaplan's (1972), and similar to Head's "coin—bowl" (1926) and to the "Token Test" of DeRenzi and Vignolo (1962). The initial commands are simple and short. Shutting the eyes is relatively easy for aphasic patients, even with severe apraxia. This serves to establish rapport, places the patient in a "set," and allows the examiner to ascertain that the patient understands that he is to perform commands and that he is willing to cooperate. Sequential pointing is one step beyond the pointing task employed before. Commands involve manipulation of one object to touch another, using prepositions of "with—to," "on top," "other side," "over," increasing the length of the sentence and the number of the components. Comprehension of these relational words is shown by Goodglass et al. (1970) to be particularly difficult for aphasics. In addition to the above aspects, this task assesses sentence comprehension, although not in the same detail as such tests as the Auditory Comprehension Test for Sentences, described by Shewan and Canter (1971). The last sentence is similar to Pierre Marie's three paper test, involving three objects and two actions, yet only using a single, 15 word sentence, to avoid memory and intellectual components. Scoring is carefully standardized and credit is given for partial response if the underlined portion of the sentence, representing action or an object, was appropriately performed. This task is given more weight than either the "yes—no" or the word recognition task, because of its difficulty and specificity for comprehension disturbances. Some aphasics (Broca's), who do very well on the auditory recognition tasks, will have difficulty with sequentially presented items. This task has been variously called auditory retention span or auditory sequencing. It is powerful in detecting slight degrees of comprehension deficit; it has even been suggested that one only need test sequential comprehension to screen for aphasia.

The issue of difficulty of the comprehension tasks is a much debated one and touches on the controversy regarding the essence of aphasic impairment. Some, like Pierre Marie, contend that intellectual impairment is the most important underlying phenomenon and, therefore, it is just a matter of testing comprehension in enough detail before this can be detected. As an example of how far this can be carried, some of the comprehension tasks used by Weisenburg and McBride are clearly tests of verbal intelligence, which are not appropriate for aphasic patients, as normal or nonaphasic, brain damaged patients will show a high rate of failure on them. Using these test scores, one cannot be certain whether the patient failed the test because of a lack of language competence or lowered intelligence, provided these are accepted to be distinct in one's conceptual framework. The view, which regards performance on these tasks as a continuum between aphasics and normals, or brain damaged patients, does not allow for the important practical considerations of diagnosing and discriminating aphasics from those patients who have no clinical aphasia. The "Token Test," designed to detect mild comprehension disturbances, was found to be frequently abnormal in nonaphasic, left hemisphere damaged and even, in right hemisphere, brain damaged patients, by Boller and Vignolo (1966). It was also found to be too difficult for moderate to severe impairment in aphasia, by Needham and Swisher (1972). The importance of using sequential commands beyond the difficulty level encountered in the comprehension of words has been emphasized by DeRenzi and Vignolo (1962), Schuell (1964), and Goodglass and Kaplan (1972). This seems to be intricately tied in with the factor of comprehension of grammar, as a dichotomy seems to emerge between aphasics who have difficulty understanding concrete words and those who have problems with grammatical relation words. The actual duration of the sequence, or what Schuell called the auditory comprehension span, could be related to short-term memory factors, but there is some evidence that this may not explain all the difficulty that aphasics have with longer sequences (Kreindler et al., 1971).

Intense psycholinguistic research has been undertaken to determine some of the factors in comprehension in the last 15 years. The significance of phonemic discrimination in the comprehension of aphasics is controversial (Blumstein et al., 1977). On reviewing the literature, it appears that impairments in phonemic discrimination are not universal; semantic and syntactic aspects of comprehension are more important. Schuell et al. (1961) related the comprehension of words to their frequency of occurrence. The role of semantic categories was investigated by Goodglass et al. (1966). Wernicke's aphasics, for instance, had more difficulty naming body parts. Semantic discrimination of words has been tested in detail by Pizzamiglio and Appicciafuoco (1971). They found that Broca's and amnesic aphasics scored well on this task, in contrast to Wernicke's and global aphasics. Goodglass et al. (1970) found that anomic aphasics were poor on a picture-vocabulary task, Broca's aphasics on point span, and Wernicke's aphasics on a preposition-preference task. Increasing the vocabulary and syntactic difficulty, but not the sentence length, increased the comprehension deficit of all aphasic groups (Shewan and Canter, 1971). These groups were different in their initial level of comprehension. Syntactic errors are made by normal controls as well as aphasics with good comprehension, indicating that the deficit measured at a certain difficulty level is not specific for aphasics or certain types of aphasia. Gardner et al. (1975) studied the comprehension of words under various conditions of presentation, such as spoken singly, in various sentences, with various speeds. Comprehension was facilitated by speaking slowly and providing redundant, semantically related information in the sentence and worsened by inserting detractor words not related semantically. Residual comprehension was evidenced in severely affected aphasics, who produced more gestures of refusal and quizzical expression when presented with foreign language or jargon than with meaningful material (Boller & Green, 1972).

It is obvious that the many factors in comprehension cannot be entirely separated and testing would have to account for them to some extent. The unity of comprehension remains a debated issue. For further reviews of psycholinguistic research the reader is referred to Lesser (1978) and Boller (1978).

REPETITION

Repetition is tested by most batteries, although often under such categories as verbal expression, oral agility, and imitation. Our repetition task in the WAB, utilizes single words [all A or AA Thorndike—Lorge frequency (1968), except "banana," with a Thorndike rating of 13], composite words, numbers, word—number combinations, high probability sentences ("the telephone is ringing"), low probability sentences ("the spy fled to Greece"), and sentences of increasing length and grammatical and phonemic complexity. We did not go beyond a nine word span or a single sentence level, hoping to avoid short-term, verbal memory disturbances.

Goodglass and Kaplan (1972) added the new dimension of low and high probability sentence repetition, which is extremely sensitive to mild aphasic disturbances, introducing a significant advance in the testing of repetition. Alajouanine et al. (1964) found a higher frequency of literal than verbal paraphasias in conduction aphasia. Boller and Vignolo (1966) also showed that repetition of conduction aphasics contained many more literal paraphasias than transcortical sensory aphasics who repeat well but have many semantic paraphasias in spontaneous speech.

Strub and Gardner (1974) investigated a patient with conduction aphasia, whose performance was improved with longer intervals between stimuli. Recalling the stimuli was superior to ordering them. The repetition of single nonsense words and the production of paraphasias could not be attributed to memory defects. They considered that impaired repetition derives from a difficulty in producing a target word with precision rather than from a failure to recall it. It seems that memory and linguistic processing are intricately related and not mutually exclusive. Shallice and Warrington (1977) distinguished between the repetition of a single, relatively infrequent, polysyllabic word (to be called reproduction) and of a number of unconnected, short, familiar words (to be called ''repetition''), and suggested that reproduction is a speech production process and repetition involves auditory short-term memory, relating to speech comprehension. The once so popular tongue twisters are of doubtful validity, as they will baffle normals often enough, although most testers tend to include them. I like Dr. Geschwind's sentence of ''no if's, and's or but's,'' consisting specifically of short grammatical words, without any content, which is difficult for most aphasics, but especially those with conduction aphasia.

Most clinicians agree on the importance of testing repetition and that no test is complete without it. One encounters, from time to time, most interesting language disturbances, where repetition, in fact, remains intact, yet no comprehension is evident although, obviously, the word has been heard and processed through language mechanisms since it is spoken again. Such disconnection from association areas has been commonly called transcortical sensory aphasia. Similarly, patients who cannot initiate speech spontaneously, but repeat and comprehend well, are called ''transcortical motor aphasics.'' Repetition is regarded as a function of the intact speech area alone; Geschwind, Quadfasel, and Segarra (1968) presented anatomical evidence to support this concept. When repetition is impaired above other language functions, the diagnosis of conduction aphasia is considered. A repetition task is essential to distinguish conduction and transcortical aphasics from other syndromes with impaired comprehension and expression. The terms ''transcortical'' or ''conduction'' are used as traditional descriptive labels for complex clinical phenomena, rather than to imply established anatomical or physiological mechanisms. To separate these cases from the larger group of sensory and motor aphasics has a valid foundation in clinical experience, as attested by our data, regardless of the theoretical implication of disconnection of speech region from other association areas.

NAMING

Naming is another major item in aphasia testing, which has gone through stages of refinement, from the very simple, bedside task of visual presentation of objects to the patient, to include such tests of word finding as sentence completion, responsive speech, and exploring word finding under specified linguistic conditions. Our naming tasks, used for all subjects, include:

1. Object Naming—60 percent of the naming score. Twenty common objects are presented visually. In case of no response or an incorrect response, the patient is allowed to palpate it and if still wrong, a phonemic or, if it is a composite word, a semantic cue is given. About 20 seconds are allowed for all of this, for each item. The score of 3 is given for correct naming, 2 for

recognizable phonemic paraphasia, and one if a phonemic or tactile cue is required. The naming task requires little, if any comprehension, provided the patient understands the initial instructions and stays with the "set." The objects were selected for their availability and handy size but variations of the shape, the category of the objects, and difficulty level were introduced deliberately. The level of expectation or frequency of occurrence was controlled on the Thorndike−Lorge scale (1968): three objects were in the category of occurring more than 100 million words used (AA), six in the 50−100 (A), and 11 in the 1−40 category.

2. Word Fluency—20 percent of the naming score. Word fluency is another test of word finding, where words in a category are to be listed within a certain time, such as names of animals or words beginning with a certain letter. The latter is certainly much more difficult for aphasics and even normals, and probably less suitable for aphasia testing. We found that these tests of word fluency, although very sensitive to aphasic word-finding disturbances, are often impaired in nonaphasics and also measure a more general, cerebral impairment. There is a significant difference in the word fluency performance of normals of various intellectual abilities. Anxiety and distractability clearly interfere with it, to a greater extent than any other language task. Nonaphasic word-finding difficulty is a well-known phenomenon. It is impossible to eliminate it entirely from any tests of naming but its role is greater in the word fluency task.

3. Sentence Completion—10 percent of the naming score.

4. Responsive Speech—10 percent of the naming score. Responsive speech, as well as sentence completion, requires auditory comprehension, but the word finding is facilitated by the context of the preceding sentence. These responses are much easier than the other word-finding and naming tasks, as the stimulus context is prepared so that the answers should be unequivocal, almost automatic. These items correspond to similar ones in the BDAE and NCCEA.

The universality of naming difficulty has led to numerous investigations of the various characteristics of the stimuli. The differences among various semantic categories of stimuli has been demonstrated by Goodglass et al. (1966). Objects were more difficult to name than letters for fluent aphasics, but this was not the case in Broca's aphasia. This was considered to be related to phonological complexity. The categories of colors, actions, geometric forms, and numbers contributed little, if any, to the differences between the major diagnostic groups. We deleted these other categories (the same as used in the pointing task of comprehension), but retained object naming and tightened the scoring criteria (see below). Letter naming is featured in our reading task, considering its dependence on literacy and probably a different mechanism of acquisition. Individual cases of category specific anomia, body parts, etc., are continuing to be described (Dennis, 1976). Differences between the level of abstraction, the pictureability of stimuli (Goodglass et al., 1969), and whether it is manipulable or nonmanipulable have been demonstrated by various authors. Naming ability was also correlated with the frequency of the stimulus in language (Newcombe et al., 1965), as well as the length of the word. Rochford and Williams (1962) showed that the naming of various objects by aphasics and children have a similar order of difficulty. The modality of presentation is also important; some studies involved a tactile presentation in addition to the visual one, especially if there were difficulties in the visual area. A failure to name could be related to either a universal linguistic problem of naming difficulty or a more specific visual agnosia if tactile naming can be accomplished. There was no significant difference between various modalities of presentation in the studies of Goodglass et al. (1968) and Spreen et al. (1966) when visual or auditory agnosia were excluded. Many clinicians utilize tactile naming only optionally, even though simultaneous multimodal presentation of stimuli may facilitate naming. We incorporated tactile naming in our sequence of object naming, as discussed above.

There is disagreement in the method of scoring, in the administration of naming tasks, even varying as to whether the patient should be timed or allowed to look at the stimulus at leisure. Also, supplying cues is a frequently used method by some and is strictly forbidden by others. We found that cueing is an important aspect of language examination and it may be important from the point of view of therapists. Therefore, we have a separate scoring category for objects named with cueing or after multiple modality presentation. We also distinguish between semantic and phonemic cueing. Semantic cueing can be used in composite words, such as eyeglasses. Naming is found to be fairly consistent and the number of items does not need to be as numerous as in the comprehension task, cutting down the need for lengthy naming tasks of various semantic categories.

READING

Literacy is much more universal now in our society than it was 50 years ago. However, the degree of reading and writing skills differ sufficiently that premorbid reading and educational achievement will influence the results of testing. We therefore tried to restrict our reading comprehension task to a moderate level of intelligence and limited attention span. Since most reading tests, such as the Gates–MacGinitie, etc., were standardized for school children, we decided to adapt and modify some of the reading tests of Goodglass and Kaplan (1972) from the BDAE, some from Schuell (1964), and construct some of our own. The test is administered to start with the most difficult items—reading comprehension of sentences and the reading of commands. If the patient reads well on these tasks, that is, the combined score is over 50, the test is discontinued and the subsequent items are prorated.

1. Reading Comprehension of Sentences consists of the first eight items from the BDAE reading task, which utilizes the technique of sentence completion with a four-way multiple choice. The answers were placed one above another, a modification of the original, to avoid the effect of hemianopia or visual field neglect so important in some alexic patients. The possible answers include several wrong responses, which are associatively related to words in the stimulus material. There is less chance to guess the answer than in a true−false paradigm. The patient is read an example and then instructed to read each sentence silently or aloud, and to point to the missing word from the choice. The sentences range in complexity, from three words to a small paragraph of two sentences and 34 words. Large, 0.5-cm print is used to eliminate problems of visual acuity.

2. Reading Commands is scored for reading aloud and for doing what the card requests, separately. This test was designed for the occasional patient who can read without comprehending. It is also a test of praxis, from written stimulation, and a test of reading comprehension of sentences.

If the combined score of items 1 and 2 is below 50, as mentioned above, the test is continued at the word level.

3. Written Word Stimulus—Object Choice Matching is tested with the printed names of six common objects, 3−11 letters in length. The patient is asked to point to the object from a choice of six.

4. Picture Stimulus—Written Word Choice Matching. The pictures of a flower, girl, horse, dog, tree, and boy are shown in sequence. The patient must choose from the six words printed below each other.

5. Written Word Stimulus—Picture Choice Matching is the exact reverse of item 4.

6. Phonetic Association is a task from the BDAE. The patient must select from a multiple choice of five written words, the one spoken by the examiner. This test is designed to examine auditory−visual phonetic associations without necessary comprehension or verbalization by the patient. Some of the wrong choices are connotatively, and some phonetically similar to the correct word. The occasional patient may respond with a connotative, rather than a phonetic, mismatch.

7. Letter Discrimination. Six individual letters are spoken by the examiner and the patient chooses from the printed choice of six.

8. Spelled Word Recognition is a task of auditory decoding of spelling, a task which is said to differentiate among various forms of alexia. Failure occurs in aphasic alexia, but performance is excellent in "pure" or "agnosic" alexia (Benson and Geschwind, 1969). The longest word is nine letters.

9. Spelling. Six common stimulus words are spoken, 2−10 letters in length, and the patient is asked to spell them. Although this is not a reading task, strictly speaking, the importance of spelling in reading and writing indicates the need for this subtest.

WRITING

The writing tasks are divided into the standard subtests used by most examiners, such as writing on request, dictation and copying. The patient's nonparalyzed hand, or, if there is no paralysis, his dominant hand is used. It is noted whether this is the left or the right. The patient is encouraged and, if necessary, the pen is placed in his hand. Anagram letters may be used if there is no written response.

1. Writing on Request. The patient is asked to write his name and address. This is very overlearned; the next subtest is more difficult and revealing of agraphic disturbances.
2. Written Output. The patient is asked to write as much as he can in sentences about the same picture that was shown for the spontaneous speech subtest. This narrative is scored according to the number of correct sentences and words, and deductions are made for paragraphic errors.
3. Writing to Dictation. "The quick brown fox jumps over the lazy dog." If the combined score of 40 is achieved on these three subtests, the rest of the writing tasks are omitted and prorated.
4. Writing of Dictated or Visually Presented Words. If the patient fails to write the name of one of the objects dictated, the actual object is shown, and the patient is encouraged to write the name. If he still fails, the word is spelled by the examiner and the patient is asked to write it. The last alternative is to have the patient spell the word using anagram letters made of cardboard.
5. Recall of Written Symbols. The alphabet and serial numbers up to 20 are requested.
6. Writing of Dictated Letters and Numbers. Six letters and six numbers are dictated.
7. Copying of words of the test sentence in item 3.

The scoring system does not fully reflect the quality and structural aspects of writing, since these are complex and variable features. We are presently reviewing this aspect of writing of aphasics, in order to categorize the various defects, such as slanting, neglect, extra loops, superimposition, perserveration, etc.

PRAXIS

Twenty commands are given for upper limb, buccofacial, instrumental (transitive), and complex performances. The patient is scored 3 for acceptable, 2 for approximate performance, 2 for imitation only, and 1 for approximate performance on imitation or if performed with the actual object. The details and rationale of assessing praxis are discussed in Chapter 13.

CALCULATION

The calculation task utilizes one or two digit numbers, three items for each of addition, subtraction, multiplication, and division. These tasks are presented visually, on cards, as well as the examiner speaking the numbers and the requested arithmetical operation. The multimodal presentation is aimed at overcoming comprehension or reading deficit and assessing arithmetical ability only.

DRAWING

The patient is asked to draw a circle, square, Christmas tree, cube, clock, house, and person, and also, to bisect a line (to quantitate visuospatial neglect). Scoring considers completeness, perspective, and quality, and penalizes perseveration, disconnected lines, inappropriate angles, and neglect.

BLOCK DESIGN

The first three items and a demonstration item from the Wechsler Intelligence Scale Block Design Test (Koh's blocks) are used, with a modified scoring system (see Chapter 14).

RAVEN'S COLORED PROGRESSIVE MATRICES

Sets A, A_B, and B are used to assess visuospatial perceptual function and nonverbal intelligence. See Chapter 14 on aphasia and intelligence for further details.

SUMMARY

The requirements for aphasia testing and the pitfalls of test construction are discussed. The Western Aphasia Battery and its rationale are presented in detail. The reason for selecting certain subtests, their administration, and scoring is described. Emphasis is placed on assessing fluency, comprehension, repetition, and naming, in the light of recent psycholinguistic research. The test intends to bridge a gap between clinical and research needs.

4

The Aphasia Quotient: Populations, Controls, Standardization and Validation

Introduction
1. Aphasic and control populations of the first standardization
2. The classification criteria
3. The difficulty level of subtests and the aphasia quotient
4. The mean and standard scores and aphasic profiles
5. The separation of aphasics and controls (criterion validity)
6. Correlation of WAB and NCCEA (construct validity)—intertest reliability
7. Internal consistency
8. Correlation of WAB subtests
9. Intrajudge reliability
10. Interjudge reliability
11. Test—retest reliability
12. Aphasic and control populations of the second standardization
Summary

The reasons for their popularity [The Wechsler Adult Intelligence Scales] . . . the scales were objective, they were standardized and they had demonstrable clinical utility.

Benton, AL: Problems of test construction in the field of aphasia
Cortex 3:32, 1967

INTRODUCTION

In order to consider a test valid for research or clinical use, the test should be standardized on subjects representative of the population the test intends to study. Preferably, several populations entering the differential diagnosis should be contrasted. The variation in test scores related to the presence or absence of various phenomena to be measured, and the cutoff points between impaired and nonimpaired individuals need to be determined (criterion validity). The test needs to be correlated with other tests acknowledged to measure the same phenomena (construct validity). The components of a test should contribute evenly to the measurement of disability (internal consistency). A test should yield the same results when the same subject is examined, provided there is no change in the disability (test−retest reliability). The same examiner should be able to score the same subject at different times (intrajudge reliability) and various examiners should reproduce the same results on the same subjects (interjudge reliability). A significant technological advance, the use of the videotape, enabled us to carry out these standardization procedures to a level of higher accuracy, until recently not available to researchers, without causing discomfort to our aphasic patients. Some of this work was done in collaboration with Cynthia Shewan, Ph.D., who contributed materially to this chapter, especially to the sections on construct validity, internal consistency, intrajudge, and interjudge reliability.

APHASIC AND CONTROL POPULATION OF THE FIRST STANDARDIZATION

The first standardization of the Western Aphasia Battery (WAB) was performed on a population of 150 consecutively examined aphasics and 59 controls (Kertesz and Poole, 1974). The majority of patients (84) were from St. Joseph's Hospital, representing an acute aphasic population. There were 37 patients from a Veteran's Hospital neurological unit and 29 patients from another general hospital. Our criteria for admission to this study were that the patient was clinically considered aphasic by a physician or speech pathologist, and well enough to be tested. This material, including recent patients, is more comprehensive and representative of the whole scope of aphasia than previous studies on chronic patients in rehabilitation units, heavily populated with hemiplegics with global or Broca's aphasia. The great majority of the patients had cerebral infarction and were neurologically and pathologically stable. Next in frequency were tumors, followed by trauma, hemorrhage, aneurysm, and degenerative disease (Table 4-1). Mentally retarded and psychotic patients, or those with a language barrier, were not included.

The sex ratio was heavily weighted—99:51—in favor of males, a difference explained mainly by the veteran population in the sample (37). Handedness was determined by questioning the patient or relative about hand preference for (1) writing, (2) throwing, (3) cutting, (4) drawing, (5) brushing, and (6) using a spoon, with four out of six items deciding. One hundred and forty-six were right-handed, and four were left-handed. The controls consisted of

1. A group of "normals," that is, 21 non−brain-damaged neurological patients with spinal cord disease, peripheral neuropathy, blackouts, tics, vertigo, ataxia, etc.

Table 4-1
Distribution According to Diagnosis

Diagnosis	Aphasics	Controls (with Brain Damage)
CVA	114	20
Tumor	14	4
Trauma	9	—
Degenerative	4	5
Aneurysm	4	—
Hemorrhage	2	1
A–V Malformation	1	2
Abscess	1	—
Uncertain	1	—
Parkinson's	—	3
Korsakoff's		3
Total	150	38

(Adapted with permission from the Canadian Journal of Neurological Sciences 1:10, 1974.)

2. 17 patients with nondominant hemispheric lesions ("comparable brain damage")
3. 21 patients with diffuse or dominant hemisphere or subcortical brain damage, but clinically, no aphasia.

The controls had similar educational (average grade VIII) and language backgrounds to the aphasics. The population was not controlled for intelligence as the test was designed to measure language and minimize the effect of intelligence.

THE CLASSIFICATION CRITERIA

The criteria to classify aphasics were arrived at after reviewing the first 150 patients (Table 4-2). These numbers represent ranges of scores chosen to classify all aphasics unequivocally. A fluency score of 4 or below separates the aphasias with significant motor involvement: global, Broca's isolation, and transcortical motor aphasia. A comprehension score of 4 or better on our battery separates Broca's aphasia from global aphasia, and transcortical motor from isolation aphasia. A score of better than 5 repetition distinguishes isolation syndrome from global aphasia, and a score of 8 or greater discriminates transcortical motor from Broca's aphasia. Among the fluent aphasias, the anomic and conduction aphasics have been than 7 comprehension, in contrast to Wernicke's and transcortical sensory aphasics, with comprehension below that. Repetition poorer than 7 separates conduction aphasics from anomics. Interestingly, some of the conduction aphasics appear to have excellent naming scores. A naming score

Table 4-2
Criteria for Classification

	Fluency	Comprehension	Repetition	Naming
Global	0–4	0–3.9	0–4.9	0–6
Broca's	0–4	4–10	0–7.9	0–8
Isolation	0–4	0–3.9	5–10	0–6
Transcortical Motor	0–4	4–10	8–10	0–8
Wernicke's	5–10	0–6.9	0–7.9	0–9
Transcortical Sensory	5–10	0–6.9	8–10	0–9
Conduction	5–10	7–10	0–6.9	0–9
Anomic	5–10	7–10	7–10	0–9

below 9.0 was arbitrarily chosen as a cutoff point, to separate anomic aphasics from nonbrain damaged controls; otherwise, the naming scores did not distinguish between subgroups (see criterion validity).

THE DIFFICULTY LEVEL OF SUBTESTS AND THE APHASIA QUOTIENT

The scoring of subtests was designed to represent equal difficulty levels at various language tasks and modalities; the subtests were chosen to represent equally important language functions. The means and standard deviations of scores of 150 aphasics for each subtest were compared (Figure 4-1). The difficulty level for each test is quite similar. For further data on the equivalence of the tests contributing to the main factor in a principal component analysis, see Chapters 6 and 7. We also selected language items that a nonaphasic adult would pass regardless of memory or intellectual deficit (see Chapter 3).

The sum of scores was called the Aphasia Quotient (AQ) because it is expressed as a percentage of a maximum (normal) score of 100. The scores of subtests are scaled $1-10$ and the AQ can be calculated simply by multiplying by 2 the sum of subscores—fluency, information content, comprehension, repetition and naming—requiring no further statistical manipulation by the clinician. The scoring of fluency and information are on a $0-10$ scale. The other subtests consist of test items with maximum scores adding up to 200 for comprehension (divided by 20 for scaling for AQ) and 100 for repetition and naming (divided by 10 for scaling).

THE MEAN AND STANDARD SCORES AND APHASIC PROFILES

The patients were grouped according to the criteria detailed above and in Table 4-2. The number of patients, their mean age, mean scores by subtests, and

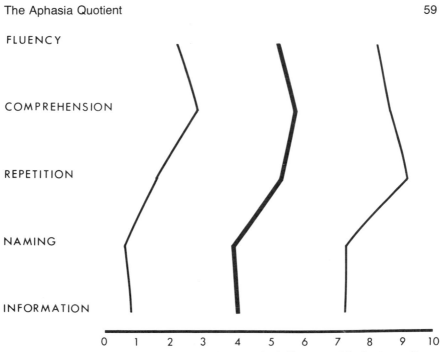

FLUENCY

COMPREHENSION

REPETITION

NAMING

INFORMATION

| 0 | 1 | 2 | 3 | 4 | 5 | 6 | 7 | 8 | 9 | 10 |

Fig. 4-1. The profile of performances using standard (Z) scores (abscissa): nonfluent aphasics on the left, fluent ones on the right. (Reproduced with permission from the Canadian Journal of Neurological Sciences 1:10, 1974.)

their standard deviations and the AQ are summarized in Table 4-3. The groups are ranked in the order of their severity as determined by their AQ.

1. *Global aphasia* is the most severe form. It is commonly seen (26)—mean AQ = 10.5. These patients are severely affected in all language functions. Their spontaneous speech is nonfluent, and lacks information; they have poor comprehension, repetition, and naming. They may produce variable amounts of stereotypic utterances, and at times, well pronounced and even long (2−3 words) phrases of emotional charge, often swear words.

2. *Broca's aphasia* is characterized by impaired speech output with relatively well-preserved comprehension. They speak little, with great effort, often showing frustration, but convey some information. Phonemic paraphasias and agrammatisms are common. Repetition and naming are impaired but at times, better than spontaneous speech output. Twenty-four cases were seen, with a mean AQ of 31.7.

3. *Isolation aphasia* or speech isolation syndrome is an infrequent entity, with little or no spontaneous speech, comprehension, or naming, but excellent repetition. Only five partial or incomplete examples were encountered— mean AQ = 34.3.

4. *Wernicke's aphasia* is characterized by fluent, paraphasic speech with impaired comprehension, repetition, and naming. Some of these patients have a

Table 4-3

The Number, Mean Ages, Mean Scores of Subtests and AQs and their Standard Deviations of the Subgroups and the Total of 150 Aphasics and 59 Controls

Number	Type of Aphasia	Age	Fluency		Comprehension		Repetition		Naming		Information		AQ	
		X̄	X̄	SD	X̄	SD	X̄	SD	X̄	SD	X̄	SD	X̄	SD
26	Global	65.0	1.0	1.2	2.2	1.7	0.9	1.5	0.5	1.3	0.6	0.9	10.5	9.2
24	Motor (Broca's)	57.3	2.5	1.7	5.9	1.5	3.3	3.1	2.4	2.4	1.8	1.8	31.7	16.6
5	Isolation	65.6	3.0	1.7	2.5	1.0	7.8	1.7	2.1	1.7	1.8	1.1	34.3	11.9
28	Sensory (Wernicke's)	60.3	6.9	1.1	3.5	1.9	3.7	3.0	2.1	1.8	3.3	2.3	39.0	12.8
4	Transcortical Motor	67.0	3.5	1.0	6.2	1.3	9.2	0.9	4.3	2.4	3.5	1.0	54.4	8.4
8	Transcortical Sensory	51.3	6.9	1.4	4.9	1.3	9.3	0.5	4.0	2.5	4.6	1.3	59.6	5.5
15	Conduction	62.2	6.1	1.2	8.3	0.9	5.0	1.9	5.2	2.6	5.7	2.2	60.5	12.7
40	Anomic	60.3	8.0	0.9	9.0	0.8	9.1	0.9	7.8	1.2	7.7	1.7	83.3	7.8
150	Total X̄	61.1	5.2	3.0	5.7	2.9	5.3	3.8	3.9	3.3	4.0	3.2	48.2	28.2
	Controls													
21	I Nonbrain Damaged	59.2	10.0	0.0	9.9	0.2	9.8	0.3	9.5	0.3	10.0	0.0	98.4	1.0
17	II Nondominant Hemisphere	59.4	10.0	0.0	9.7	0.4	9.8	0.2	9.1	0.4	9.9	0.3	97.1	1.9
21	III Mixed Group	58.6	9.7	0.7	9.5	0.6	9.6	0.5	8.9	0.6	9.2	1.3	93.8	4.7

(Adapted with permission from the Canadian Journal of Neurological Sciences 1:10, 1974.)

great amount of neologistic paraphasias, under pressure at times, and often without too much awareness of their disability. (These patients are often misdiagnosed as psychiatric disturbances.) We consider neologistic jargon aphasics a distinct group; but, for the purposes of this study, they are combined with the others because their performance on the verbal subtests is similar. "Pure" word deafness, meaning impaired comprehension but otherwise intact speech, repetition and naming, was seen in two patients, but only transiently, 28 cases belonged to Wernicke's group, with a mean AQ of 39.0.

5. *Transcortical motor aphasia* is an interesting entity characterized by good comprehension and excellent repetition, but the patient speaks very little on his own. This is more often seen transiently and by the time the patients are tested, there is often only slight anomia left or even that has recovered. Four cases were considered to represent this group with a mean AQ of 54.4.

6. *Transcortical sensory aphasia* is fluent with good repetition but poor comprehension and naming. This can also be regarded as the sensory component of the speech "isolation syndrome." Eight cases were seen—mean AQ = 59.6.

7. *Conduction aphasia* is distinguished by very poor repetition with relatively fluent but paraphasic speech and good comprehension. This group of aphasics is most interesting and has been inconsistently reported in the literature until recently. One reason is that they resemble other aphasics and repetition has to be tested specifically to identify them. There were 15 patients with a mean AQ of 60.5.

8. *Anomic or amnestic aphasia* is common. These patients have fluent, often circumlocutory speech, associated with good comprehension and repetition but impaired naming. Some patients included in this study performed near normally on naming tasks, in spite of word-finding difficulty. There were also a few patients whose spontaneous speech was very near normal but who had significant impairment of naming on visual stimuli. These may represent a pure stimulus–response defect. They were rechecked on a control subtest involving naming by palpation, to see if there was significant difference between the two input modalities for naming, to rule out visual agnosia. Forty cases were seen, with a mean AQ of 83.3.

A profile of performance for each aphasic subgroup was drawn using standard (Z) scores (Fig. 4-2). This illustrates the outstanding features of each aphasic group. Nonfluent aphasics are grouped separately on the left for the illustration. They are further distinguished by their performance on comprehension and repetition. Fluent aphasics on the right of the profile diagram also show further separation on comprehension and repetition. With the exception of Wernicke's aphasia they tend to be milder on the severity scale than their nonfluent counterparts. The advantage of using standard scores is to allow the comparison of the performance of an individual on each subtest with other subtests and other

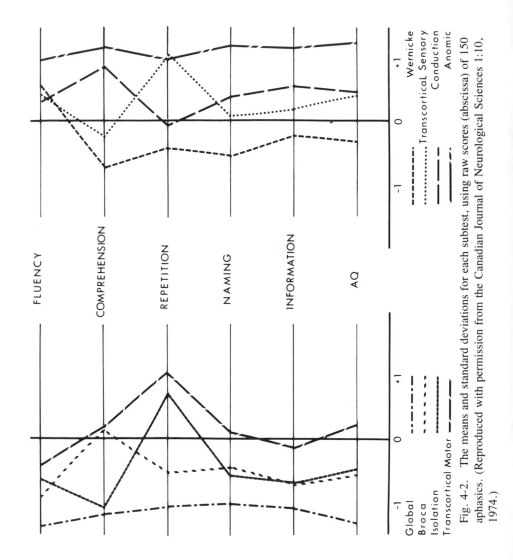

Fig. 4-2.   The means and standard deviations for each subtest, using raw scores (abscissa) of 150 aphasics. (Reproduced with permission from the Canadian Journal of Neurological Sciences 1:10, 1974.)

FLUENCY

COMPREHENSION

REPETITION

NAMING

INFORMATION

AQ

Global
Broca
Isolation
Transcortical Motor

Wernicke
Transcortical Sensory
Conduction
Anomic

individuals. However, the test items and scoring were designed to have approximately equal difficulty level for each subtest as discussed above. This and the use of the criteria for classification (Table 4-2), eliminates the need for transforming the observed scores to standard scores by the clinician.

THE SEPARATION OF APHASICS AND CONTROLS (CRITERION VALIDITY)

One of the problems that a clinician may face is to determine whether the patient is aphasic or normal. The researcher may also need a criterion or a cutoff point to define aphasic and normal language performance. Criterion validities indicate the extent to which a test may be used to estimate an individual's standing in respect to the disability.

All our aphasics differed from the "non−brain-damaged controls" in that either their fluency scores were below 10 or their naming fell below 9.0. (There was one mildly anomic patient whose fluency was scored as 10 but his naming on confrontation was only 7.9.) The lowest naming score for the nonbrain damaged controls was 9.1. The controls were comparable in age and since they were taken consecutively from the same hospital population, probably for other socioeconomic factors as well. The control of educational levels would be more important in the reading and writing tasks, which were not included in the initial study. The majority of patients was tested on Raven's Colored Progressive Matrices, also a nonverbal test of intelligence. The performance of aphasics was comparable to the controls, suggesting that the population was matched for intelligence as well (Kertesz and McCabe, 1975).

The ages of various aphasic and control groups were subjected to a one-way analysis of variance and were found not significantly different from each other ($F = 1.35$ at 10 and 198 df at $p \leqslant 0.05$).

Overlapping scores were observed with the third group of controls examined on the battery. The border appeared indistinct between this group and recovering mild anomic aphasics. A comparison with aphasics seemed to be worthwhile because of the problem of drawing the line between diffuse brain damage affecting language and aphasia. The group consisted of three cases of Parkinson's disease with dementia, three cases of Korsakoff's psychosis, five cases of subcortical or brainstem infarcts, three cases of presenile dementia—two presumed to be Alzheimer's disease clinically—one proven Jakob−Creutzfeldt on autopsy, two left hemisphere tumors—one parietal glioma (Gerstmann syndrome without aphasia)—one parasagittal meningioma, one postconcussion syndrome, one postencephalitic, and three patients with diffuse, dominant hemisphere or subcortical brain damage and no obvious difficulty with language. Some of the presenile dementias, of course, involve the speech areas sooner or later in the course of the disease, although they are not as likely to present with aphasia. The implication of verbal memory loss in Korsakoff's disease as a factor in the mild anomia seen, at times, is of theoretical interest to the mechanism of anomia. This group had a higher mean AQ (93.8−SD = 7.8) than anomic aphasia (83.3−SD = 4.3), the least severe of aphasic groups. The difference is very significant at $p \le 0.0005$ level, using Student's "t" test ($t = 5.7$ at 58 df).

The determination of the AQ seems useful to distinguish between aphasic and nonaphasic, control patients. An operational definition of aphasic score may be provided by the above control scores. The patient may be considered normal or nonaphasic if the AQ is 93.8 or above. This is the mean AQ of the diffuse or subcortical brain damaged control group. The most useful, single subtest seems to be the fluency rating, where all the undamaged controls achieved a score of 10.

There is a group of recovered or mild aphasics, whose word-finding difficulty or the occasionally uttered paraphasias would justify regarding them with the aphasic group clinically but their performance on the battery is in the normal range, as defined above. For the purpose of this study, we did not include them in the aphasic group, although for some individuals, this so-called "normal" performance was probably below their usual language ability. Since they were referred to us as either questionable aphasics or known-but-recovered aphasics, we could not include them in the normal group either. Subsequent to our first standardization, we established a fourth "control" group consisting of recovered aphasics, as we found that many of our previously aphasic patients have reached our operational criterion of recovery. For some studies, this separation was desirable but on other occasions, such as the taxonomic analysis of chronic patients, they were treated as part of a continuum of language behavior. The mean AQ of these 21 recovered patients is 97.47, with a standard deviation of 4.47. We also examined 18 patients since the first standardization, who were referred to us as either questionable aphasics or had a left hemisphere lesion which was considered potentially aphasia producing. Their AQ was above our cutoff point of 93.8 and we did not include them in the aphasic population. Their mean AQ was 97.17 with a standard deviation of 1.46. The right hemisphere lesion control group ($N = 17$) on the first standardization had an AQ of 97.1 with a standard deviation of 1.9. Since then, we examined 60 other nonaphasic right hemisphere lesion patients with the WAB. This group had an AQ of 94.26 with a standard deviation of 5.31. Twenty of these patients had an AQ of below our arbitrary cutoff of 93.8. A high false positive rate of 30% indicates that the AQ alone cannot be used to label whether a brain damaged patient is aphasic, although it can be used as a cutoff point between aphasics and normals. Many patients with deep subcortical right hemisphere lesions are dysarthric, which makes it difficult for them to use full and complete sentences, and lowers their fluency scores. They tend to speak telegraphically and their repetition score may be decreased. Patients with large, posterior, right hemisphere lesions also exhibit striking neglect. This neglect interferes with their performance on the auditory comprehension tasks requiring pointing to objects, pictures, letters, etc. Their reading and writing may also be impaired for this reason. However, this rarely, if ever, gives rise to a false positive diagnosis. The examiner can alter the array of stimuli to compensate for hemianopia and neglect and the qualitative features, such as the good naming and sentence comprehension on sequential commands, as well as the lack of paraphasias, distinguish these nonaphasic patients with a lower AQ from those aphasics achieving the same or higher AQ.

CORRELATION OF WAB AND NCCEA (CONSTRUCT VALIDITY)—INTERTEST RELIABILITY

Construct validity is the ability of a test to measure a concept. This is often determined by comparing it to an accepted measure of the same concept, in this case, aphasia. The Neurosensory Center Comprehensive Examination for Aphasia (NCCEA) appeared to be the most suitable for an intertest comparison. The Western Aphasia Battery (WAB) and the NCCEA by Spreen and Benton (1968) were administered to 15 aphasics at the same time, mostly on the same day and, at the most, two weeks apart. These patients represented a fair sample in terms of severity and types of aphasia. Five were severe, six moderately, and four mildly affected aphasics, of anomic (8), Broca's (3), Wernicke's (2), global (1), and conduction (1) varieties.

All subtests and test totals correlated to a significant degree ($p \leq 0.0001$). The subtests which were considered to correspond sufficiently to establish a correlation are summarized with their correlation coefficients in Table 4-4.

This then indicates a high degree of construct validity and interest validity as measured against a well-standardized and recognized battery which forms the basis of a planned international aphasia test (Benton, 1969).

INTERNAL CONSISTENCY

The measurement of the stability of a test instrument, whether various parts of the test contribute in a consistent manner to the total score, is referred to as internal consistency. The scores of 140 aphasics who had the complete test including reading, writing, praxis, calculation, drawing, block design, Raven's matrices, as well as the language tasks, were used to measure internal consistency, using Cronbach's alpha coefficient (Nunnally, 1967), which uses a random half correlation procedure. The coefficient for the WAB was 0.905 ($p \leq$ 0.001), indicating high internal consistency. Nunnally (1967) considered a Cronbach α of 0.80 acceptable. The WAB consists of a number of components which are combined to yield a composite score. Bentler's coefficient theta (θ) is a measure of internal consistency, specifically designed for such tests. It is a

Table 4–4
WAB–NCCEA Correspondence Correlation

WAB	NCCEA	Pearson *r*
Spontaneous speech	Description of use	
fluency	Sentence construction	
content		0.8173
Comprehension	Identification by name	
yes–no question	Identification by sentence	
word discrimination		
sequential commands		0.9513
Repetition	Sentence repetition	0.8802
Naming		
object naming	Visual naming	
word fluency	Word fluency	
sentence completion		
responsive speech		0.9040
Reading	Oral reading (names)	
	Oral reading (sentences)	
	Reading names for meaning	
	Reading sentences for meaning	0.9188
Writing	Visual graphic naming	
	Writing names	
	Writing to dictation	
	Writing from copy	0.9049
Total WAB–NCCEA Correlation		0.9635

The subtests that appeared to measure the same language parameters were correlated. For details of the reading and writing task, see Chapter 3. The Pearson *r* values are all significant at 0.01.

measure of how well the composite score reflects each of the components. The obtained coefficient θ of 0.974 *(p $\leq$ 0.001)* demonstrates that the components of the WAB are highly consistent internally.

CORRELATION OF WAB SUBTESTS

The correlation matrix for the WAB subtests is shown in Table 4-5. Few of the correlations are below 0.6 and these appear on the fluency subtests and repetition. The lower correlation with comprehension is probably explained by the nonfluent aphasics who comprehend well (Broca's, transcortical motor). On the other hand, fluency correlates well with information content, naming, and repetition parameters of language output. Information content correlates highly with all language subtests and it has the highest correlation with the AQ (the

Table 4–5
Correlation Matrix for the Subtotal Scores on the WAB

Subtest scores	Information content	Fluency	Auditory comprehension	Repetition	Naming	Reading	Writing	Praxis	Construction
Information content	1.000								
Fluency	0.787	1.000							
Comprehension	0.729	0.506	1.000						
Repetition	0.774	0.703	0.677	1.000					
Naming	0.875	0.704	0.783	0.848	1.000				
Reading	0.769	0.584	0.835	0.687	0.852	1.000			
Writing	0.648	0.530	0.659	0.593	0.706	0.753	1.000		
Praxis	0.690	0.563	0.815	0.679	0.707	0.739	0.607	1.000	
Construction	0.640	0.462	0.791	0.549	0.697	0.790	0.770	0.711	1.000

total score), as well. Auditory comprehension correlates best with reading, praxis, and naming. Further evidence for this is supplied in the chapters on alexia and apraxia in this book. Naming correlates best with information content; both are a general measure of the severity of aphasia. Information content is dependent, to some extent, on the ability to find names for the information requested. Reading and writing correlate highly in the aphasic population. Construction, which includes calculation, drawing, block design, and Raven's matrices, correlates well with reading, probably reflecting the role the dominant parietal lobe plays in these functions.

INTRAJUDGE RELIABILITY

To measure the consistency with which the test is applied by the same individual to the same subject, three examiners scored twice, several months apart, the videotaped tests in ten patients. In other words, each judge scored the same language behavior twice. The time interval and the number of intervening tests ensured that the judges did not remember the scores from the first time. The correlation between the two sets of scores for the ten patients, a measure of intrajudge reliability, was very high as displayed in Table 4-6. The correlations were computed for each judge separately and coefficients were obtained for each subtotal score, as well as AQ and CQ (the cortical quotient or the total of all scores).

INTERJUDGE RELIABILITY

The scoring system of the WAB allows relatively little interjudge variation in the subtests where the patient's response per item is recorded as correct or incorrect. More variation can occur conceivably in the subtests requiring judgmental scoring, such as the fluency of spontaneous speech (with possibilities $0-10$) or praxis $(0-3)$. To measure variation between examiners, ten patients of various types and severity were videotaped during the administration of the WAB.

Eight judges (five speech pathologists, two psychometricians, and one neurologist) familiar with the WAB, scored the same tapes at their convenience. The writing and drawing were available for direct scoring. The scores were correlated in a matrix of interjudge comparisons for each subtest. The average intercorrelations between judges were very high, as illustrated in Table 4-7. Relatively, the lowest correlation is seen in the spontaneous speech fluency subtest which requires a judgmental score as predicted. However, even the lowest individual interjudge correlation of 0.759 was significant at the 0.05 level and the overall average correlation for this subtest was high enough (0.98) to consider the fluency scale reliably reproducible by various examiners.

Table 4-6
Intrajudge Reliability Correlations

	Judge 1	Judge 2	Judge 3
Spontaneous speech content	0.94	0.95	0.92
Spontaneous speech fluency	0.79*	0.98	0.94
Comprehension	0.99	0.99	0.98
Repetition	0.99	0.99	0.99
Naming	0.99	0.99	0.99
Reading and writing	0.99	0.99	0.98
Praxis	0.98	0.98	0.98
Construction	0.99	0.97	0.98
AQ (total language)	0.99	0.99	0.99
CQ total	0.99	0.99	0.99

*Significance at 0.003 and the rest are at 0.001 level.

Each judge rescored the same videotaped interview, three or more weeks apart in ten patients. Correlations for each subtest per judge are documented.

TEST–RETEST RELIABILITY

To consider a test as a valid measure of aphasic impairment, consistency from one administration to another has to be established. This is particularly difficult to do with aphasics because of the effect of recovery on the performance. For this reason, we chose 22 chronic aphasics in whom the tests and retests were done one year after onset, observing little if any recovery taking

Table 4-7
Interjudge Reliability

Subtests	Average Intercorrelation*
Spontaneous speech content	0.998
Spontaneous speech fluency	0.984
Comprehension	0.998
Repetition	0.999
Naming	0.999
Reading and writing	0.996
Praxis	0.997
Construction	0.997
AQ (language total)	0.999
CQ (all test total)	0.999

*All intercorrelations were significant at $P \leq 0.001$

place beyond that time. This assumption was fully supported by the very high test−retest reliability [Pearson r correlation coefficient = 0.992 (df = 20), significant at $p \leq 0.01$], and the very low mean difference between tests−retests (a negligible value of 0.9).

A second group of stable, chronic aphasics were examined twice on the WAB ($N = 35$). The mean postonset time of the first test was 2.05 years and the second, 3.91 years. Table 4-8 shows the means of both tests for each parameter, and the correlation between them. The means were subjected to t test for repeated measures, and for the majority of the subtests no significant difference was found. Exceptions were word fluency, object naming, and naming total, and to a lesser extent, reading and writing, where the change was slightly significant. Correlation between the tests was high, and these results confirm reproducibility of the test or, in other words, a high test−retest reliability. Since the same examiner did not always administer the test on both occasions, this is probably a conservative estimate of the temporal stability.

Table 4-8
Test Retest Reliability

	Means			Pearson r*
	1st Test	2nd Test	N-Pairs	(Test 1–2)
Information content	5.00	5.20	35	0.95
Fluency	5.45	5.28	35	0.93
Yes–no questions	47.57	49.62	35	0.76
Auditory word recognition	41.11	40.51	35	0.85
Sequential commands	51.08	49.20	35	0.90
Comprehension total	7.05	6.97	35	0.88
Repetition	5.57	5.35	35	0.97
Object naming	30.02	33.25	35	0.94
Word fluency	5.11	6.28	35	0.89
Sentence completion	6.17	5.94	35	0.88
Responsive speech	5.48	5.60	35	0.96
Naming total	4.67	5.12	35	0.96
Aphasia Quotient	55.36	55.48	35	0.97
Reading	63.30	63.30	30	0.92
Writing	53.37	57.22	24	0.95
Praxis	78.29	78.11	17	0.45
Drawing	16.64	17.20	25	0.79
Block design	7.20	7.26	15	0.89
Calculation	17.58	18.00	24	0.81
Raven's Colored Progressive Matrices	21.61	22.19	26	0.89

*All significant at $p \leq 0.01$.

APHASIC AND CONTROL POPULATIONS OF THE
SECOND STANDARDIZATION

Since the first standardization in 1974, we have added 215 aphasics and 63 controls to our population, who had the complete language portion of the WAB. These patients were unselected, consecutive referrals to our aphasia laboratory, a population comparable to that of the first standarization. Our active interest in recovery from stroke may have resulted in more strokes than other etiologies in the sample. However, the infarcts are analyzed separately from other etiologies in this population. The means and standard deviations of subtotal scores and the AQ are summarized per types of aphasics for infarcts, and the totals are similarly shown for infarcts and other etiologies separately in Table 4-9. The controls, consisting of ten normals (age matched, hospital staff) and 53 nonaphasic patients with right hemisphere damage, are also summarized. The types are grouped with the four nonfluent aphasics on top, fluent ones below. AQs (total language scores) are on the right. The results are quite similar to the first (excepting that the different scaling for comprehension leaves the values out of 20 instead of 10). When the infarcts and other etiologies (tumor: 34, trauma: 25, miscellaneous: 15) are compared, the noninfarct patients show slightly higher scores across subtests, attributable to the younger posttraumatic aphasics in this group—$N = 25$, mean age = 44, SD 19. When the first and second standardizations are compared, there is an increase in the number of transcortical aphasics, with a significant decrease of Wernicke's aphasics in the infarct group. This correlates with slightly higher overall comprehension and repetition scores in the second standardization. These differences seem to relate to the higher portion of transcortical aphasics in the acute stroke population, and the higher numbers of Wernicke's aphasics in other etiologies.

To obtain the overall incidence of various aphasic types, we combined both standardizations to arrive at the following distribution:

Global	16%
Broca's	17%
Wernicke's	15%
Anomic	29%
Conduction	9%
Transcortical Motor	4%
Transcortical Sensory	7%
Isolation	3%

This is similar to the estimates of Vignolo as mentioned by Boller (1978) and Benson and Geschwind (1971).

Table 4-9

Second Standardization Group—Means and Standard Deviations of Subtest/Groups

Type of Aphasia	N	Age		Information		Fluency		Comprehension		Repetition		Naming		AQ	
		$\bar{X}$	SD	$\bar{X}$	SD	$\bar{X}$	SD	$\bar{X}$	SD	$\bar{X}$	SD	$\bar{X}$	SD	$\bar{X}$	SD
Global	20	64.3	11.3	0.2	0.4	0.7	1.1	3.1	2.3	0.2	0.6	0.06	0.1	6.2	5.3
Broca's	26	59.3	15.3	2.5	2.3	2.2	1.7	13.3	3.2	3.5	2.8	2.6	2.6	35.2	20.4
Isolation	3	81.0	6.2	1.6	2.8	3.0	1.0	4.8	2.5	6.8	1.7	2.0	2.3	31.8	16.4
Transcortical Motor	7	67.5	6.9	5.7	1.8	4.1	0.38	13.7	2.4	8.6	0.62	5.6	1.6	62.0	8.2
Transcortical Sensory	13	66.9	9.6	5.3	2.0	7.7	0.93	10.7	2.9	9.1	0.70	4.3	2.5	63.8	9.5
Conduction	12	64.8	11.1	5.9	2.2	6.2	1.4	15.9	1.6	4.9	1.6	5.2	1.9	60.6	12.1
Wernicke's	16	69.6	13.0	3.5	2.8	7.0	0.99	7.3	4.0	3.6	3.0	2.7	2.4	41.4	16.2
Anomic	44	66.1	12.0	8.5	1.1	8.2	1.3	17.8	1.6	9.1	0.79	8.1	0.8	85.5	7.0
Aphasics with infarcts	141	65.3	12.5	4.8	3.4	5.4	3.1	12.4	5.8	5.8	3.7	4.5	3.3	53.5	29.9
Aphasics other etiology	74	54.4	17.0	5.5	3.0	6.5	2.7	12.4	5.6	6.5	3.4	4.6	3.0	59.0	26.5
Controls Normals	10	61.0	6.3	10.0	0	10.0	0	20.0	0	9.9	0.1	9.8	0.1	99.6	0.3
Nondominant	53	64.7	10.8	9.2	1.4	9.4	1.3	18.7	2.1	9.5	0.5	8.8	1.4	92.9	8.0

The comprehension scores are from a maximum of 20, twice the scale of the others.

SUMMARY

The Western Aphasia Battery (WAB) is standardized on four populations.

1. 150 patients of all etiologies (the first standardization) and 59 controls.
2. 141 patients with stroke, and 74 with other etiologies, and 63 controls (the second standardization).
3. 127 patients overlapping the second aphasic population group, who had all subtests, including the nonverbal, optional portion of the test (internal consistency).
4. 21 recovered aphasics, who scored above the cutoff criterion and 18 nonaphasics, according to this criteria, who were referred as possibly aphasic (criterion controls).

The language test results on this population of 365 aphasics and 161 controls are described. The criteria for classification of aphasics and the definition of the aphasia quotient is derived from scoring. Evidence for comparable difficulty levels and internal consistency is presented. The significance of the correlation of subtests is discussed. Criteria for differentiating aphasics from controls is validated. High construct validity, test—retest reliability, and intrajudge and interjudge reliability is shown.

5

Numerical Taxonomy

We must start by observing a set of similar individuals and consider what elements they have in common . . . to define and divide one need not know the whole of existence

Aristotle (Analytica Posteriora)

INTRODUCTION

Numerical taxonomy is a recently emerged quantitative science of classification and systematics. It has been used and developed primarily by biologists, botanists, and zoologists, and it is beginning to be applied to psychology and medicine. Much of the subsequent description of numerical taxonomy is derived from the work of Sneath and Sokal (1973). The fundamental steps of numerical taxonomy are:

1. The characteristics of organisms (patients in our case) are chosen and recorded.
2. The resemblances between organisms are calculated.
3. Taxa (groups) based upon these resemblances are established.
4. Generalizations may be made about these groups, such as inferences about the evolution of groups (phylogeny) and the evolution of individuals (ontogeny).

75

5. Discriminatory characteristics for subsequent identification of individuals are
    chosen.

Estimation of resemblance is the most important step in numerical
taxonomy. For the method to be reliable, many characters are needed. It is
important to guard against the exclusion of pertinent material by including possibly atypical or unsatisfactory characters, as an insurance against an unrepresenta-
tive study. Language parameters, in our case, were most important, but in the
future, localization, size, and recovery data will be included in our studies.
While trying not to introduce bias into the choice of characters, meaningless
characters must be avoided also. Hence, some selection by the taxonomist is
virtually inevitable. An earlier section (Chapter 3) discusses the rationale for the
character selection used in the studies of aphasics reported here. The numerical
evaluation of relationship is called cluster analysis, in which the most similar
individuals are paired. Then these pairs are fused into successively larger groups,
on the basis of mutual similarity, until a hierarchy is obtained. This permits the
definition of groups in an objective manner. The number of groups to be defined
is arbitrary; the clusters can be selected at a lower or higher level of resemblance.
Boundaries for taxonomic groups can be represented as the intersections, or
horizontal transects, across the branches of the tree like diagrams of relationships
(dendrograms—see Fig. 6-1). Transects of a lower level of resemblance would
create taxa of higher taxonomic rank. Too many boundaries would provide too
fine a classification; too few would leave much structure unrevealed. The position and number of the boundaries are arbitrary, but they must be based on
comparable criteria in all regions of the taxonomic space studied. The representation of taxonomic relationships on a scatter diagram of individuals in a space of
two, three, or several dimensions, is called ordination (see below). In Fig. 5-1, a
flowchart of numerical taxonomy, as applied to our data by Dr. James Phipps is
displayed.

The advantage of numerical taxonomy, lies in objectivity and reproducibility. It also has been used to integrate data from a variety of sources, such as
behavior, linguistic analysis, and neurological signs, in our field of study. Quantitative methods are more sensitive in discriminating groups, and the process can
be automated to a great extent. An added advantage is that the creation of a data
base for taxonomy forced us to reconsider the methods of examination and
description of characteristics of patients. The method has led to the reexamina-
tion of other biological concepts and hopefully, it will have the same heuristic
value in the field of language – brain relationship.

THE PURPOSE AND PHILOSOPHY OF CLASSIFICATION

Empirical taxonomy bases classifications on observation and not on theoretical assumptions. In theoretical classifications, variances and exceptions often

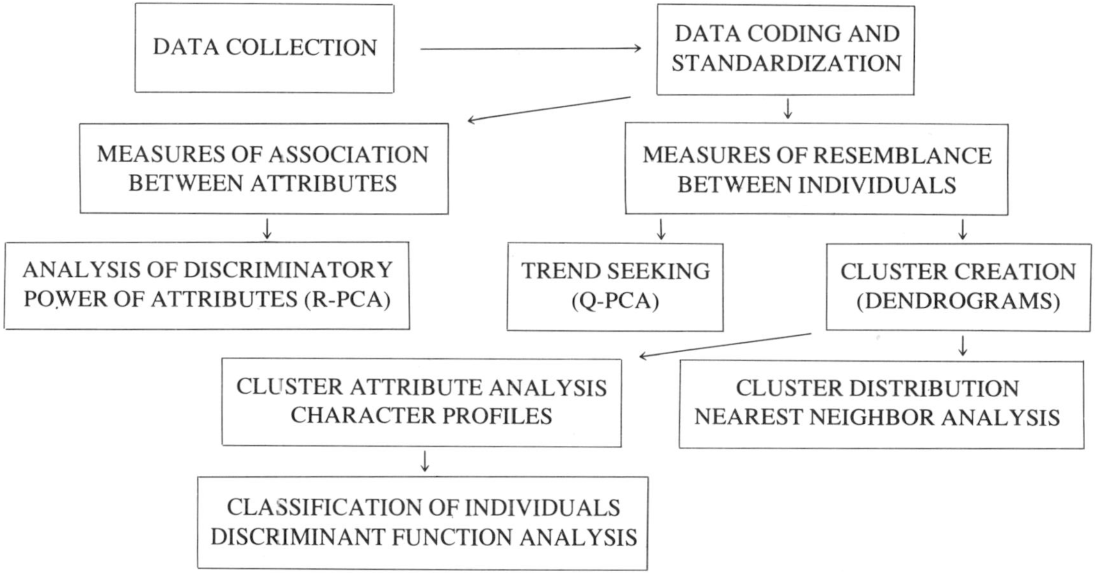

Fig. 5-1. Flow diagram of numerical taxonomy.

The boxes in the flow diagram, in reading order, contain:

- DATA COLLECTION
- DATA CODING AND STANDARDIZATION
- MEASURES OF ASSOCIATION BETWEEN ATTRIBUTES
- MEASURES OF RESEMBLANCE BETWEEN INDIVIDUALS
- ANALYSIS OF DISCRIMINATORY POWER OF ATTRIBUTES (R-PCA)
- TREND SEEKING (Q-PCA)
- CLUSTER CREATION (DENDROGRAMS)
- CLUSTER ATTRIBUTE ANALYSIS CHARACTER PROFILES
- CLUSTER DISTRIBUTION NEAREST NEIGHBOR ANALYSIS
- CLASSIFICATION OF INDIVIDUALS DISCRIMINANT FUNCTION ANALYSIS

give rise to contorted explanations to allow them to conform to the confinement of theories. Instead of considering variations as embarrassing exceptions to general principles, a descriptive method is emphasized by numerical taxonomy.

In Aristotelian logic, the essence of things or groups is expressed in axioms which give rise to properties that are inevitable consequences. However, biological systems do not lend themselves to Aristotelian logic, since properties of such systems cannot be inferred from definitions if taxonomy is to be a "natural" one (as contrasted to an arbitrary system). A monothetic system is formed by a unique set of features; the possession of these features is both sufficient and necessary for membership in this group (see our Table of Criteria in Chapter 4). Such a system carries the risk of misclassification of an individual who has an aberrant character, which is used to make the primary division (such as repetition in our study). As a result, such an individual will be moved to a taxon (group) away from its "natural" position, even though it is identical with its congeners in every other way. A polythetic group consists of organisms that have the greatest number of shared characters but no single character is essential or sufficient for membership in that group. Beckner's (1959) definition of a polythetic group is that:

1.   Each individual possesses a large number of characters in a certain set.
2.   Each character in the set is possessed by a large number of individuals.
3.   No character in the set is possessed by every individual.

If condition 3 is fulfilled, the class is said to be fully polythetic.

The advantages of polythetic groups are that they are "natural," have a high content of information and flexibility. However, they may partly overlap one another, and they cannot be used to identify each individual unequivocally. Wittgenstein emphasized the importance of polythetic concepts in language and philosophy, ideas implied by the words "meaning," "description," "referring."

Gilmour (1937) pointed out that the nature of taxonomy depends on its purpose. For a restricted purpose, arbitrary classifications are created, e.g., for the purpose of localization of lesions in the brain, a different system is used than for the purpose of neurolinguistics, although they both deal with aphasics. Natural classifications are intended for a general purpose, but they may not be as useful for a specific use.

The quality of any classification system is measured by its stability when further information is added. On the other hand, variation induced by new characters, for instance, recovery data, may have a biological reason and by themselves could be useful. External criteria may confirm the validity of a classification, such as an agreement between clustering patients according to their language deficit and the size of the lesions producing it.

DESCRIPTION AND DEFINITIONS

Operational taxonomic units. OTUs are the lowest ranking entities for which data is obtained in a given study. In our case, these would be individual patients. Each of these units have characters or attributes which are defined as "any observable feature which may vary from one OTU to another." For instance, the comprehension of yes—no questions is a character or an attribute of the taxonomic units as patients. A state of a character is its manifestation by a given individual. This can be a qualitative or quantitative variation. Many of these characters can be further subdivided, but for the purpose of each study, certain unit characters are chosen. The character, feature, or attribute is also called a *unit character,* when according to the principles of information theory, it can be defined as an attribute, providing a single piece of information.

Number of characters. The number influences the stability of classifications. As the number of characters increases, the value of similarity coefficients between two OTUs becomes more stable. One can express the resemblance between OTUs as a proportion of characters matching out of the total number being compared. Investigators in biology recommend using as many characters as feasible (Sneath and Sokal, 1973).

Weighting of characters. Weighting is used in the identification of individuals, but this is not recommended before classification is started. Characters are initially accorded equal importance or weight, since no *a priori* weighting methods avoid subjective bias. Character complexes are not considered equally, however. When broken down into unit characters, the amount of these in each complex will provide the weight in proportion to the complexity of a certain set of characters.

Coding and scaling. These are steps that convert the data into a form suitable for analysis. An example is the expression of characters as proportions to avoid effects of gross size. Another kind of transformation equalizes the variability of characters. There are methods to code *one state* (all or none) characters, or *multistate* (quantitative) characters. Scaling is used to reduce to equal range otherwise incomparable characters. Such a standardization method is, for instance, the use of z scores (to express values as units of standard deviations from the means). The effect of coding schemes can be large, particularly on clusters derived from correlation coefficients. This is of more than ordinary importance in aphasiology, where appropriate coding and scaling are not always obvious.

Taxonomic distances seemed to provide clusters in better accord with clinical diagnosis than did correlation coefficients.

Similarity matrix. The resemblance or similarity matrix is a comparison of every OTU with every other OTU. This is followed by *pattern recognition,* which is a description of the distribution of OTUs in A space (configuration or constellation). *A space* means the spatial distribution of *A*ttribute factors. *I space,* on the other hand, means *I*ndividual space, and contains OTUs. The observed dispersion pattern is compared against alternative null hypotheses, such as regular distribution and random distribution.

Clusters. These are defined as sets of OTUs that are mutually close in A space, and exhibit neither random nor regular distribution patterns. The center of a cluster may be represented by the average organism or *centroid,* whose coordinates are the mean values of each character, or by a hypothetical median or modal organism. However, an actual OTU (or patient, in our case) can be used as the *centrotype.* This is the OTU with the highest mean resemblance to all other OTUs of the cluster. It is nearest to the centroid for Euclidean distance models. Other aspects of the cluster, such as density, variance, dimension, connectivity, and number of members contribute to its definition, as well as the gaps separating it from other clusters. For the actual mathematical methods of clustering, the reader is referred to the detailed descriptions of Orloci (1967), Phipps (1971), and Sneath and Sokal (1973).

Ordination. This is the placement of OTUs in an A space of dimensionality. Only two- or three-dimensional ordinations can be represented by conventional methods. *Principal Component Analysis* (PCA) is a vector analysis of variance. The principal axis is the dimension along which there is greatest amount of variance in the sample. The second axis is that axis orthogonal to the first that accounts for the second largest amount of variance. Quite often, only as few as three principal axes will be responsible for most of the variance. Q technique PCA illustrates similarity between OTUs (rows in the data matrix) and the R technique refers to the study of similarity between characters (columns in the data matrix).

REPRESENTATION OF TAXONOMIC STRUCTURE

Taxonomic structure may be represented by dendrograms (phenograms), skyline plots, linkage diagrams, nearest neighbor networks, contour diagrams, two- or three-dimensional ordinations, etc. In our study, dendrograms, two-dimensional ordination of Q, PCA, and nearest neighbor networks are utilized.

IDENTIFICATION AND CLASSIFICATION OF INDIVIDUALS

Identification keys and discriminant functions are being developed for the purpose of assigning individuals to taxonomic groups. Characters can be weighted for identification by various mathematical means. Identification may be one of two kinds: (1) sequential, by diagnostic keys, or (2) simultaneous, by discriminant functions. A Synoptic Table is a table of classification criteria. We have used it in Chapter 4 and throughout our studies. For a few close groups, in which identification must be as certain as possible, discriminant analysis is recommended (Sneath and Sokal, 1973).

VALIDITY OF APPLICATION IN APHASIA

There is a danger that the logic and methods of classifying biological specimens may not be applicable to patients who represent deviation from nature, in a sense. Classification work in psychology has been dominated by factor analytic methods and much less has been done on cluster analysis (Cattell and Coulter, 1966). It is difficult to choose objective sets of characters for psychometrics (Hawkins, 1964). A factor analysis of aphasia tests by Schuell et al. (1962) produced a factor which was interpreted by them as a general language factor, crossing all language modalities. A similar factor, which was interpreted as severity, was found in a factor analysis used by Goodglass and Kaplan (1972), for the Boston Diagnostic Aphasia Examination, and confirmed by us (Kertesz and Phipps, 1977). The clusters appearing on the inspection of the intercorrelation matrix of all the subtests corresponded to the factors in the principal components factor analysis by Goodglass and Kaplan (1972). They drew attention to the basic limitation of the factor analytic technique which is not responsive to the independent variation that can occur in only a few individuals.

The use of a hierarchical clustering scheme to study the relatedness of words in the speech of aphasics and normals by Zurif and Caramazza (1976) is an application of taxonomy in psycholinguistics. The relatedness judgments of the control subjects were constrained by the surface syntactic properties of sentences, while that of the aphasics were not.

An individual cluster analysis was used by Hecaen and Kremin (1976) on data concerning the reading disorders of 38 left hemisphere damaged patients of various etiologies. The average linkage technique distinguished the three cases of pure alexia and another group of five, with characteristics of a dominant parietal syndrome. Principal components analysis was used to study the clustered variables of recognition and reading.

We published the first numerical taxonomy of aphasics based on the language parameters of 200 patients examined on the WAB (Kertesz and Phipps, 1977.) Further details of this study will be described in Chapter 6. Crockett (1977) analyzed the rating scales of fluency, naming, grammar, and understanding in 57 aphasics with a "hierarchical grouping" program of Ward (1963). The four groups so derived showed multivariate differences on the basis of their performance on the Neurosensory Center Comprehensive Examination for Aphasia. The subtests showing significant differences among the four groups were: visual naming, description of use, sentence repetition, repetition of digits, reversal of digits, identification by sentence and oral reading of sentences. Crockett concluded that at least four varieties of aphasia should be distinguished, and that the fluency-nonfluency dichotomy and the severity dimension were most important. Ammon and Godehardt (1978) used cluster analysis to study paraphasics in a naming paradigm, among various types of aphasics. They found a homogenous group of mild aphasics with good comprehension and naming, mainly anomic and Broca's aphasics, with low paraphasia rating, in contrast to the rest of the 60 patients who were more diffusely distributed. They concluded that when paraphasia ratings are used for clustering, the distinction occurs in the dimension of severity rather than among types in aphasia.

The application of objective methods of taxonomy in medicine, psychology, and linguistics is beginning to expand considerably. Disease has to be considered through its nature, etiology, as well as evolution. Discriminant function methods and Bayesian analysis can be used to predict evolution and outcome quite accurately, when adequate data are supplied. The data structure of our material suggests that the knowledge gained from biological application of numerical taxonomy can be used for clinical purposes also. Our results of taxonomy, detailed in Chapters 6 and 7, not only increase the objectivity of our classification, but have a positive effect on our methods of measurement and theoretical considerations of aphasia.

SUMMARY

This chapter introduces the reader to the method of numerical taxonomy, our special approach to the classification of aphasics. The method is briefly described as a more objective and precise one than intuitive taxonomies. The philosophy of classification is important, as the purpose affects the method considerably. Definition of the more frequently used taxonomic terms, and methods of displaying taxonomic structures, will help the reader to understand our results. The validity for studying aphasias by this method is discussed.

6

Clustering of Aphasics by Numerical Taxonomy Based on the WAB

Statistics are curious things. They afford one of the few examples in which the use, or abuse, of mathematical methods tends to induce a strong emotional reaction in non-mathematical minds.

Hill AB: Principles of Medical Statistics
New York, Oxford University Press, 1971

INTRODUCTION

The classification of aphasics has been usually based on clinical experience. This has a long and rich history, which is reviewed in detail in Chapter 1. The process of clinical classification consists of recognizing the similarities between certain patients on the basis of their behavior and language parameters. Numerical taxonomy provides us a tool, whereby we can streamline and quantitate this process and increase the objectivity, precision, and stability of classification. Most workers in the field of aphasia agree on the need for a workable, clinically accurate, yet objective classification, even though there is a minority opinion that aphasia is an indivisible phenomenon, and classification introduces artifact.

The results of any classification process depend on the parameters used or measured. In order to measure aphasic performance, a standardized, comprehensive, yet reasonably practical, test, such as our WAB (see Chapter 3), is essential. Clinical impressions only may result in impressionistic, biased, or idiosyncratic

83

classifications. Most clinicians will use some sort of aphasia test; however, often, only certain subtests are selected for the actual need in any instance. Many tests are too large to use consistently in every patient, preventing reliable comparisons. Often, even research workers are satisfied to form groups on the basis of one or two parameters, such as the fluency—nonfluency or severity—mildness dimensions. It is clear that the accuracy of classification will increase if a comprehensive, clinically relevant test is used, covering the most important aspects of language impairment. Idiosyncratic tests, based on purely theoretical considerations, will produce inapplicable results. Mechanically constructed tests, using every input and output modality in all combinations, introduce too much noise into the system, and, similarly, decrease the usefulness of the method. Disregarding clinical aspects for the sake of objectivity has often resulted in meaningless abstractions in aphasia testing and classifications. A careful selection of the important parameters from the complex language impairment of aphasics, and measuring these with a standardized test, will provide the optimum data base for meaningful taxonomy.

TAXONOMY OF UNSELECTED APHASICS

Our first numerical taxonomic study published used 200, consecutively examined aphasics for a data base (Kertesz and Phipps, 1977). Since etiology plays an important role in the clinical picture of aphasia, the 142 infarcts in this population were separately analyzed. The rest included 18 tumors, 16 trauma, 12 intracerebral hemorrhages, five degenerative disease (Alzheimer's dementia), five aneurysmal subarachnoid hemorrhages, and two of uncertain etiology (probably degenerative). This representative sample was obtained from three general hospitals and one veterans hospital. The patients had an average age of 60.6, with SD 10.1 and a range from 19—87. The sex ratio M:F = 129:71 is strongly skewed towards males due to the veteran population in the study. The average educational level was grade 9.9 with SD of 1.0 and range of 0—18.

All patients were tested on the 17 tasks of the "Western Aphasia Battery" (WAB) (Kertesz and Poole, 1974) similar to the "Boston Diagnostic Aphasia Examination" (Goodglass and Kaplan, 1972). We selected, for this study, only the spoken language tasks (see Chapter 3):

1. Fluency, judged by a list of criteria (scale: 1—10)
2. Comprehension, measured by (a) yes—no questions, (b) auditory discrimination or pointing, (c) auditory sequencing with relational words (scale: 1—200)
3. Repetition of words, numbers, and high and low probability sentences (scale: 1—100)
4. Naming: (a) visual confrontation naming of objects, (b) word fluency, (c) sentence completion, (d) responsive speech

5. Information content of replies to standardized conversational questions (scale: 1—10).

We termed, for the purpose of this study, the data for 10 individual tests as "subscores" and the pooled results for each of the five main areas (e.g., fluency, comprehension, etc.) as "set totals." These are, in fact, character complexes (see discussion in Chapter 5).

A minimum variance clustering algorithm, called the sum of squares agglomeration (Orloci, 1967a) on the Euclidean distance matrix of dissimilarities, was used. This is a "tight" or high center-of-gravity clustering technique that is especially valuable for beginning explorations of taxonomic structure. Like all clustering algorithms, it imposes structure on the group and extrinsic tests of the significance of the groups formed are required. The clustering results are displayed in dendrograms.

The groups recognized were subjected to a cluster attribute analysis, which produced character profiles for each group. A further analysis of group intercentroid distances was conducted to obtain information on the proximity and validity of the distinctiveness of the groups so far recognized.

Ordination was carried out by principal components analysis (Cooley and Lohnes, 1962) of the correlation matrix. Both Q and R strategies were employed (Orloci, 1967b), the former being used to depict the patients in the most efficient two space, while the latter provided us with information about the contribution of the different attributes to the spatial arrangement of the entities (patients).

RESULTS OF TAXONOMIC ANALYSIS OF APHASICS DUE TO INFARCTS

The dendrogram of 142 infarcts (language area set totals) clearly generates ten groups at the 2.5% level of total variance, as shown in Fig. 6-1. The proportion of various clinical types, as defined by previously published, clinical, taxonomic criteria (See Table 3-2), was determined for each cluster (Table 6-1).

When subjected to attribute analysis, the average values and standard deviations for each of the ten recognized clusters provided a meaningful profile for each group (Fig. 6-2). This allowed us to relate most clusters to traditional terminology, although there were important exceptions to this. The terms used for each cluster are tentative approximations although quite often the overlap between the objective cluster and intuitive classification is complete or nearly so. The first cluster showed low values on all scores (this group can be called global aphasia). Cluster two was very similar, except for a much higher rating for character two (comprehension), and corresponds to Broca's aphasia. The third group had moderately high repetition but low fluency (nonfluent, echolalic, sensory aphasia or "isolation syndrome"). Cluster four had higher scores, with low fluency, and high repetition and comprehension (transcortical motor aphasia). The small fifth cluster scored well on characters three and one (repeti-

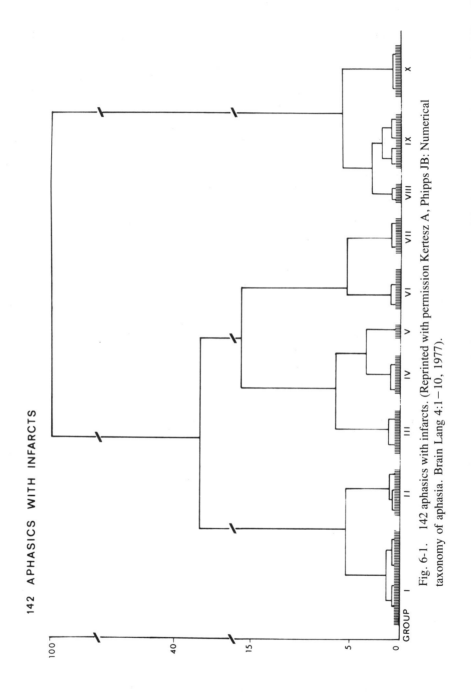

142 APHASICS WITH INFARCTS

Fig. 6-1. 142 aphasics with infarcts. (Reprinted with permission Kertesz A, Phipps JB: Numerical taxonomy of aphasia. Brain Lang 4:1–10, 1977).

Table 6–1
Cluster Composition of Infarcts

Cluster	Number of Patients	Percentage of Clinical Types of Aphasia	
I	30	97%	Global
II	15	86%	Broca's
III	12	25%	Global
		25%	Broca's
		25%	Isolation
IV	13	54%	Broca's
		23%	Isolation
		23%	Transcortical motor
V	4	100%	Transcortical sensory
VI	12	58%	Conduction
VII	11	100%	Wernicke's
VIII	7	57%	Conduction
XI	18	63%	Anomic
X	20	100%	Anomic

(Reprinted with permission Kertesz A, Phipps JB: Numerical taxonomy of aphasia. Brain Lang 4:1-10, 1977).

tion and fluency), and moderate−low on the others (transcortical sensory aphasia). The sixth cluster had low repetition, naming, and comprehension, but high fluency (we called this "afferent conduction aphasia"). The seventh cluster had lowish scores, not unlike clusters one and two, but differed in having a high value for fluency (this group corresponds to Wernicke's aphasia). Cluster eight had scores slightly higher than median, but differed from cluster six, in having a high value for character four (naming), but a relatively low score for fluency (we took the liberty of calling this "efferent conduction aphasia"). Clusters nine and ten represented a moderately high and a near normal set of scores (anomic aphasia). The relatively low standard deviation for each attribute, in each cluster, supported the significance of the groups detected.

It proved interested to subject the ten clusters to a nearest neighbor network analysis, in which intercentroid distances were computed, and deviations along the intercentroid axes established (Fig. 6-3). This is essentially an extension of the method presented by Sneath and Sokal (1973, pp. 286). There are four pairs of mutually closest clusters—(I, II), (IV, V), (VI, VII), and (IX, X). If the summed deviations on the intercentroid axes are more than the intercentroid distance, then the clusters are not significantly different statistically. The only example of this situation is cluster pair (I-II). Inspection of the cluster attribute analysis for this group confirms the similarity of these two clusters and also the

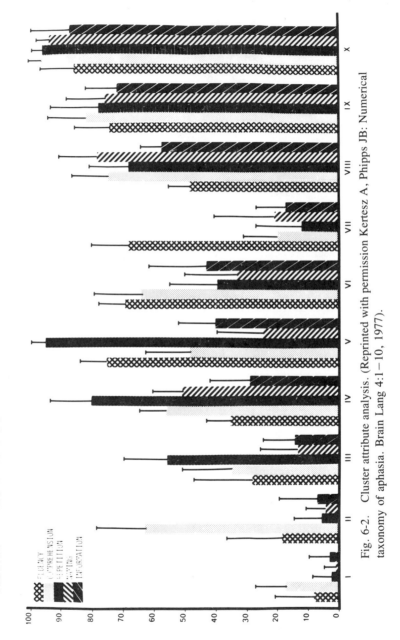

CLUSTER ATTRIBUTE ANALYSIS

Fig. 6-2. Cluster attribute analysis. (Reprinted with permission Kertesz A., Phipps JB: Numerical taxonomy of aphasia. Brain Lang 4:1–10, 1977).

NEAREST NEIGHBOR NETWORK ANALYSIS

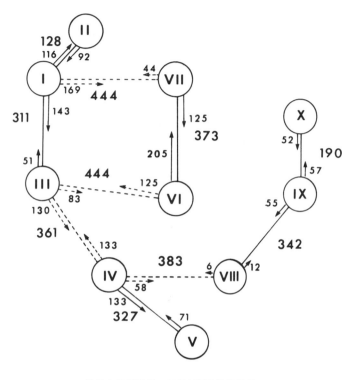

———————— NEAREST NEIGHBORS
– – – – – – – 2nd NEAREST NEIGHBORS

Fig. 6-3.   Nearest neighbor analysis. (Reprinted with permission Kertesz A, Phipps JB: Numerical taxonomy of aphasia. Brain Lang 4:1–10, 1977).

attribute which makes them distinct clinically—comprehension. Cluster pairs (IV-V), (VI-VII), and (I-III) are also quite close, but each member of the pair, nevertheless, constitutes a distinct cluster. It is noteworthy that when second nearest neighbors have to be utilized to complete the network, e.g., by forming the bond (IV-VIII), the dispersions do not remotely approach the intercentroid distances. Thus, we may conclude that at least nine statistically distinct groups are present.

The Q-type PCA is essential in interpreting the general trends of variation observed (Fig. 6-4). The main scatter of groups is along the first factor which, significantly, accounts for 82% of the total variation. This underlines the fairly strong degree of correlation among all the attributes (tests) measured. It also means that the tests contribute to this factor (severity of aphasia) evenly. Some

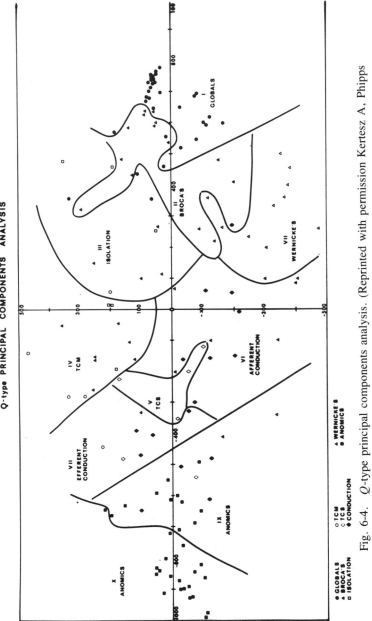

Fig. 6-4. Q-type principal components analysis. (Reprinted with permission Kertesz A, Phipps JB: Numerical taxonomy of aphasia. Brain Lang 4:1–10, 1977).

groups, however, e.g., (III and VII), (IV and VI), are separated principally on the second factor, which accounts for about 9% of the total variation, and our results from the attribute analysis or the R-type PCA indicate in which characteristics they differ.

The R-type PCA ranks the characteristics according to their discriminatory value on the Q-type PCA factors (Table 6-2). It illustrates a fairly even significance (i.e., high correlation) of characters on the first root (this is why axis 1 accounts for so high a percentage of the variation), but on root 2, characteristics 1 (fluency) and 2 (comprehension) have by far the most differentiating power, while on root 3, repetition is the most important discriminant.

THE TAXONOMY OF POSTTRAUMATIC APHASICS

Twenty-five aphasics who were tested within 35 days of head injury were subjected to clustering on the basis of all the subtests of the WAB. A portion (16%) of these patients had surgery for subdural hematoma and the others (84%) had closed head injuries with contusion only. There were no penetrating injuries; the group was characteristic of the usual civilian population with closed head injuries that were mostly the result of auto accidents. All subtests, including reading, writing, drawing, calculation, block design, and Raven's matrices, were used in the clustering. This should be taken into consideration when the results are compared with the stroke population discussed above, where only the language subtests were utilized. This population is comparable, however, to the acute stroke population analyzed for all the subtests in Chapter 7.

The posttraumatic groups on the dendrogram at 4% of the total variance were: (1) Global ($N = 4$), (2) Wernicke's ($N = 1$), (3) Transcortical Sensory (TCS = 2, Wernicke's = 1), (4) Isolation ($N = 1$), (5) Broca's ($N = 2$), (6) Efferent Conduction (TCM = 1, Conduction = 1, Anomic = 2), (7) Afferent

Table 6–2
r-Type Component Analysis of 142 Infarcts

	% of Total Variation	Percentage of Characteristics Contributing to Each Root				
		Fluency	Comprehension	Repetition	Naming	Information
Root 1	82	17.5%	18.6%	21.8%	23.2%	18.8%
Root 2	9	52.0%	38.3%	1.9%	2.7%	5.0%
Root 3	7	2.7%	2.1%	56.1%	.6%	38.6%
Root 4	3	1.9%	.9%	16.7%	60.9%	19.6%
Root 5	0	23.1%	34.6%	13.4%	17.0%	11.9%

(Reprinted with permission Kertesz A, Phipps JB: Numerical taxonomy of aphasia. Brain Lang 4:1–10, 1977).

Conduction (Conduction = 1, Anomic = 4), (8) Anomic (N = 5) (Fig. 6-5). These objectively formed groups are small but similar in composition and number to the taxonomic groups in stroke.

Our observations differ from those of Heilman et al. (1971) who found only Wernicke's and amnesic aphasia after closed head trauma. The N's are comparable, but differences in patient selection and classification may account for the discrepancy. Although anomic aphasics are numerous, global, Broca's, isolation, conduction and transcortical sensory aphasics are also represented. Nonfluent aphasics constituted almost a third of the population. Considering the diffuse nature of closed head injury, the relatively large anomic group is not surprising, since lesions in anomic aphasics are the least localizable (see Chapters 8 and 9). Broca's, Wernicke's, transcortical motor and conduction aphasia are more likely to result from focal damage to the dominant hemisphere.

THE TAXONOMY OF APHASICS WITH NEOPLASM

Thirty-four aphasics with neoplasm were seen at the time of the discovery of their tumor. This represents a variable time from the onset of their aphasia and along the spectrum of progression of their illness. Tumor patients as a rule present a different clinical picture which tends to change in the direction of worsening. We were specifically interested in the taxonomy of the tumor group as we felt that the lesions were likely to be more randomly distributed and the clustering would be less likely to be homogeneous or clinically useful.

The dendrogram of 34 tumor patients reveals 6 groups at 6% level of variance (Fig. 6-6). The first group had 1 global, 1 Broca's, 2 Wernicke's, 1 isolation, and 1 transcortical sensory aphasic, a rather unusual mixture. The second group had 2 global and 1 Wernicke's patient. The third group consisted of 2 Broca's and the fourth group of 3 Wernicke's and 2 transcortical sensory aphasics. The fifth group is a mixture of conduction (3), transcortical motor (2), transcortical sensory (1), and anomic (2) patients. The sixth group is entirely anomic (10).

These groups are quite dissimilar to the stroke or the posttraumatic aphasics. The prominent global group is absent, reflecting the fact that global aphasia is seen only at a rather advanced stage of tumor growth. The small Broca's and Wernicke's group indicates the rather low frequency of these classical types of aphasia in tumors, and the large anomic group indeed confirms our clinical impression that tumors often and most commonly present with anomic aphasia, regardless of their location in the brain. There are other studies in the literature concluding more or less the same from autopsy and surgical material (Kanzer, 1942).

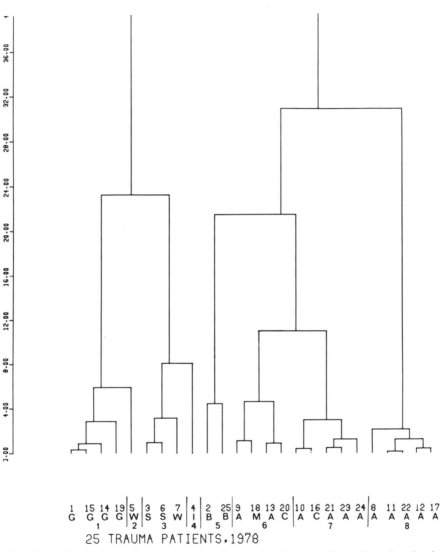

Fig. 6-5. Dendrogram of post-traumatic aphasics. The letters underneath each patient's number represent the type of aphasia: G, global; W, Wernicke; S, transcortical sensory; M, transcortical motor; I, isolation; B, Broca; C, conduction; A, anomic; Z, recovered. The taxonomic groups are separated by vertical lines.

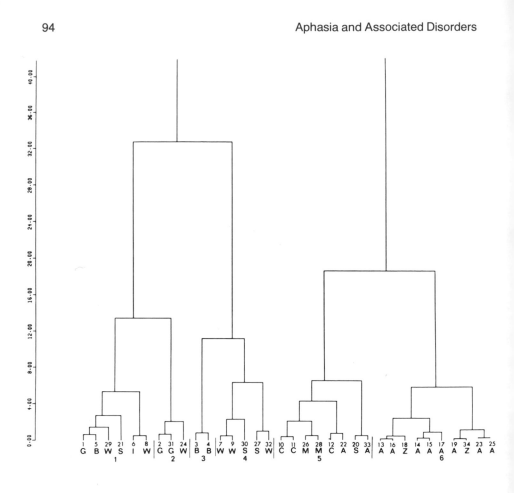

34 NEOPLASM PATIENTS, 1978

Fig. 6-6.   Dendrogram of tumor patients (see legend, Fig. 6-5).

RESULTS OF TAXONOMY OF ALL APHASICS

The dendrogram of all the 200 aphasics language totals depicts a somewhat different group structure from that for the infarcts alone. There are six larger, less homogenous clusters (Fig. 6-7). In the first, 67% of 41 patients in the cluster are global; 72% of 38 globals of the total sample belong to this cluster. In the second ($N = 31$), 59% are Broca's; 56% of the 32 Broca's aphasics are in this cluster. In the third ($N = 33$), 37% are Wernicke's and 36% of the 37 Wernicke's aphasics are there. In the fourth ($N = 32$), 44% are "conduction"; 58% of the 24

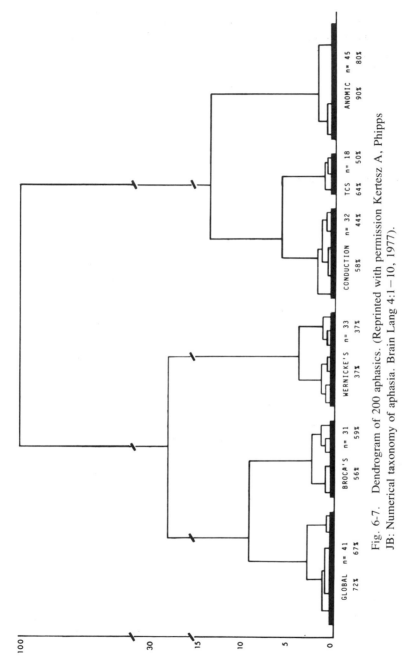

DENDROGRAM OF 200 APHASICS

Fig. 6-7. Dendrogram of 200 aphasics. (Reprinted with permission Kertesz A, Phipps JB: Numerical taxonomy of aphasia. Brain Lang 4:1–10, 1977).

conduction aphasics are in this cluster. In the fifth ($N = 18$, 50% are transcortical sensory; 64% of the 14 transcortical sensory aphasics belong in this cluster. In the sixth ($N = 45$), 80% were anomics; 90% of the 40 anomic aphasics are in this sample. The least homogenous, third group contained 100% of the isolation, 37% of Wernicke's, and 35% of the transcortical sensory aphasics—a low scoring receptive group. The fourth group, although predominantly conduction patients, had a fair share of Broca's aphasics, indicating the validity of the "efferent motor aphasia" as a cluster.

COMPARISON AND DISCUSSION

The reason for the lower specificity of clustering in the larger group of aphasics is partly due to the nature of the lesions. In the larger group, in addition to the 142 infarcted patients, a number caused by tumors, trauma, and hemorrhage were included. Anatomically, only the infarcts produce similar lesions repetitively, by virtue of a similar territory of arterial supply being involved, and with less variation than might occur with neoplasms or trauma. Analyzing the infarcts alone seems to yield more precise and detailed clustering.

The similarity between infarct groups I and II is not surprising, since the clinical criteria to separate Global from Broca's aphasics, is their comprehension. There is an obvious overlap in the other scores. The third group is an interesting mixture of various types, a low scoring with higher repetition group, including three Global aphasics with relatively better repetition, three "isolation" patients, who are like Globals, except for their better repetition, three low scoring Broca's, one Transcortical Motor aphasic, and even two Wernicke's aphasics, who repeated relatively well. This cluster approaches, in a broad sense, what has been described clinically as the speech area "isolation syndrome" (Geschwind et al., 1968). The widely ranging composition is seemingly paradoxical, but this is the result of the difference between the objective, polythetic, numerical taxonomy, and the arbitrary, intuitive criteria, applied in the previous classification.

One of the most interesting findings was the emergence of two distinct clusters, in which the so-called conduction or central aphasics were bimodally distributed, confirming the long-established doubts of clinicians about the homogeneity of this aphasic group. Cluster VI had seven "conduction" and five Wernicke's aphasics. Common to this cluster were high fluency and relatively low comprehension and repetition scores; these were "afferent conduction" aphasics. Cluster VIII, on the other hand, had conduction patients with lower fluency and higher comprehension, along with a few Broca's and transcortical motor patients, indicating the existence of an "efferent conduction" group. Rating of paraphasias may further clarify the distinctness of these groups.

The homogeneity of some of the clusters is striking. The first and tenth represent the two most clearly defined and largest of aphasic groups (globals and anomics). These occupy the opposite extremes in the component analyses and dendrograms, as well as the severity scales. There is general agreement in the literature about the existence of these groups. However, pure clusters (by previously established criteria) can be found elsewhere. In the seventh cluster, the seven patients were all Wernicke's, and in the fifth, all were transcortical sensory aphasics. Even the large, second cluster turned out to be overwhelmingly (86%) a Broca's group.

The degree of correspondence of most of the computer-generated clusters with clinically recognizable groups was surprising. We had been prepared to discover many alternative groupings to the classical ones, but the two major deviations were the distinct bimodality of conduction aphasia and the splitting of the anomic group. The new cluster, between the predominantly Wernicke's and anomic clusters, had a higher proportion of subjects with a somewhat impaired comprehension. Perhaps, the old term "semantic aphasia" may be used here, although it is being resurrected in a somewhat different, more traditional sense, by Jason Brown (1972).

The spatial distribution of the clustering and the degree of separation or similarity of individual aphasics is, of course, due to those characteristics which were examined and subjected to analysis. The Q-type principal component analysis provides a two-dimensional picture, where separation along the horizontal axis (root 1 in Table 6-2) derives from all characteristics just about evenly. The summary of these characteristics is the "Aphasia Quotient" or the severity scale. Therefore, distribution on the horizontal axis depends on the severity of aphasic impairment. Fluency and comprehension are the main contributions to positioning in the vertical axis (root 2). The visual display of further discriminating characteristics has not been undertaken, due to the graphical complexity of superimposing information pertinent to third and fourth dimensions in the scatter diagram. These data are, however, made explicit in Table 6-2.

Some of these patients were examined in a more chronic state than others. The acute ones were well enough to be tested, but some of them undoubtedly changed categories in the course of recovery. For instance, some global aphasics evolve into the Broca's group, and anomic aphasia is a common endstage for the conduction, Wernicke's, and transcortical groups. In another study, we have shown how certain aphasias evolve, and what changes are likely to occur (Kertesz and McCabe 1977). In chapter 7 the acute and chronic groups are separated.

SUMMARY

This study attempts to provide objectivity and precision for clinical classification, which are very much needed for reliable research in aphasia. Infarcts were separately classified as the most homogenous group. The ten major clusters, revealed by numerical taxonomy of infarcts, corresponded more or less to recognizable clinical groups of aphasics. "Conduction" aphasics distributed bimodally into clearly separated clusters. There was an extra cluster, not belonging to Wernicke's or anomic's, but in between, labeled "semantic" aphasia. The total aphasic group separated into six major clusters, which are less specific.

7

Taxonomies of Aphasics in Acute and Chronic Stroke Populations

Introduction
Discussion

Only a particular period in the course of the disease should be considered if one is to diagnose aphasia correctly.

C. Wernicke (1874)

INTRODUCTION

The significant recovery in a substantial portion of aphasics is well documented in the literature (see Chapter 15 on Recovery). The extent of recovery is better known than the variation in aphasic types produced by the evolution of language impairment. The evolution of aphasics follows a regular pattern, as documented by us previously (Kertesz and McCabe, 1977). Often global aphasia evolves to Broca's aphasia; Broca's, conduction and Wernicke's aphasics usually become anomic aphasics when recovery reaches a plateau. When such patterns are reversed, other etiologies, such as brain tumors, should be suspected. The knowledge of these patterns has significant diagnostic and prognostic value. It is this evolution of the individual aphasia which gives rise to variations in the composition of aphasic populations, depending on whether they are examined before, during, or after recovery. It is likely that the classification of acute and chronic populations would yield substantial differences. To test this hypothesis, we decided to examine separate clusters of acute and chronic aphasics, due to infarcts. James Phipps, Ph.D., contributed generously by coding our data, generating the various clusters and providing the methods to display the results.

CLUSTERING OF ACUTE APHASICS DUE TO INFARCTS—LANGUAGE SUBTESTS ONLY

Sixty-four right-handed aphasics, who had a WAB within $14-45$ days $(2-6$ weeks) from the onset of their stroke, were included in this cluster analysis. Excluded were 69 aphasics, who had tests in the first two weeks from the date of onset because of the rapid, physiological changes in this period, and 38 patients who had their first test after six weeks from onset, in order to examine a relatively stable but acute segment in the evolution of aphasia. Dendrograms were constructed on the basis of language subtests only (Fig. 7-1). Groups were formed at maximum 5.8% of variance (the ordinate). The clusters have a remarkable overlap with the clinical classification. Cluster I consists of 15 global aphasics. Cluster II has five Broca's aphasics. Cluster III has 12 members, almost all Wernicke's aphasics, with one Broca's and one conduction aphasic included $(N = 12)$. Cluster IV is a mixture of four Broca's and two conduction aphasics reminiscent of the "efferent conduction" cluster in Fig. 6-1 $(N = 6)$. Cluster V has three conduction aphasics and one anomic patient, the "afferent conduction" cluster $(N = 4)$ (see Fig. 6-1). Cluster VI consists of two isolation aphasics, well apart from the rest of the aphasic population $(N = 2)$. Cluster VII has three transcortical sensory, two Wernicke's, one conduction, and one transcortical motor aphasic $(N = 7)$. Cluster VIII has a great majority of 11 anomics and two transcortical sensory aphasics $(N = 13)$.

The cluster attribute analysis (Table 7-1) for Cluster I reveals very low scores throughout (global aphasia). In Cluster II, comprehension is much better, compared to the rest of the scores, as would be expected from a pure cluster of Broca's aphasics, and Cluster III has good fluency scores but poor performance in other subtests, as one sees in Wernicke's aphasia. Cluster IV, a relatively nonfluent group with good scores otherwise, is not easily categorized, but high comprehension suggests a mild motor aphasia. Cluster V has a low repetition score as the outstanding feature (conduction aphasia); Cluster IV is the opposite, with repetition being the only high score, quite characteristic of the "isolation of the speech area" syndrome. Cluster VII has good repetition and fluency, and

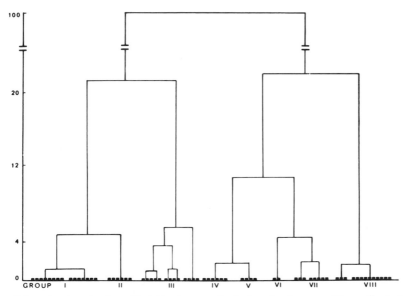

Fig. 7-1. Acute aphasics with infarcts on a clustering dendrogram. The ordinate (percentage of variance) is broken for display. Each individual is represented by a square.

Table 7–1

Attribute Analysis for Language Clusters of acute Aphasics

Cluster	Information		Fluency		Comprehension		Repetition		Naming	
	$\bar{x}*$	SD	$\bar{x}*$	SD	$\bar{x}*$	SD	$\bar{x}*$	SD	$\bar{x}*$	SD
I	121.3 ± 45.9		153.4 ± 71.2		229.1 ± 103.8		100.0 ± 0.0		100.0 ± 0.0	
II	116.0 ± 32.0		117.8 ± 35.6		689.4 ± 130.6		164.0 ± 78.4		117.8 ± 35.6	
III	346.7 ± 177.3		662.8 ± 122.2		433.3 ± 187.1		226.7 ± 147.7		211.2 ± 126.3	
IV	526.7 ± 59.6		455.7 ± 88.7		788.8 ± 61.8		606.7 ± 37.7		544.3 ± 72.3	
V	680.0 ± 103.9		633.0 ± 109.0		837.0 ± 63.0		580.0 ± 56.6		744.3 ± 38.5	
VI	180.0 ± 80.0		278.0 ± 178.0		247.0 ± 21.0		660.0 ± 80.0		189.0 ± 89.0	
VII	397.1 ± 110.8		684.1 ± 114.9		569.1 ± 94.0		740.0 ± 165.6		417.7 ± 104.6	
VIII	752.3 ± 98.5		879.5 ± 37.5		793.2 ± 112.8		795.4 ± 48.5		783.6 ± 94.9	

Cluster profiles in each horizontal line show scaled mean values and standard deviations for each attribute.

101

relatively poor comprehension and information content, quite compatible with transcortical sensory aphasia. Cluster VIII has uniformly high scores (anomic aphasia), with slightly lower information content (empty, circumlocutory speech).

A nearest neighbor network analysis depicts the intercentroid distances and the extent of the deviation from the center of the clusters (Fig. 7-2). This method illustrates the taxonomic structure of acute aphasia exceptionally well. The three clusters on the bottom are the low scoring global (I), Broca's (II), and isolation (VI) aphasics, with a secondary link to Cluster VII, the transcortical sensory group, which is, in turn, neighbor to Wernicke's (III) and conduction aphasia (IV). The latter is linked to V (the mixture of mild Broca's and conduction aphasia) by the shortest intercentroid distance, which, in turn, connects to VIII (anomic aphasia). The deviations from the centroids in the clusters are small, indicating a significantly tight clustering. (The small numbers near the clusters indicate the extent of deviation or dispersion.)

The R-type component analysis indicates the roots of variation, the percentage of each root accounted for by the attributes (character), and the percentage of variation accounted for by each root. This is similar to a factor analysis. Roots are best understood as factors in dispersion. The roots and their contributing characters are shown in Table 7-2. The various characters or language scores contribute evenly to root 1, which suggests that this is, in fact, a general language

ACUTE   APHASICS — LANGUAGE

NEAREST   NEIGHBOR   NETWORK   ANALYSIS

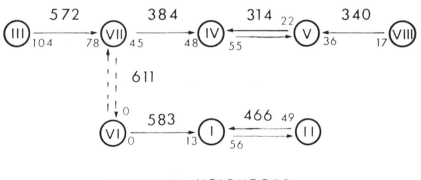

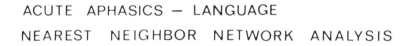

—————— NEAREST   NEIGHBORS

- - - - - - - - 2 nd NEAREST   NEIGHBORS

Fig. 7-2.   Nearest neighbors among aphasic groups with acute infarct. The arrows point towards the direction of the nearest (solid line) or the second nearest (interrupted line) neighbor. The large numbers are intercentroid distances and the small ones indicate the extent of dispersion from the centroid.

Table 7–2

R-Type Principal Components Analysis
64 Acute Aphasics, Language Subtests

	Percentage of matrix/root	Percentage of root accounted for by characters				
		Information	Fluency	Comprehension	Repetition	Naming
Root 1	81%	22.17	18.49	15.66	21.19	22.48
Root 2	12%	6.84	46.76	41.99	1.98	2.41
Root 3	5%	3.99	0.17	0.74	69.40	25.67
Root 4	2%	3.33	27.68	33.94	10.59	24.44

The *r*-type PCA displays the percentage of matrix which accounts for each root in the left column and in each horizontal row following. The extent to which characters are contributing to each root is indicated.

or a severity factor. This root accounts for an overwhelming 81 percent of the dispersion. Root 2 has a high loading on fluency and comprehension, the most important factors separating aphasics into groups, besides the severity of aphasia. They are responsible for 12 percent of the dispersion. Root 3, which is mainly accounted for by repetition, contributes 5 percent to dispersion. Root 4 accounts for 2 percent of dispersion and has a moderate loading on comprehension, fluency, and naming. Naming, as a character on which clustering is based, contributes rather evenly and modestly to all roots; therefore, it seems to have less discriminatory function than the other attributes. This confirms the clinical impression of many, that anomia is a nonspecific component of most aphasic syndromes.

CLUSTERING OF CHRONIC APHASICS DUE TO INFARCTS—LANGUAGE SUBTESTS ONLY

Eighty-three right-handed aphasics, who had the WAB 330 days or more after an infarct, constitute the subjects for this study. The same methodology is used as for the acute group. The clusters are displayed on the dendrogram (Fig. 7-3), and the cluster attribute analysis in Table 7-3. The first cluster includes five severely affected Broca's aphasics, in addition to ten global patients. The improvement in their comprehension was not enough to place them in a different group. Cluster II is made up of two Wernicke's aphasics, close to global's because of their severity, but quite distinct by their fluency. This also underlines the clinical experience that severe Wernicke's aphasia persists relatively infrequently. Cluster III is a pure Broca's group (*N* = 6), and Cluster IV has two cases of isolation, one transcortical motor, and one Broca's aphasic. Cluster V

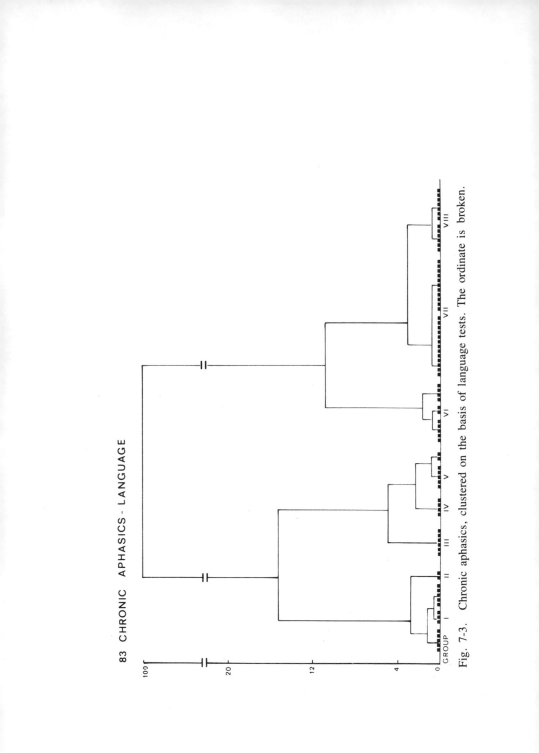

83 CHRONIC APHASICS - LANGUAGE

Fig. 7-3. Chronic aphasics, clustered on the basis of language tests. The ordinate is broken.

Table 7–3

Attribute Analysis for Language Clusters of Chronic Aphasics

Cluster	Information		Fluency		Comprehension		Repetition		Naming	
	$\bar{x}^*$	SD	$\bar{x}^*$	SD	$\bar{x}^*$	SD	$\bar{x}^*$	SD	$\bar{x}^*$	SD
I	148.0 ± 64.0		206.7 ± 80.9		282.5 ± 114.9		121.3 ± 45.9		111.9 ± 44.4	
II	100.0 ± 0.0		700.0 ± 40.0		205.5 ± 105.5		100.0 ± 0.0		144.5 ± 44.5	
III	220.0 ± 61.1		286.7 ± 99.8		654.3 ± 98.6		206.7 ± 59.6		218.7 ± 42.0	
IV	280.0 ± 87.2		380.0 ± 69.3		458.0 ± 109.2		620.0 ± 120.0		278.0 ± 0.0	
V	408.6 ± 79.2		442.9 ± 140.0		683.3 ± 85.7		431.4 ± 79.2		417.9 ± 44.0	
VI	606.7 ± 105.0		533.3 ± 144.1		742.2 ± 96.1		620.0 ± 132.7		692.3 ± 104.8	
VII	843.3 ± 43.1		833.3 ± 37.7		866.8 ± 34.2		833.3 ± 44.2		855.5 ± 51.4	
VIII	740.0 ± 83.0		776.9 ± 67.4		764.1 ± 72.4		783.1 ± 74.4		722.0 ± 60.5	

Cluster profiles for chronic aphasics language tasks. See Table 7–1.

has four Broca's, one Wernicke's, and two conduction aphasics. Cluster VI is a mixed group, which is difficult to relate to our intuitive taxonomic system. They are all milder aphasics, with relatively low fluency. The exception is a Wernicke's aphasic, who has a fairly high comprehension, almost like the other conduction aphasics in the group. Cluster VII has 24 anomic aphasics, some with scores high enough to consider them recovered, if our criteria or the mean AQ (93.8 percent) of the nonaphasic brain damaged control group, is used. Cluster VIII consists of 12 anomic and one conduction aphasic.

Cluster attribute analysis of chronic aphasics (Table 7-3) shows the first cluster to have uniformly low scores, the second has very good fluency (Wernicke's aphasia), and the third good comprehension (Broca's aphasia). The fourth has good repetition (isolation and transcortical motor) and the fifth, good comprehension with generally better overall performance (''the afferent'' conduction aphasia). The sixth cluster has higher scores, especially comprehension, but relatively lower fluency. The seventh cluster differs from the eighth only in the uniformly higher scores.

The R-type component analysis of chronic aphasics (Table 7-4) indicates that the various scores or characters contribute to root 1 equally (probably a severity factor). Root 1 also provides 81 percent of the dispersion factor in the matrix. Root 2 is accounted for mainly be comprehension and fluency, and it amounts to 8 percent of the dispersion. Root 3 is a repetition, and to a lesser extent, naming factor, amounting to only 1 percent of total dispersion factor. This is quite similar to the rPCA of acute aphasics.

A nearest neighbor network was constructed for the eight clusters of 83 chronic aphasics. The three neighbors in the bottom, separated by the longest distances, are globals (I), Broca's (III), and Wernicke's aphasics (II). Broca's group (III) is second neighbor to ''afferent conduction'' (V), which is next to but distinctly separate from isolation (IV) aphasics. The other three groups are con-

Table 7–4
R-Type Principal Components Analysis
83 Acute Aphasics, Language Subtests

	Percentage of matrix/root	Percentage of root accounted for by characters				
		Information	*Fluency*	*Comprehension*	*Repetition*	*Naming*
Root 1	87%	18.79	16.73	15.72	23.29	25.45
Root 2	8%	17.78	32.08	48.10	0.92	1.09
Root 3	4%	60.01	37.88	0.32	1.50	0.27
Root 4	1%	0.33	1.18	0.35	58.24	39.88

The *r*-type PCA for chronic aphasics indicates the same roots of dispersion and attributes accounting for each root, as in Table 7–2 for acute aphasics.

nected only through a secondary link between afferent conduction (V), and a mixed group of mild aphasics (VI), which in turn is connected to anomics (VIII), and to a nearly recovered group (VII) (Fig. 7-4).

ACUTE APHASICS CLUSTERED ON ALL SUBTESTS

In order to increase the objectivity of clustering, parameters which do not obviously contribute to the clinical classification were also included in this analysis. The subtests used as characters remained within the area of cognition and language related disorders. Including the color of the eyes or the height of the patients in the classification of aphasics would be clearly nonsensical, but we

CHRONIC APHASICS — LANGUAGE
NEAREST NEIGHBOR NETWORK ANALYSIS

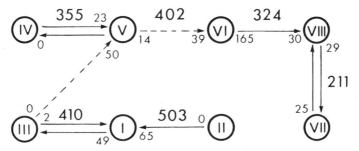

Fig. 7-4.   Chronic aphasics: Language. Nearest Neighbor Network Analysis.

have included nonlanguage tasks which have bearing on the cognitive behavior of aphasics. Reading, writing, praxis, block design, drawing, calculation, and Raven's colored matrices were measured with the language subtests to provide 17 parameters for clustering. There is evidence that some of these allegedly nonverbal functions are impaired in aphasia. Including them for the clustering of aphasics is not without rationale. It was hoped that more objective and stable clustering can be achieved by increasing the characters without preselection. The contribution of these nonverbal tasks, as well as reading, writing, calculation, and praxis, to clustering is an important issue in the classification of aphasics.

This is the same population as in the section on acute aphasics due to infarcts clustered on language only. The 64 aphasics were tested within 2−6 weeks from onset. Nine groups were formed on the dendrogram at 4 percent of the variance (Fig. 7-5). The first (N = 11) had mainly global, except for two Wernicke's aphasics. The second group (N = 7) also all global, with one isolation syndrome. The third cluster (N = 7) had all Broca's, except one conduction aphasic. Group 4 (N = 5) was a mixture of transcortical motor, sensory, and isolation aphasics. Group 5 (N = 6) consisted of three Wernicke's, two conduction, and one transcortical sensory aphasic. Group 6 (N = 5) had all Wernicke's aphasics. The seventh cluster (N = 9) was an interesting combination of conduction (4), Broca's (4), and anomic (1) aphasia (efferent conduction). Group 8 (N = 5) consisted of mainly anomic, with a transcortical sensory and a

64 ACUTE APHASICS − ALL TESTS

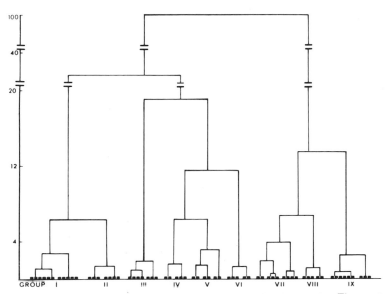

Fig. 7-5. Dendrogram for acute aphasics clustered on all subtests. See Figures 7-1 and 7-3.

Wernicke's aphasic. Group 9 was all anomic, except for one conduction aphasic ($N = 9$). The q-type PCA, displayed in a scattered diagram (Fig. 7-6), indicates the dispersion of the groups along two main axes. This does not account for a third or fourth dimension, but the extent of the contribution to these roots can be appreciated from the R-type PCA.

The cluster profiles for the acute aphasic groups on all subtests are seen in Table 7-5. These are complex and difficult to review at a glance. A narrative description and clinical deductions are as follows:

1. Cluster I is characterized by low language and performance scores.
2. Cluster II has the same low language scores but better nonverbal performance.
3. Cluster III is clearly distinguished by better comprehension subtests and also relatively good performance scores (Broca's aphasia).
4. Cluster IV is more fluent, with high repetition but poor performance scores.
5. Cluster V has higher fluency but lower comprehension and performance scores than Cluster III.
6. Cluster VI has relatively better performance but poorer language scores, with the fluency an exception (suggesting a profile of Wernicke's aphasia).
7. Cluster VII is characterized by less fluency but high comprehension and performance.
8. Cluster VIII is unique in its low writing, reading, and performance scores, associated with high repetition and fluency scores, and some comprehension deficit (alexia and agraphia with mild speech disturbance).
9. Cluster IX has uniformly high scores in both language and performance areas.

The nearest neighbor network analysis (Fig. 7-7) shows Clusters I and II, the Global groups, the closest. They only differ in the better nonverbal scores of Cluster II, which is second nearest neighbor to Cluster VI or Wernicke's aphasics, with poor language comprehension and performance. This in turn is next to Cluster V, a similar, high frequency, low comprehension group, with poor nonverbal scores, occupying a "nodal" or central position connected to Cluster III (a nonfluent group with good comprehension and performance) by a longer distance, and to Cluster IV (good repetition and poor comprehension and performance) by a shorter distance, and to Cluster VIII (poor reading and writing with high repetition and fluency). Cluster VIII is another nodal cluster connected to Cluster VII (less fluent but higher comprehension with better performance) and to Cluster IX (with good language and performance scores).

The r-type principal component analysis (rPCA) of acute aphasics for 17 subtests indicated that root I accounted for 64 percent of variance (Table 7-6). Auditory word recognition, repetition, object naming, responsive speech, sentence completion, and the other language tasks contribute rather evenly to this root, with relatively smaller inputs from reading, writing, and calculation, and

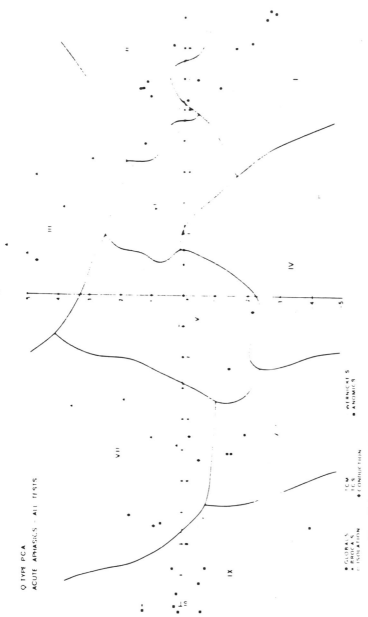

Fig. 7-6. *Q*-type PCA for acute aphasics on all subtests displays the factors of variance in two dimensions. Some of the dispersion has to be imagined perpendicular to the plane of the diagram. The clinical diagnosis for each individual is coded.

Table 7-5
Cluster Profiles for Acute Aphasics—All Subtests

Cluster (N) / Character	I (11) X	SD	II (7) X	SD	III (7) X	SD	IV (5) X	SD	V (6) X	SD	VI (5) X	SD	VII (9) X	SD	VIII (5) X	SD	IX (11) X	SD
Information content	121	49	134	58	157	70	276	32	446	119	484	192	588	115	596	106	802	62
Fluency	245	197	138	64	227	176	580	132	662	98	722	97	524	137	846	43	890	27
Yes–no comprehension	456	216	442	258	711	89	700	80	684	117	484	137	806	62	748	68	851	31
Auditory word recognition	136	44	103	9	675	153	476	156	524	128	278	151	834	97	668	123	864	47
Sequential commands	172	105	120	21	661	127	380	126	525	163	260	147	735	121	572	127	781	137
Repetition	121	68	168	167	180	95	788	156	526	188	180	87	597	50	756	93	793	53
Object naming	100	0	105	9	151	53	355	102	484	168	276	138	719	119	670	75	858	42
Word fluency	100	0	100	0	100	0	112	24	223	154	161	123	353	110	469	67	729	103
Responsive speech	100	0	122	55	157	110	660	143	340	80	132	64	668	133	772	64	882	50
Sentence completion	100	0	100	0	100	0	516	239	340	153	132	64	722	159	644	217	900	0
Reading	143	92	267	149	423	121	319	87	481	174	431	53	591	100	421	199	752	80
Writing	143	75	198	111	357	43	222	133	294	153	267	83	440	153	277	68	683	190
Praxis	344	203	512	168	625	142	558	126	654	63	546	52	649	126	589	17	798	120
Drawing	224	135	395	78	564	124	322	133	375	106	432	55	582	145	400	63	544	126
Block design	220	146	407	0*	486	158	206	66	240	140	631	194	573	257	416	19	534	288
Calculation	141	111	488	0*	698	144	260	171	533	239	375	144	624	252	517	58	796	151
Raven's matrices	156	101	432	0*	608	163	322	166	379	267	527	99	610	154	366	133	555	130

*Indicates low relevance (data missing).

Cluster profiles for acute aphasics—all subtests. The means and standard deviations of the scaled values of each attribute in each cluster are shown. The characters or attributes are in the left column. Minimum scaled score is 100, maximum is 900.

NEAREST NEIGHBOR NETWORK

ACUTE APHASICS ALL TESTS

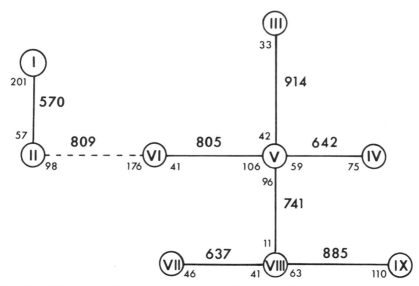

Fig. 7-7.   Nearest neighbor network for acute aphasics on all subtests shows the clusters, intercentroid distances (large numbers), and the deviation from the centroid (small numbers). Nearest neighbors are indicated with solid, second nearest neighbors with interrupted lines.

negligible performance component. On the other hand, root 2, accounting for 16 percent of the variation, and substantial performance components. Root 3 (5 percent of the variation) is most influenced by fluency and comprehension.

CHRONIC APHASICS CLUSTERED ON ALL SUBTESTS

Chronic aphasics, due to infarct, were clustered on all subtests. This population is the same as the one clustered on language only, consisting of patients who had a test at least 330 days after their stroke. We were interested in the acute versus chronic population differences, when nonverbal subtests were also used in clustering. The dendrograms generated nine clusters at 3.5 percent of the variance (Fig. 7-8). The first cluster has five Global, five Broca's, and one Wernicke's aphasic. The second group is a mixture of six Globals, one Isolation, one Wernicke's and one Broca's aphasic. The third cluster has seven Broca's, seven Conduction, and one Wernicke's aphasic. The fourth cluster has two Conduction, one Isolation, one Broca's, and one Transcortical Motor aphasic. The fifth group consists of five Broca's, three Conduction, one Transcortical Motor, one

Table 7-6

r-Type Principal Component Analysis of Acute and Chronic Aphasics on all Subtests

Character	Root 1		Root 2		Root 3		Root 4	
	Acute 64%	Chronic 73%	Acute 11%	Chronic 8%	Acute 5%	Chronic 3%	Acute 4%	Chronic 3%
Information content	6.8	9.6	0.7	1.0	7.5	3.1	1.9	1.0
Fluency	7.0	5.8	6.7	2.1	28.5	21.3	2.6	7.0
Yes–no comprehension	2.1	1.4	0.3	0.1	6.4	9.8	0.1	0.3
Auditory word recognition	10.7	5.9	3.3	1.0	16.7	23.6	2.4	0.3
Sequential commands	7.0	6.8	4.7	2.5	15.2	21.5	0.0	0.5
Repetition	9.1	9.8	8.7	4.1	0.1	3.6	27.4	4.6
Object naming	11.1	11.6	2.1	2.5	0.4	1.2	2.7	2.4
Word fluency	4.6	3.5	0.1	0.0	1.9	4.1	4.7	6.5
Responsive speech	12.7	11.3	8.6	4.9	0.1	0.0	5.0	26.6
Sentence completion	14.2	17.0	7.8	7.3	1.1	0.0	6.7	1.5
Reading	3.8	4.6	1.6	7.3	0.3	3.0	11.7	3.0
Writing	2.5	4.1	1.4	25.2	0.6	0.2	8.6	8.7
Praxis	1.6	1.1	1.4	2.7	0.4	0.3	1.7	5.4
Drawing	0.7	1.0	5.6	10.6	0.0	2.7	1.8	5.8
Block design	0.9	0.8	13.2	11.6	17.4	2.0	11.1	0.3
Calculation	4.2	4.6	19.1	6.8	0.7	3.7	6.0	15.5
Raven's matrices	1.1	1.2	14.1	10.1	1.4	0.0	5.9	10.6

r-Type principal component analysis, acute and chronic aphasics—all subtests. The roots of variance are in the top horizontal row. The percentage of contribution of each character is in the column under each root.

83 CHRONIC APHASICS – ALL SUBTESTS

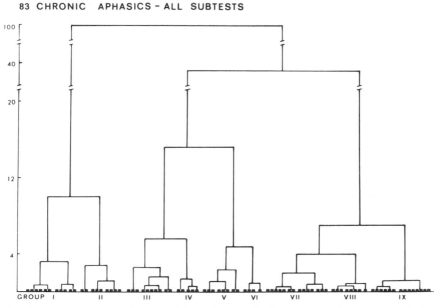

Fig. 7-8. Chronic aphasics on all tests. The ordinate (the percentage of variation) is broken for display. Each individual is represented by a block.

Wernicke's, and one Anomic patient. The sixth cluster has only four Anomics. The seventh group has all Anomics (12), except one Conduction aphasic. The eighth ($N = 8$) and ninth ($N = 13$) clusters are all Anomic or recovered patients, according to our previously discussed cutoff point.

The cluster attribute analysis throws further light on the cluster profiles (Table 7-7). Cluster I is characterized by low language and performance scores, in contrast to Cluster II, with equally low language but better performance scores. This is probably related to the low relevance (missing data) of those attributes, as some severely affected patients were not given the test. Average scores were assigned to missing data, in order to allow the individual to participate in the PCA Cluster III. Low fluency but a high comprehension language pattern showed better performance scores. Cluster IV, with low fluency and somewhat less comprehension than Cluster III, has higher performance also. Cluster V has slightly better comprehension, but interestingly, poorer performance than Cluster IV. This is, clinically, the least homogenous group. Cluster VI is distinguished by poor writing, reading, drawing, and Raven's scores, with relatively intact language. Clusters VII, VIII, and IX all had good language scores, but Cluster VIII had somewhat poor performance (low Raven's scores), and IX had better scores in all subtests.

The q type principal component analysis (Fig. 7-9) shows the individuals in A-space. The horizontal and vertical axes are different from the analysis by

Table 7–7

Cluster Profiles for Chronic Aphasics—All Subtests

Cluster (N)	I (11)		II (9)		III (10)		IV (5)		V (8)		VI (4)		VII (13)		VIII (8)		IX (15)	
Character	X	SD	X	SD	X	SD	X	SD	X	SD	X	SD	X	SD	X	SD	X	SD
Information content	150	70	153	65	340	101	468	164	530	88	620	40	758	71	820	40	857	39
Fluency	274	159	277	187	388	156	404	128	480	111	740	138	733	106	820	40	841	35
Yes–no comprehension	515	109	497	232	773	78	759	42	800	82	841	20	820	76	862	37	871	37
Auditory word recognition	342	145	215	106	720	102	692	104	810	77	746	107	842	47	891	13	894	9
Sequential commands	285	146	181	84	641	146	478	144	677	127	772	56	754	155	872	33	875	51
Repetition	129	38	171	152	340	123	580	143	600	124	800	34	770	86	840	34	825	45
Object naming	157	88	148	68	372	127	489	161	678	134	780	97	783	74	865	14	892	10
Word fluency	100	0	100	0	196	56	218	86	268	101	426	80	336	75	484	97	706	117
Responsive speech	165	101	224	210	372	124	676	163	760	124	740	195	838	77	900	0	900	0
Sentence completion	114	45	117	50	356	178	260	143	800	111	860	69	887	42	900	0	900	0
Reading	224	129	443	209	519	109	580	137	649	182	562	260	747	89	815	63	856	66
Writing	212	143	450	187	429	123	559	126	498	115	120	13	734	114	720	157	833	82
Praxis	420	216	739	0*	709	107	757	70	758	98	775	75	815	75	813	96	859	62
Drawing	364	160	457	194	488	150	603	117	555	95	253	57	632	117	588	58	717	119
Block design	427	212	659	40*	706	78	748	96	581	198	520	165	759	130	598	114	873	61
Calculation	142	71	640	2*	496	141	661	195	635	145	700	105	792	87	817	77	859	58
Raven's matrices	217	131	550	32*	498	108	608	89	574	117	370	94	661	92	489	156	718	101

Cluster profiles for chronic aphasics—all subtests. See Table 7–5 for comparison and explanation.

*Indicates low relevance (data missing).

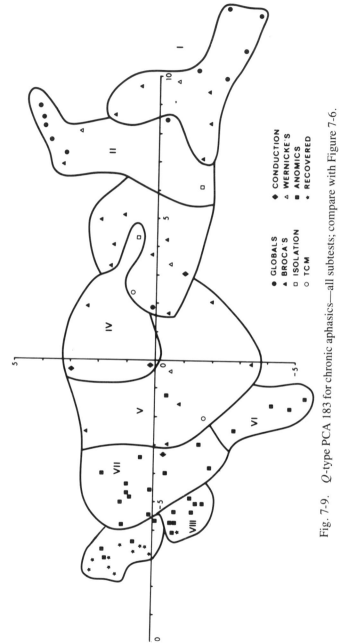

Fig. 7-9. *Q*-type PCA 183 for chronic aphasics—all subtests; compare with Figure 7-6.

115

language subtests only. The differences are explained by the r-type principal component analysis (see below). The vertical axis is predominantly a performance factor, adding to the complexity of disperson.

A nearest neighbor network analysis of intercentroid distances and deviations (Fig. 7-10) revealed that Clusters VII, VIII, and IX were close (mostly mild aphasics with variations in nonverbal performance). The next pair of clusters, V (better comprehension but poorer performance) and VI (good language but poor reading and writing), were secondarily connected with the recovered, mild group and the next two clusters—Cluster IV (a mixed group with low fluency, good comprehension, but better performance) and Cluster III (low fluency, good comprehension but poorer performance). Quite a long secondary connection is seen from Cluster III to II (low language, better performance scores), and its nearest neighbor—I (poor language and performance).

The r-type principal component analysis (rPCA) for chronic aphasics, clustered on all subtests, indicated sentence completion, responsive speech, object naming, repetition, and spontaneous speech content were the most important contributors to root 1, which accounted for 74 percent of the variance (Table 7-6). Sentence and word comprehension and fluency were of secondary importance in this factor, which seems to be somewhat different from the general

NEAREST NEIGHBOR NETWORK
CHRONIC APHASICS-ALL TESTS

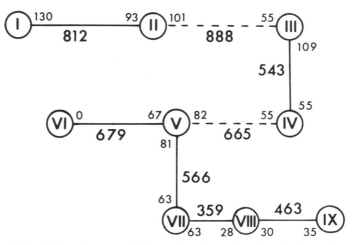

Fig. 7-10.   Nearest neighbor network for chronic aphasics—all subtests; compare with Figure 7-7.

language factor of acute aphasics. Root 2 (8 percent of variance) is again clearly a performance factor, with writing and the nonlanguage tasks of drawing, block design, and Raven's matrices contributing to it most. Root 3 (3.3 percent of variance) is accounted for mainly by fluency and comprehension, the features most important in clinical taxonomy. The fourth root (2.7 percent of variance) is loaded with the factor of information content, as it accounts for 27 percent of it.

APHASICS WITH BOTH ACUTE AND CHRONIC LANGUAGE TESTS

There were 17 aphasics who belonged to both the acute and chronic group. The Q-type PCA was used to display the changes of these individuals in the attribute space in the course of a year (Fig. 7-11). The individual numbers $18-34$ are in the acute state, and $1-17$ in the chronic state, superimposed in the same scatter diagram, allowing the reader to trace the changes made by individuals from one cluster to another. The greatest gains were made by a global and a Broca's aphasic, who then became anomic, a major shift along the horizontal axis. Similarly, large shifts were seen in another Broca's aphasic, who remained Broca's, another who evolved towards anomic aphasia, and a Wernicke's aphasic who became a conduction type. There were two clusters at the ends of the scatter diagrams that did not seem to move much. With the exception of two cases, the shift appeared to be from right to left (from the more severe to the milder impairment), and upwards (from nonfluent to fluent and from low comprehension to better comprehension). The two exceptions were a Wernicke's aphasic who deteriorated, and another who had fluent mumbling, interpreted as jargon initially, which was probably stereotyping, since she became less fluent as her comprehension improved. This illustrates the occasional misclassification that can occur when one crucial parameter is not interpreted or measured correctly.

DISCUSSION

The comparison of acute and chronic groups yields important differences. It is evident from the dendrograms that the acute and chronic clusters are different in composition. One of the most striking differences is a large, acute cluster of Wernicke's aphasics and a small ($N = 2$) Wernicke's group in the chronic population. This confirms the clinical experience of considerable recovery in Wernicke's aphasia, and the less frequent persistence of this entity to the chronic stage. Among the acute clusters, efferent and afferent conduction, isolation, and transcortical sensory aphasics feature in different groups, but in the chronic population, these do not appear in significant enough number to form distinct

17 LANGUAGE PATIENTS. ACUTE + CHRONIC DATA.RUN AS 34 PAT

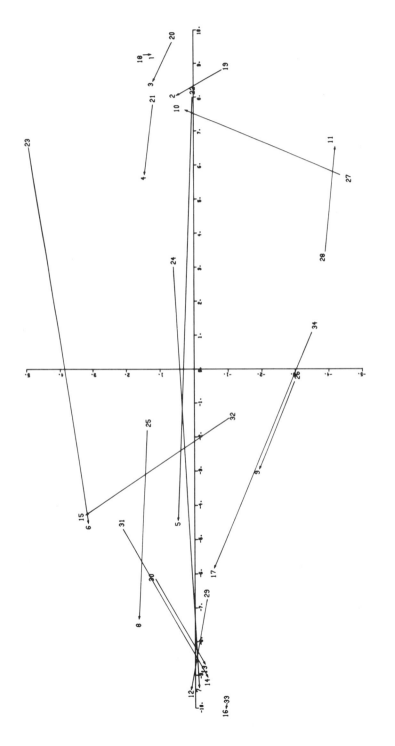

Fig. 7-11. *Q*-type PCA for 17 aphasics in the acute and chronic state. This scatter diagram represents the changes of individuals from acute to chronic state in the language attribute space. The right to left shift represents an improvement in severity, and vertical shift, changes in comprehension and fluency. The arrow points from the acute towards the chronic state of the aphasic.

clusters. In the chronic population, there is a larger group of anomic and recovered patients, evolved from other varieties of aphasia, forming two large clusters.

There are features which are common to both acute and chronic groups. There are large numbers of global aphasics in Cluster I and anomic aphasics in Cluster VIII, in both populations. There are pure clusters of Broca's aphasia both in the acute and chronic populations. The r-type PCA reveals the same roots or factors of variance for acute and chronic aphasics. The first root, accounting for most of the dispersion on the horizontal axis of the Q-type PCA, is a general language or severity factor, as all language subtests contribute to it evenly. The second factor of variation for both populations is mainly comprehension and fluency. The third root is mainly repetition; naming contributes to all roots, in both acute and chronic groups, indicating the low discriminatory value of the naming task between types of aphasia.

The rPCA was quite different in the classification involving nonverbal parameters. The first root was a similar, general language factor, as in the previous analysis, based on language tests only, but had a more substantial contribution from the naming tasks (object naming, sentence completion, responsive speech). The high number of anomic aphasics in the chronic sample may explain the importance of naming tasks in this first factor. The second factor clearly related to a performance component.

The inclusion of not obviously language tasks of cognition redefined the clusters in both populations. Even though the number of factors increased, the clustering appeared to remain clinically relevant. Higher performance in the low scoring language groups alters the clustering and suggests that performance measurements may have a role in the classification of aphasics. Better performance scores may be helpful in identifying those global aphasics who will show more recovery than others. An example of this was actually seen in a patient who had been followed for a year, from global scores to good functional recovery. His initial performance scores were relatively high.

The performance scores often correlated best with comprehension in the cluster attribute analysis; on the other hand, fluency and performance seemed to be independent. A clearly distinct cluster, characterized by low reading, writing, and performance scores, with relatively high language scores, corresponded to the syndrome of alexia with agraphia.

8

Localization of Lesions by Autopsy, Stimulation, Surgery, Arteriography, and Electroencephalography

To locate the damage which destroys speech and to localize speech are two different things . . .

Hughlings Jackson (1878)

INTRODUCTION

The conceptual and philosophical background of localization of function in the central nervous system is complex and controversial. The seductive speculation of nineteenth century mosaicism, an offspring of phrenology, that each behavior corresponds to an area in the brain, influenced the theoretical basis of describing centers of language, as clinical symptoms were correlated with lesions found at autopsy. There is no doubt that Broca's discovery (1861) of the association of aphasia with left hemisphere lesions, and Wernicke's introduction (1874) of the anteroposterior, motor−sensory dichotomy, and the connections of language areas, were turning points in correlating language function with brain structure. Around the same time, Fritsch and Hitzig (1870) discovered that stimulating areas on the cerebral cortex of a dog will produce discrete movement. Mapping of the cerebral cortex yielded the best results for primary motor and sensory function. Although the motor mosaic is not as sharply defined as was originally believed and a great deal of overlap exists, Penfield's homunculus (1950) remains a clinically valid concept. The wide open mouth of the grotesque figure reminds us of the wide area on the surface of the brain from which vocalization can be elicited. The physiology and columnar organization of cells in the primary somatosensory cortex of the cat were explored with the microelectrode technique by Mountcastle (1960), and the hierarchies of simple to hypercomplex visual receptors were established by Hubel and Wiesel (1965). The gap between the discovery of the physiology of primary receptors and complex human behavior is yet to be bridged. The careful, accurate, and measurable observation of a patient with a damaged brain remains a powerful source of information, though the method has been subjected to much criticism and even, irrational neglect by modern workers. Much of our current knowledge about higher order brain function is based on this method. Jackson's (1878) warning, nevertheless, still stands: "Speech and words are physical terms; words have, of course, anatomical substrata or bases, as well as other states have. We must as carefully distinguish betwixt words and their physical basis as we do betwixt color and its physical basis; a psychical state is always accompanied by a physical state, but nevertheless, the two things have distinct natures."

AUTOPSY MATERIAL

The end of the last century saw the publication of several hundreds of clinicoanatomical correlations. This extensive literature is summarized in the monumental work of Henschen (1922), who abstracted 1337 cases of aphasia and related disorders with autopsy material. His own 60 cases were also included and formed the largest individual series. Although he drew rather definite conclusions, the lack of uniformity of clinical examination and recorded symptomatology, combined with the variable quality and extent of the postmortem descriptions, cast doubts on these interpretations. After Jackson (1876) postulated that the minor hemisphere swears and the left "propositionizes," Henschen further pointed out that when the major hemisphere was destroyed, the minor one could take over. He showed that when recovery had taken place after a stroke on the left side, and another lesion destroyed the right third frontal convolution, speech was lost without further recovery! He also demonstrated this for disturbances of comprehension. Bilateral temporal lesions were accompanied by persisting word deafness without alexia or agraphia, and mildly paraphasic and anomic speech. Among his own cases, a hemorrhage in the angular gyrus caused alexia and anomic aphasia. Other angular gyrus lesions were characterized by word blindness (alexia). Only five cases were found restricted to this area, but the gyrus was involved in 250 larger lesions. Two cases of sensorimotor aphasia with frontal and angular gyrus lesions had alexia and agraphia. Henschen promoted the second frontal gyrus as Exner's writing center.

Foix (1928) outlined the vascular territories of the brain, and noted aphasia with lesions of the posterior territory of the middle cerebral artery:

1. Total softening of posterior territory resulted in severe sensory aphasia
2. Parietoangular gyrus softening produced moderate sensory aphasia and alexia
3. Temporoangular gyrus lesion sensory aphasia

Another similar clinicopathological correlation is by Davison et al. (1934), who selected 48 cases with "adequate" clinical information and without multiple lesions from 200 infarcts at autopsy. Among the complete middle cerebral artery occlusions, only two cases of motor aphasia without comprehension deficits were found, and these had spared the temporal convolutions. Seven others had global aphasia. In partial, middle cerebral artery occlusions, the third frontal, precentral opercular, insular, and first temporal convolutions were often involved. Motor aphasia was present in ten cases, global in four. Among the cortical branch occlusions, only one sensory aphasia was found. Deep branch occlusions also caused aphasia: the left lenticulostriate artery occlusion resulted in transient motor aphasia. Unfortunately, such a series exemplifies the problem of surveying pathological material: the lack of clinical information to provide confidence about the nature of language deficits described.

Global Aphasia

Cases of global or total aphasia have excited much less interest among localizationists than have other aphasic syndromes. Liepmann (1915) emphasized that although the lesion occurs in the whole region of speech, comprehension may recover, and, subsequently, the clinical picture of Motor aphasia predominates. Nielsen (1946) presented 18 cases of Henschen's and one of his own to demonstrate that patients who survive large lesions may, in time, be able to recover some function subserved by the other cerebral hemisphere. Kleist (1962) presented a case of his own and another of Jolly's as examples of word deafness, but the clinical descriptions indicated global aphasia and the brains had large perisylvian lesions. It is difficult to understand why the severely impaired, stereotypic speech production is put aside and the comprehension deficit is discussed as if it were a specific form of aphasia. We have pointed out in our localization studies that when global aphasics are retested at a later date, they may fall into Broca's category (Kertesz et al., 1973, 1977). The 15 autopsied cases, presented by Mohr (1978) as representative of Broca's aphasia, were initially global. Details of subsequent language performance and pictures of the brain are given for one case only, indicating recovery toward the picture of Broca's aphasia. Clinical information for the remainder of these cases seems to be restricted to the examiner's impression; but for two of the cases, which were published previously, recovery of some comprehension was evident at three months (Mohr, 1976).

Broca's Aphasia

Broca's first case, Leborgne (Tan), was 51 when he died, and lost his speech at 30 (it is not known whether gradually or suddenly). He understood everything but he only answered "tan, tan" rather expressively. He would lose his temper and supplement his vocabulary with expletives. He had gradually increasing right arm and leg paralysis, ten years after the onset of the illness. Broca examined him on several occasions, and noted erroneous responses; these he attributed to impaired intelligence, due to his expanding cerebral lesion (a stroke in evolution?) or his fever (he was admitted with cellulitis of his right leg). Broca predicted that a slowly progressive, chronic softening would be found in the left frontal lobe, with extension into the corpus striatum (because of the hemiplegia). The autopsy showed a cyst over the left sylvian fissure. When this was punctured, an egg-sized cavity was found, separating the frontal and temporal lobes, representing the loss of cerebral substance. Softening extended beyond the limits of this cavity and a considerable portion of the left hemisphere had been gradually destroyed by this process. The posterior half of the third frontal convolution (F3), and the second frontal convolution (F2), the inferior marginal convolutions (T1), and the insula had been eroded. Broca stated that the loss of the third frontal convolution amounted to nearly half of the total loss. He went on to say that the brain appeared to be soft beyond the described cavity. He said that the striatum was softened but the thalamus spared (the cavity was connected with the ventricles). The brain had not been sectioned, and it has disappeared since from the Dupuytren Museum. Broca assumed that the illness progressed in a biphasic manner: first one of the frontal convolutions, "probably the third," was affected (loss of speech), then other areas as well (paralysis). He then said that generalized atrophy was responsible for the disorder of intellect.

Pierre Marie (1906) attacked Broca's doctrine 45 years later with his dramatic paper proclaiming that "the third frontal convolution plays no special role in the function of language," right in the title. He examined the brains of Broca's cases and emphasized that Leborgne's brain showed lesions of the frontal, parietal, and temporal lobes, and Lelong's brain only showed diffuse atrophy. Dejerine (1907) defended Broca's description as correct. Nielsen (1946), who also reviewed Broca's cases, claimed that Lelong, his second case, who understood language but could only say a few words perseveratively, had only a small hemorrhage, subcortical to the second, and third frontal convolutions (F2 and F3). This, then, would be an example of Broca's aphasia in Broca's area, described by Broca! Marie and his pupil, Moutier (1908), reviewed other cases of aphasia without F3 lesions, and lesions of F3 without aphasia. Only temporary motor aphasia accompanied the cases of Tuke and Fraser (1872) and Bramwell (1898), with Broca's area lesions. Moutier (1908) reported a case with bilateral F3 lesions and another one with complete lesion in the left, and a partial one in the right side, without permanent aphasia. Monakow (1914) had two cases of F3 lesions, with initial aphasia, but relatively rapid recovery.

Among the lesions restricted to F3, 22 were corticomedullary, 20 medullary, and seven cortical, with the clinical symptom of "aphemia" or mutism in Henschen's collection. Twenty cases of bilateral F3 lesions all had "aphemia." Bilateral atrophy without softening, however, was compatible with speech. Eighty-five cases had aphemia (nonfluent aphasia) with F3 lesions on the left side. Seventeen contradictory cases were also recorded six definitely so), where there was no aphemia with F3 lesions on the left; three of these did not have enough time after the injury to invoke the right hemisphere to take over. Kleist (1934) stated that severe and persistent "word dumbness" indicated involvement of the deeper white matter, including callosal and other association fibers. Nielsen (1946) considered the time and extent of clinical recovery in his review of published cases, but failed to do so in one of his own cases of Broca's area infarct. Another of his cases was an example of persisting Broca's aphasia with a lesion in Broca's area. The patient was able to understand, but could say only "yes" and "no." He had a small lesion in the left third frontal convolution and, also, a small lesion in the anterior portion of the first temporal convolution.

Goldstein (1948) called the cases of transient, milder, mostly articulatory motor disturbances "peripheral motor aphasia," and noted that good, rapid recovery was compatible with the destruction of Broca's area in the left hemi sphere. Hecaen and Consoli (1973) found 19 lesions relatively limited to Broca's area. Two were congenital and had no aphasia, five only had articulatory and mild writing disturbances, seven cases. had persistent language disorder with some comprehension disturbance and severe agraphia. Four milder cases were left-handers and another case, with a slowly growing tumor, only had anomia. The mild cases were superficial lesions and the severe ones more extensive. The authors felt that the findings were in keeping with Dejerine's view that lesions of Broca's area can produce either "pure" motor aphasia or Broca's aphasia. More recently, Mohr (1976) reviewed the literature and presented his own experiences of F3 lesions producing rapidly ameliorating motor aphasia on one hand, and larger lesions of the upper division of the middle cerebral artery producing the syndrome of persisting Broca's aphasia, on the other. He presented four autopsied cases of F3 lesions, all with rapidly ameliorating motor aphasia. Although he did not define the type of aphasia quantitatively, from the qualitative description, one obtains the impression of variable language deficit associated with Broca's area infarct. His four cases would probably be classified by our taxonomy as having mild Broca's aphasia (3), and transcortical motor aphasia (1), the one with good repetition.

Wernicke's Aphasia

Sensory aphasics have been described before Wernicke, but the first important anatomical contribution came from Meynert (1866) (cited by Meyer, 1974). He described a case with lack of comprehension and paraphasic speech, but without hemiplegia, associated with an infarct of the posterior insular artery.

Wernicke (1874) presented two autopsied cases of sensory aphasia. One had softening of the first temporal convolution (T1) on the left, as well as generalized atrophy, the other a left temporal lobe abscess. An excellent early review from the literature of 50 autopsied cases of Sensory aphasia was carried out by Starr (1899). He excluded large tumors from his survey to eliminate the effects of increased intracranial pressure. Starr recognized the limitations of the method of his contemporaries and wrote: "The pathology of Sensory aphasia rests more upon forcible assertion and the analysis of ingenious diagrams than it does upon the collation of reliable evidence." He also perceived that "a considerable modification of symptoms occurred after the first few weeks and conclusions would be unreliable from pathology which is obtained very soon after the onset." In seven cases of "pure" word deafness the lesion was limited to the posterior two-thirds of the first and second temporal convolution. He recognized that word blindness (alexia) and paraphasia often accompanied "word deafness" and that the lesions often included the inferior parietal convolutions and the occipital lobe as well. He tried to tabulate the actual language functions tested in the cases in his review. He concluded that temporoparietal lesions resulted in the combination of word deafness (sensory aphasia) with word blindness (alexia), and that parieto-occipital lesions produced the combination of word blindness (alexia), psychic blindness (visual agnosia), and hemianopsia. Difficulty in recalling the names of objects (anomia), although tested uniformly, was not found to be a reliable localizing index. There was no constant pathological difference between the cases of sensory aphasia with and without paraphasia.

Liepmann and Storch (1902) reported a case of *pure word deafness* with a subcortical lesion in the left temporal lobe, isolating the auditory association area. Similarly, unilateral cases in addition to bilateral temporal lesions have appeared in the literature since (see review by Goldstein, 1974).

Henschen (1922) went as far as to postulate that the posterior part of T1 is related to sentence agrammatism, whereas defects of the middle portion produce word agrammatism. The word sounds are registered in the middle portion and then arranged in sentences in the posterior portion. Supporting this idea of differential functioning were the findings of O. and C. Vogt (1910): that the middle portion myelinized earlier and more extensively. In Henschen's series of the 35 cases of temporal lesions without alexia, 20 had "word deafness," demonstrating the independence of auditory from visual comprehension, which is contrary to Wernicke's theory.

Kleist (1962), in his monograph on sensory aphasia and amusia, presented the myeloarchitectonic divisions of the temporal lobes by Beck and Hopf. He also provided clinical and pathological details on eight patients with sensory aphasia. One of them (Be) appeared to be actually a global aphasic and was mentioned previously. A case (De) with severe comprehension deficit, paraphasias, and neologisms, but relatively intact sentences and small words, had lesions in the deep white matter of the left temporal lobe, subcortical white matter of T_2 and T_1. Another patient (Döl), with neologistic speech and comprehension deficit, had lesions in the subcortical white matter of the transverse gyri and the planum temporale, as well as in T_1 and T_2. A right posterior T_1 lesion with deep white matter lesion to the ventricle produced almost "complete speech deafness" in a fourth case (Rit). Kleist concluded that there were no obvious clinical differences between cortical, subcortical, and transcortical lesions. *Word deafness* with literal paraphasias and anomia (Wernicke's aphasia in our terminology) was seen with lesions of the planum temporale and the posterior third of the first temporal convolution, and the adjacent inferior parietal lobule (case Papp). A second lesion in the right hemisphere prevented recovery in this case, according to Kleist. *Word sense deafness,* equivalent to semantic jargon with verbal paraphasias and comprehension deficit, was produced by a small, irregular lesion between the posterior ends of the first and second temporal gyrus (case Bayr). *Sentence deafness,* in another case (Seuf), appeared to be equivalent to severe, semantic jargon, with long, irrelevant but constructionally normal replies to questions. Repetition was not detailed in the published protocol. The patient was able to appreciate musical tone quality but could not reproduce melodies. Contusion of the second and posterior quarter of the first temporal convolution and the supramarginal gyrus was found. Although the anatomical and clinical descriptions are extensive, no attempt was made to quantify the clinical and linguistic features. The distinction between the terms "word," "sound," and "sentence deafness" seems arbitrary and fanciful. In some patients, the disturbed repetition was used as an important classifying feature (conduction aphasia); in others, it was not documented.

A well-documented case of *auditory agnosia* for non-verbal sounds, without aphasia, and with normal hearing—a unique dissociation—was described by Spreen et al. (1965), with a large infarct involving the right superior temporal, angular, inferior parietal, inferior and middle frontal, and insular regions, in a right-handed man. Sound agnosia in association with sensory aphasia, on the other hand, is common (Vignolo, 1969). A recent case with bilateral temporal infarcts was documented by Oppenheimer and Newcombe (1978).

We have published ten cases, five of them autopsied, of *neologistic jargon aphasia* with clinicopathological correlations (Kertesz and Benson, 1970). Each of these patients produced copious, fluent, prosodically correct speech, resembling English syntax and inflection, and had significantly impaired auditory comprehension, repetition, naming, reading, and writing. In each case, the most posterior portion of the first temporal convolution and the supramarginal gyrus and the underlying white matter was involved. In three cases, the lesion was limited in size and location to the posterior end of the Sylvian fissure; however, this syndrome has been seen with larger lesions extending parietally, posteriorly, and temporally, inferiorly. In two of the cases, the temporal lobe was minimally involved. Transverse sections showed the involvement of the temporal operculum, planum temporale, and the parietal operculum and underlying white matter, representing the arcuate fasciculus, in each case.

Lhermitte et al. (1973) published a complex case with coexisting segments of meaningless jargon and meaningful but nonfluent output. This patient had multiple, bilateral infarcts, of various ages, in Broca's area, insula, temporal operculum, supramarginal gyrus, etc. One could only postulate that the reason for the curious language behavior was the irregular recovery and compensation of various language modalities.

Conduction Aphasia

The original cases Wernicke presented as conduction aphasia did not have impaired repetition recorded, and are not equivalent to the modern usage of the category. Central aphasia, which was Goldstein's term for conduction aphasia, was considered an incomplete receptive syndrome by Stengel and Patch (1955), with lesions in the posterior part of the insula and the supramarginal gyrus in three cases. Kleist (1962) also presented two cases with significant temporal lobe destruction, in whom comprehension recovered but repetition remained poor (conduction aphasia). He assumed that the right temporal lobe took over the functions of comprehension in ambidextrous patients. His third case of "conduction aphasia" spared the first temporal gyrus, and he concluded that the second temporal gyrus was critical for repetition of speech. The associated damage to the inferior parietal regions was explained by the common blood supply rather than by functional connections. Geschwind (1965) and Brown (1972) discussed the variable anatomical correlations. Benson et al. (1973) have recently reviewed the literature on autopsy-proven cases of conduction aphasia and have added three cases of their own. The two patients with severe apraxia had entirely suprasylvian lesions, involving the white matter deep to the parietal operculum; the nonpraxic subject had a lesion in the posterior third of the first temporal convolution, under Heschl's gyrus and the parietal operculum. They accepted

Kleist's idea of the right hemisphere assuming the function of comprehension in the latter patient. Although most of the cases involve the arcuate fasciculus, in one report it was shown to be spared (Howes and Green, 1972). Green and Howes (1977 studied 52 cases, 25 with neuroanatomical accounts from the literature. Thirteen cases involved the superior temporal and the supramarginal gyri. In 9 cases the temporal area was spared, and in 3 cases the supramarginal gyrus was spared. This indicated to the authors that the temporoparietal junction in the dominant hemisphere acts as a unit, necessary to carry on repetition, and that damage to either temporal or supramarginal gyri could produce similar disruption.

Transcortical Syndromes

"Transcortical motor aphasia" is a term that was coined by Wernicke, who used it to describe the same disturbance that Lichtheim called "central conduction aphasia." The features are mutism with good comprehension and repetition. The first anatomical confirmation of this speech disturbance found a small lesion of the white matter beneath the motor speech area (Rothmann, 1906). Goldstein (1917) discussed the mechanisms of transcortical aphasias. The motor variety may occur with damage to Broca's area or with more superior frontal lesions disrupting volitional impulses to the speech areas. Boetz and Barbeau (1971) reviewed lesions in the supplementary motor area causing speech disturbances with parasagittal tumors, ligation of the anterior cerebral artery, callosomarginal arteriovenous malformation, and frontal lobectomy. Difficulty initiating speech, decreased volume and amount of speech, and transient mutism were the main clinical features.

An "isolation syndrome" with pathological confirmation was published by Geschwind et al. (1968). This patient, who for ten years showed no spontaneous speech or comprehension, but could repeat complete sentences and learn new songs, had an intact speech area isolated from the rest of the brain by widespread, carbon monoxide induced necrosis. A case of mixed transcortical aphasia or isolation syndrome, with presenile dementia, was described in detail by Whitaker (1976). The pathological findings showed severe atrophy in the frontal and inferior temporal regions, with relative sparing of the perisylvian speech area.

Anomic Aphasia

Anomia or word-finding difficulty is the least specific but most universal linguistic feature of aphasia; anomic aphasia, where this is the only or predominant feature, has the least constant localization. Most modern workers agree that the evidence for a "naming center" in the inferior temporoparietal region, as proposed by Mills (1895), is insufficient. Tumors in the frontal, temporal, or parietal regions are equally liable to present with anomic aphasia (Kanzer,

1942). Anomic aphasia alone is less frequent in localizable (large) infarcts, but it is often seen after recovery from other syndromes, with lesions in the frontal or temporal speech areas. Botez and Barbeau (1971) stated that anomia associated with frontal lesions is qualitatively different from anomia in conjunction with posterior lesions of the dominant hemisphere. Suter (1953) reviewed the localization of cases with anomic aphasia and found 13 out of 20 cases to have localizable lesions in the left temporoparietal region. Nine of these were noted to be alexic and 12 had hemianopia. Three cases showed only diffuse lesions. Goldstein (1948) thought that anomic (amnesic) aphasia may indicate generalized damage, but that if it occurs as a localized lesion, it usually concerns the temporoparietal regions.

There has been a great vacuum in the modern literature of clinicopathological correlation of higher cortical functions. The reasons for this are multiple.

1. The rarity in obtaining an autopsy in those cases who were examined in detail.
2. The usual lack of clinical detail in autopsied material.
3. The variability and distance effects of tumor and trauma and the tendency of strokes to be multiple and to occur in aged, atrophied brains.
4. The skepticism, disinterest, lack of agreement, and technical difficulties in cytoarchitectonics and myeloarchitectonics, the variability of the surface anatomy of gyri, and the limited correlation of cytoarchitectonics and surface anatomy.
5. The unfavorable attitudes toward localization of higher nervous functions.

A handful of neurologists, linguists, neuropathologists, and psychologists are beginning to take up the slack. The process is bound to be slow because of the limitations imposed by the first two factors. Large stroke populations, examined in systematic detail and followed with improved methods of analyzing autopsy material, will provide significant new information. Technological improvements in cytoarchitectonics or physiology may improve functional–anatomical correlation.

POSTTRAUMATIC LOCALIZATION (SKULL DEFECTS)

A younger population, with circumscribed destruction of the brain without generalized atrophy and widespread vascular disease, was seen in both World Wars. Investigators on both sides of the conflict were able to examine a large number of cases. The limitations of this technique are well recognized.

1. The skull defect does not reflect the extent or the location of the injury in many cases.
2. The injury is often multiple or diffuse.

3. The interval between the initial injury and detailed examination is often too long in a rapidly recovering illness.

Marie and Foix (1917) distinguished anterior anarthric syndrome and posterior aphasic syndromes on the basis of skull defects. They further subdivided the anarthric group into: (1) nearly complete recovery, (2) isolated dysarthria, (3) some aphasia, (4) slow speech and ideation; and related these varieties to the depth, intensity, and site of the damage. They noted that the more posterior lesions were associated with more "aphasia." Despite Marie's earlier dictum, that there is only one "true" aphasia, they went on to distinguish (1) temporal aphasia, (2) supramarginal gyrus syndrome, (3) posterior angular gyrus aphasia with alexia, (4) minor aphasic syndromes with superficial lesions (no cases documented), and (5) global aphasia. It is interesting to see that his "anarthric zone" is located over the third frontal convolution and the foot of the ascending gyrus, and his "temporal zone" over Wernicke's area. The frontal pole, the first and anterior portion of the second convolution, were not involved in speech disturbance. His composite lateral pictures (Fig. 8-1) resemble our recent results with isotope localization (Fig. 9-20).

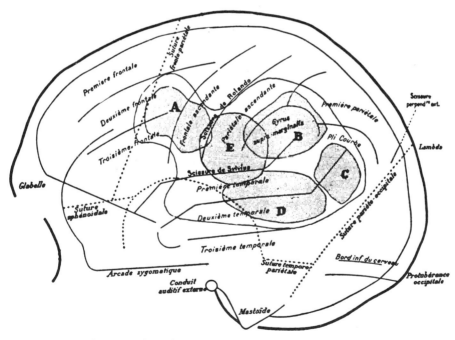

A map to show the location of the zones of Marie and Foix (1917).

Fig. 8-1.   The composite lateral view of Marie and Foix skull defect study. Note similarity to Fig. 9-20, the composite lateral of isotope scans.

Henry Head (1926), despite his well-known critique of the "diagram makers," carefully localized the lesions of 14 of 26 war injured aphasics, by using an elaborate method of reconstructing the wounds on casts of cadaver skulls. In two cases of verbal (motor) aphasia, the foot of the percentral gyrus and the inferior frontal convolution were involved. A case of "syntactical" aphasia, with fluent paraphasic speech, had an exit wound over the middle of the second temporal gyrus, with destruction of tissue above and below the superior temporal fissure. Two other cases of syntactical aphasia and jargon had lesions localized in the first temporal gyrus. Nominal aphasia, difficulty in naming objects, was localized to the left parietal lobe in two cases. Semantic aphasia, Head's novel category, which he does not define exactly, was also localized to the parietal lobe. One case with alexia, agraphia, acalculia, and constructional apraxia (paraphrasing his lengthy description of the patient) had a supramarginal lesion. It is difficult to be certain just what kind of language disturbance these patients had on the basis of descriptions such as: "inability to formulate, to recognize and to retain in his mind the exact general intention of some action requiring symbolic representation." Two other patients with a left and another with a right supramarginal gyrus lesion were considered to have Semantic aphasia.

Schiller (1947) studied 46 cases of penetrating missile wounds with a battery of tests, including examinations of spontaneous speech, comprehension, naming, word fluency, a vocabulary test of reading, writing, spelling, copying of block designs, and Raven's matrices, scoring $0-5$. The drawings of the bone defects were overlapped for each major symptom.

1. Disturbances of articulation, inflection, and speed of language were associated with wounds over the foot of the precentral, third frontal convolution.
2. Paraphasias were found with frontal and posterior sylvian lesions.
3. Disturbance of syntax and telegrammatic speech with frontotemporal wounds.
4. Perseveration and stammer with parietal lobe damage.
5. Disturbance of auditory comprehension with smaller lesions in the temporoparietal regions and with larger lesions over the whole speech area.
6. Reading problems with temporoparietal lesions (some frontally).
7. Spelling defect with parietal lobe.
8. Constructional apraxia with parietal lobe damage.

Word-finding difficulty was considered the least valuable for localization. The bulk of the brain destroyed was proportional to the severity of the disorder. Conrad (1954) had 216 aphasics with war wounds. He found that pure motor aphasia is related to perirolandic lesions. Lesions involving F3 were compatible with recovery. Persisting motor disturbance corresponded to a larger area around the rolandic and sylvian fissures. He thought that not the selective destruction of the base of F3, but the quantity and size of the destroyed substratum of the brain, if the lesion involves the motor region, decides whether or not an irreversible motor aphasia will result. Sensory aphasia is associated with lesions of T_1 and the parietal region. The lesions are dispersed widely in amnestic aphasia.

Alajouanine et al. (1957) correlated anterior suprasylvian lesions with articulatory disturbances, "phonetic disintegration," parietorolandic, and anterior temporal lesions with persistent "agrammatisms" and Broca's aphasia, and posterior temporal lesions with jargon aphasia. Alexia was associated with posterior supraslyvian lesions. Luria (1974) also localized war injuries causing aphasia. The syndrome of "efferent motor aphasia" was the result of lesions around Broca's area. "Afferent motor aphasia" was associated with inferior parietal lesions. "Linguistic−acoustic impairment" was usually seen with temporal lesions. "Semantic aphasia," a disturbance of complex simultaneous synthesis, was associated with parietotemporal lesions.

Russell and Espir (1961) studied 280 cases of traumatic aphasia and charted the skull defects from the radiographs. The defects that were associated with aphasia centered over the "lower half of the left precentral and postcentral gyrus, the supramarginal and angular gyrus, the inferior parietal gyrus, and a large part of the temporal bone." They charted the lesions in central aphasia ($N = 11$), where all language functions were impaired. Most lesions were posterior temporal and inferior parietal. Motor aphasia ($N = 13$) was associated with lesions in the foot of the Rolandic area. They found four cases with outstanding agraphia, associated with parasagittal parietal entry wounds, and three cases with alexia at the region of the angular gyrus.

SURGICAL EXCISIONS

Surgeons, from time to time, are forced to excise diseased brain from what is considered the speech area. Excision of epileptic foci removes previously malfunctioning cortex and healthy tissue adjacent to a scar. Excision of tumors is less satisfactory because of the distortion and shift of structures; the identification of gyri is often difficult. Tumors often infiltrate grossly normal tissue microscopically. Edema and increased intracranial pressure, along with vascular changes, create distance effects which interfere with function well beyond the actual tumor. The extent of excision and the precision of localization are variable. Burckhardt (1891) removed part of Broca's area, and in another case, the posterior parts of T_1 and T_2, without permanent aphasia. Walter Dandy (1931), after presenting three cases said, "Auditory speech is located in the parietal lobe, (after a temporary lobectomy), visual speech is distinct and separate from auditory speech (an occipital lobectomy involving supramarginal and angular gyrus) and Broca's area is essentially the area described by Broca, except that it is a little more posterior." Schwab (1927) with Foerster found that 14 out of 21 patients with parasagittal excisions developed transient transcortical aphasia.

Mettler (1949) claimed that bilateral removal of Broca's area does not produce aphasia, but the area was not identified by stimulation or autopsy. Jefferson (1950) also reported removal of Broca's area without aphasia, but did not give the means of identification. Zangwill (1975) presented a case of removal and another of undercutting of Broca's areas for tumors with rapid recovery.

Penfield and Roberts (1959) described aphasia after operation on the left hemisphere 144 times in 246 operations (58 percent). Limited excision of any part of the hemisphere was found to be compatible with recovery. One hematoma, removed from Broca's area, did not cause permanent aphasia. Persisting defects were associated with large lesions in previously damaged areas. The importance of speech areas was ranked as: (1) parietotemporal, (2) inferior frontal, (3) supplementary motor. The types of aphasias were not described consistently, but comprehension deficits were related to superior temporal and parietal, and motor aphasia to frontal lobe excisions.

Hecaen and Angelergues (1964), in a study of 214 cases of mostly tumor and trauma, considered the localization of various symptoms rather than types of aphasia. Disorders of fluency and articulation were associated foremost with Rolandic lesions, while comprehension and naming disturbances were associated with temporal ones.

HEMISPHERECTOMIES AND CALLOSAL SECTIONS

Total or subtotal dominant hemispherectomies in the adult are infrequently performed, usually for glioma (Zollinger, 1935; Crockett and Estridge, 1951; French et al., 1955; Smith, 1966). One is struck by the similarity of the disorder in the movies of the patients with dominant hemispherectomy, presented by A. Smith, to cases of global aphasia due to large left hemisphere strokes. More recovery of repetition and recitation was reported in a recent case of Burklund and Smith (1977). All the infrequently performed adult hemispherectomies were for gliomas and were aphasic before. The gradual increase in lesion size could contribute to the transfer of some of the functions by the right hemisphere. Early brain damage in infantile hemiplegia results in more or less complete takeover of language by the right hemisphere. Hermispherectomy in a child up to puberty will not result in aphasia (Basser, 1962).

The isolated right hemisphere has significant auditory and visual comprehension, which seems to be more than that after dominant hemispherectomy, according to studies of corpus callosum sectioned patients by Sperry et al. (1969) and Gazzaniga (1970). On the basis of one left hemispherectomy and two commissurotomies, Zaidel (1976) estimated the vocabulary of the right hemisphere to be at or above the level of a ten-year-old child. Kinsbourne (1971) produced no further deficit with Na Amytal (Wada test) in the damaged left hemisphere of aphasics, but noted speech arrest in the undamaged right hemisphere, indicating that dominance for residual language had shifted to the right.

CORTICAL STIMULATION

Jefferson (1935) reported speech arrest during and after stimulation of the angular gyrus, and Foerster (1936) noted vocalization on stimulation of the lower Rolandic region. Penfield and his associates have stimulated the cerebral cortex systematically and the results pertaining to speech are summarized in a monograph (Penfield and Roberts, 1959). They obtained composite maps of the responses to stimulation from 94 patients on the left and 20 on the right side. Electric current applied to Broca's area, the posterior parietotemporal area, and the supplementary motor area, produced arrest, hesitation, slurring, repetition and distortion of speech, confusion of numbers, inability to name, misnaming with or without perseveration, and difficulty in reading and writing. Aphasic speech arrest was produced only in the dominant hemisphere. In addition to the negative effects of stimulation, vocalization (but not formed speech) was also obtained from the rolandic and supplementary motor areas of either hemisphere. Whitaker and Ojemann (1977), in stimulation studies, have found that an individual's language zone occupies a large extent of the lateral cortex, including the parietal operculum and midfrontal and midparietal lobes. There seemed to be a marked degree of individual variation, and adjacent sites responded to stimulation quite variably. The posterior inferior frontal cortex in front of the precentral gyrus (Broca's area) was the only zone producing naming errors invariably (Ojemann and Whitaker, 1978).

THALAMIC LESIONS AND STIMULATION

Although the thalamus has not been considered an indispensable part of the language mechanism of the nervous system, Smyth and Stern (1938) reported speech disturbance with tumors of the medial and anterior, but not the ventral, nuclear group of the thalamus. Only two cases of the 24 thalamic tumors reported by McKissock and Paine (1958) had aphasia. Thalamic hemorrhage was reviewed by Fisher (1959) with few instances of aphasia. Isolated thalamic hemorrhage caused poor comprehension, paraphasic, fluent speech, but good repetition in the case of Bugiani (1969). Ciemins (1970) reported a case with reduced spontaneous speech, perserveration, impaired comprehension, but good repetition, and another one with mild aphasia. Mohr (1975) emphasized good repetition, associated with a dichotomous state of logorrheic jargon, alternating with unresponsiveness in two cases of thalamic hemorrhage, which were localized on computerized tomography. He reviewed other autopsied cases one, involving the posterior thalamic nuclei, had jargon speech; another, with only anterior involvement, had no aphasia.

Aphasia can be a complication of left ventrolateral thalamotomy, although it is usually transient. Aphasia was noted in 42 percent of operations in one series (Selby, 1967). The speech becomes hesitant but repetition is not impaired.

Dysarthria and confusion are common features and interfere with language testing. Bell (1968) considered the deficit to be similar to aphasias of frontal regions. Four of his nine aphasic cases, after thalamotomy, were persistent. An example of a ventrolateral thalamic lesion producing mild anomia was shown by Ojemann (1976). The severity of language deficit seemed to be related to the degree of degeneration in the pulvinar in lesions of the temporal and parietal lobes, according to Van Buren and Borke (1969).

In contrast to the effects of cortical stimulation, which never produces words or sentences, compulsory vocalization or "speech-like utterance" was evoked on stimulating the dominant thalamus in six of 14 patients, and the nondominant side in two of 14 patients, by Schaltenbrand (1965). Object naming is impaired when the dominant anterior superior pulvinar and ventrolateral nucleus of the thalamus is stimulated (Ojemann et al., 1968). Penfield and Roberts (1959) hypothesized that the thalamus is an integrating center between the frontal and temporoparietal speech areas.

ARTERIOGRAPHIC AND CEREBRAL BLOOD FLOW STUDIES

Kohlmeyer (1969) correlated 76 angiographically proven obstructive vessel disease cases with their neuropsychological symptoms. Orbitofrontal and Rolandic artery occlusion produced pure motor aphasia. The syndrome of orbitofrontal to the parietal artery occlusion in the left hemisphere produced global aphasia in one, pure motor aphasia in one, and predominantly motor aphasia in five. The posterior parietal and posterior temporal artery syndrome produced pure sensory aphasia in nine, global aphasia in two, mainly sensory aphasia in one, "repetition aphasia" in five, and amnestic aphasia in nine. The anterior and posterior parietal artery syndrome had 12 cases of "repetition aphasia," 11 with amnestic aphasia, and two with global aphasia. The posterior temporal artery occlusion produced pure sensory aphasia in all five cases. These patients were all paraphasic as well. An angiographic study of tumors showed that posterior lesions were fluent and anterior ones were nonfluent (Rosenfield and Goree, 1975).

Ingvar and Schwartz (1974) investigated regional cerebral blood flow (rCBF) in the left hemisphere in psychiatric patients during speech, reading, and contralateral arm movements. The typical rCBF resting pattern, with precentral high flows and postcentral low flows, changed to high flows in the premotor Rolandic and the anterior and midsylvian regions during speech. During reading, an increase in flow in the postcentral parts of the hemisphere was noted. During abstract thinking and problem solving, the rCBF showed activation of frontal and postcentral areas. Carmon et al. (1975) showed increased left hemispheric flow, especially in the frontal, anterior temporal, midtemporal, and posterior frontal regions, during a verbal memory task. Larsen et al. (1977) found increased rCBF in the premotor, upper frontal, lower Rolandic, and temporal cortical areas during speech, and in the posterior temporal and frontal regions while listening. Learning and recalling word pair associates activated the parietal and occipital regions, but only learning activated the prefrontal regions in a study by Maximilian et al. (1978). Automatic speech seemed to activate the whole right hemisphere (Larsen et al. 1978).

Kohlmeyer (1975) studied rCBF in different types of aphasia, which seemed to increase in the regions around the lesions. Maly et al. (1977) found rCBF decreased beyond the speech region in aphasics. Four out of six motor aphasics had Broca's area, and sensory aphasics had the posterior speech cortex involved. Three of five amnesic patients had Broca's area, and in the others the parietal lobe was involved. Soh et al. (1978) claimed that Broca's area was not consistently affected in their nonfluent aphasics ($N = 10$). However, one gains the opposite impression on looking at their sketches. In fact, their "sensory," "motor," and "global" overlap areas of dysfunction were very similar to ours (Kertesz et al., 1977). They emphasized the activation of the inferior Rolandic area bilaterally during speech. One of their tumor cases, in Wernicke's area, showed increased flow at rest, but during speech, the frontal and parietal regions "stole" from this region.

ELECTROENCEPHALOGRAPHY AND EVOKED POTENTIALS

The recording of electrical potentials generated by intact or diseased brain is a noninvasive method of localization. Electroencephalograms (EEG) have been used to localize cerebral lesions for nearly 50 years. Reports of EEG localization in aphasia are few (Marinesco et al., 1936; Tikofsky et al., 1960), possibly because of the low specificity. Alpha rhythm suppression in the dominant hemisphere during verbal tasks and in the nondominant side during spatial tasks was noted (Galin and Ornstein, 1972). The technique of cortical coupling, developed by Callaway and Harris (1974), attempts to assess intercortical functional communication through measuring the degree of correlation between pairs of electrodes.

Average evoked potentials (EPs) is a more recent method to study cerebral functional states and events made possible by the introduction of signal averaging computers. EPs have been studied in relation to verbal and nonverbal stimuli (Buchsbaum and Fedio, 1970), stop—consonant versus frequency of phonemes (Wood et al., 1971), speech stimuli (McAdam and Whitaker, 1971; Morrell and Salamy, 1971; Morrell and Huntington, 1971), meaningfulness of stimuli (Matsumiya et al., 1972), words versus nonsense syllables (Shelburne, 1972), and contextual meaning (Brown et al., 1973; Teyler et al., 1973). Most of these studies have sought hemispheric asymmetries. The rationale for this work is that finding EP effects to "linguistic" stimuli localized to the left hemisphere would provide evidence that the EP effects are associated with linguistic processing. Certain components of EPs with long latency (more than 300 msec) are sensitive to task relevance and expectancy. This component, called P300, is more endogenous, as it is not dependent as much on stimulus characteristics. The amplitude of the contingent negative variation (CNV), a potential preceding movement or cognition, has been found to be correlated with hemispheric dominance, as determined by the intracarotid amytal test (Low et al., 1973).

A number of artifacts from head, lip, tongue movements, respiration, muscle tension, and galvanic skin response, can influence asymmetrically speech related electrical potentials. Szirtes and Vaughan (1973) concluded that the cortical potentials associated with muscle innervation, and possibly with reauditorization of speech sounds, overshadow neural activity (related to speech production) in the dominant hemisphere.

AN AUTOPSIED CASE OF BROCA'S APHASIA

This case is presented as an example of clinicopathological correlation in Broca's aphasia. The complexity of the case is by no means unusual. It illustrates the fact that each case has typical, as well as atypical, clinical and pathological features. It is meant to caution against the acceptance of less than adequately presented case material or unwarranted conclusions from it at face value.

Table 8–1
WAB Scores of Patient 0—Onset February, 1969

Subtests	Maximum	June 1969	October 1969	April 1970
Information	/10	2.0	2.0	4.0
Fluency	/10	4.0	4.0	4.0
Comprehension	/10	7.4	8.1	8.1
Repetition	/10	7.8	7.9	8.0
Naming	/10	3.3	5.6	6.1
AQ	/100	49.0	55.2	60.4
Reading	/10	3.0	2.8	4.9
Writing	/10	2.7	3.1	3.7
Praxis	/10	5.3	—	—
Calculation	/24	22.0	16.0	14.0
Raven's	/36	1.0	—	—
Drawing	/30	11.0	16.0	15.0
Blocks	/9	8.0	9.0	9.0

Case description — Patient O, a 49-year-old man, was first examined with the WAB four months after his stroke due to a left carotid occlusion and was followed until his death 21 months later. Initially, his spontaneous speech was limited to single words and short automatic sentences. Auditory comprehension was somewhat impaired, especially for the complex commands. His ability to repeat single words and phrases was good, but he made phonemic, paraphasic errors on the more complex (*buks* for *buts*) sentences. His automatic speech and recitation were good, but his speech showed altered prosody and slurring. He was able to name only half of the objects presented. He was alexic and agraphic, being unable to write more than his name and single letters. He could copy fairly well. He had difficulty with the constructional tasks (i.e., drawing, block design). His score on the *R*CPM was only 1/36. His scores placed him in Broca's category (see Table 4-2). He received speech therapy and physiotherapy. Although he remained nonfluent, his repetition and reading scores improved. This placed him in the transcortical motor category. His paraphasic dysfluency was exemplified by this sentence, repeated 14 months after his stroke: "The bread brown flox led or the brave log docks" ("The quick brown fox jumped over the lazy dog").

Pathology. Courtesy of Dr. J. Gilbert. (Figs. 8-2−8-4):

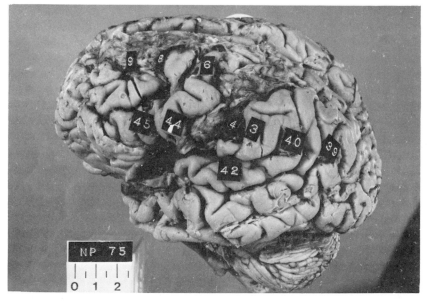

Fig. 8-2. The lateral view of O's brain. Note lesions over left parasagittal (8, 9), and rolandic areas (4). Broca's area (44) is replaced by a cavity.

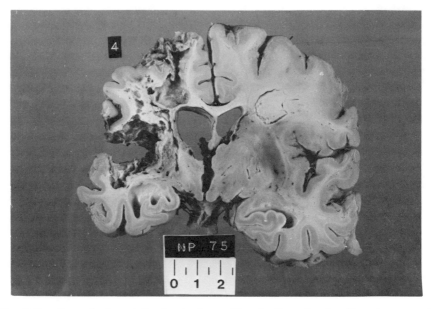

Fig. 8-3. Coronal view at the level of mamillary bodies, showing Broca's area and anterior temporal lobe involvement.

The brain shows a large old cystic infarct involving the anterior portions of brain supplied by the left middle cerebral artery. The lesion involves inferior frontal cortex, precentral gyrus (Brodman 4), supplementary motor areas 6, 8, 9, and anterior portions of the superior temporal gyrus. The cavitation affects the centrum semiovale, adjacent putamen, external capsule, claustrum, and insular cortex. The cortex of areas 44 and 45 are partially preserved. The "U" fibers are partially spared but the tissue is isolated as all the underlying white matter is destroyed. The infarct spares the parietal cortex (3), the posterior superior temporal gyrus (42), the angular gyrus (39), and the supramarginal gyrus (40). The left carotid artery showed atherosclerosis and occlusion which extended into the proximal portion of the middle cerebral artery.

Comment. This patient had persistent Broca's aphasia, yet he was atypical in his high repetition scores. These earned him the label of transcortical motor aphasia eventually when, in fact, he was not very much different clinically from the initial examination. He continued to have a significant nonfluent, agrammatic aphasia, with good comprehension, clearly conforming to most clinicians concept of a moderately severe Broca's aphasia until his death. The pathology shows multiple involvement of the left frontal lobe, allowing us only to speculate what role the supplementary speech area infarct played in his persisting neurological and speech deficit. It is possible that if only Broca's area or the supplementary area alone were involved, more rapid and dramatic recovery would have taken place. One can also conclude that persisting Broca's aphasia can result from frontal lobe infarc-

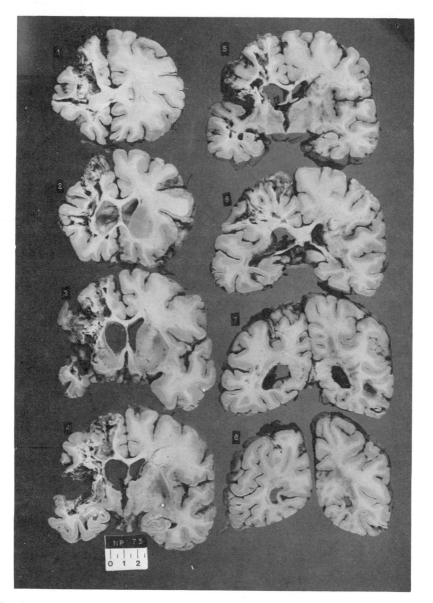

Fig. 8-4. Coronal section of the whole brain from the frontal (1) to the occipital (8) region. Note sparing of Wernicke's area on sections 5, 6, and 7.

tion only, which undercuts and partially involves Broca's area, and that the lesion of the inferior parietal region which is so often involved in the "superior division middle cerebral artery syndrome" is not necessary to produce Broca's aphasia.

SUMMARY

The evidence from autopsy material, stimulation studies, surgical excisions, cerebral blood flow, arteriograms, and electroencephalograms is reviewed and the reasons for the controversies of localization are discussed. The lack of standardization of clinical description and the limitations of available anatomical methods continue to thwart precise correlation. However, certain principles clearly emerge.

1. Only lesions causing impairment are localizable, not the impairment itself. This does not, however, justify the nihilism about the value of localization.
2. Structure and function are related, but the complexity of their variables in the brain tends to obscure the relationship.
3. The time of examination in relation to the time of anatomical confirmation, and the extent of recovery, are major variables which have not been uniformly considered in the past.
4. The lesions causing persistent global aphasia involve the whole perisylvian area.
5. Some degree of comprehension recovers, even in lesions amounting to dominant hemispherectomies, clearly mediated by the right hemisphere.
6. Lesions restricted to Broca's area (F3) often cause only mild or transient motor aphasia.
7. Persistent Broca's aphasia (severe, nonfluent aphasia with relatively good comprehension) is more often caused by larger lesions involving Broca's area (F3), the inferior Rolandic area, and a variable amount of the anterior parietal and temporal operculum, but spare the posterior Sylvian region.
8. Wernicke's aphasia, sensory aphasia (fluent, paraphasic speech with poor comprehension), is a changing and variable clinical picture, but large inferior and posterior Sylvian regions are involved in the persisting variety.
9. The lesions causing conduction aphasia are similar but smaller, and at times, more anterior and superior to those of Wernicke's aphasia. The role of the arcuate fasciculus is controversial but it is usually involved.
10. Transcortical motor aphasia is correlated with lesions either in the supplementary motor or near Broca's area; and isolation syndrome with lesions surrounding the speech area.

A personal clinicopathological correlation of a Broca's aphasia is also described.

9

Isotope Localization of Lesions in Aphasia

1. Brain scanning and aphasia
2. Isotope localization of infarcts
3. The overlap of areas producing aphasia
4. Lesion size and severity
5. Discussion
6. Correlation with CT scans
   Summary

The necessarily ill-defined parts of the speech region which border on receptive and motor cortical fields, have acquired the significance of speech centres from the point of view of morbid anatomy but not in respect of normal function; their lesions cut off one of the elements of speech association from its connexions with the others.

Sigmund Freud (1891)

BRAIN SCANNING AND APHASIA

Radionucleide scanning enabled us for the first time to outline cerebral lesions with a certain amount of precision in aphasic patients whose language was tested at the same time. Its value for tumors has been established, often giving clear-cut three-dimensional information. Benson and Patten (1967) correlated clinical prediction of the location of lesion with the scans of 27 aphasic patients (20 were vascular cases). Satisfactory agreement was obtained in 20 patients. In another study, by Benson (1967), localization of lesions in fluent and nonfluent aphasics demonstrated a clear anterior—posterior dichotomy. We reported our preliminary observations of localization of lesions in aphasia in 65 patients. (Kertesz et al., 1973). Sixty-three had isotope scans. Global aphasics had large lesions. Nine of 11 Broca's aphasics had frontal lesions and 12 of 14

143

Wernicke's aphasics had temporal lesions. Five of the ten anomic patients had tumor in the parietal lobe. Karis and Horenstein (1976) correlated speech parameters with scans in 18 stroke patients. Seven patients had decreased fluency and comprehension and the center of their lesions was posterior to the central gyrus. One patient with low fluency and high comprehension had a frontal lesion, and another with high fluency and low comprehension a "perislyvian" lesion. The syndrome of transcortical motor aphasia was locaized to two areas of the brain using isotope scans (Rubens 1976). Both anterior and cerebral territory infarct involving the supplementary motor area and Broca's area infarct could produce nonfluent speech with good repetition and comprehension. We have also seen examples of both localizations. Heilman and Valenstein (1972) used isotopes to localize lesions producing auditory, visual, and somesthetic neglect associated with hemiparesis, abnormal cortical sensation, and spatial disorientation in nine patients to the right inferior parietal lobe, and in one patient to the left frontal lobe. Verhas (1975) found a greater frequency of abnormal scans in the left hemisphere. Among those with aphasia, 87% had positive uptake and those without aphasia, only 50%. Angiograms, isotope, and CT scans were correlated with aphasic impairment in 14 patients with strokes by Yarnell et al. (1976). Fluent aphasics had posterior−parietal lesions.

ISOTOPE LOCALIZATION OF INFARCTS

We undertook to localize infarcts on the basis of radionucleide brain scans to determine the anatomical areas corresponding to various types of aphasia (Kertesz et al., 1977). We selected only the patients with a single infarct who had a positive scan within one month of being tested on the WAB, the test given within one month after the stroke. Sixty-five patients fulfilled these strict criteria. Some of these patients were observed with subsequent tests, and the evolution of their language deficit is commented on (see Chapter 15).

The rectilinear isotope scans with technetium Tc 99^m were found to be the most reliable method of localization. For the sake of objectivity, the lesions were traced on the films by a radiologist who did not know the patients and was not aware of their symptomatology. A transparent template of the left lateral surface of the brain was drawn in the manner presented in Sobotta's atlas, this was fitted on the scan, and the lesions were retracted onto these templates. For the anterior and posterior scans, the focal planes of the radioactivity collimator were determined perpendicular to the 15° above horizontal elevation of the tubes in the orbitomeatal line, and the templates were traced from a normal brain, cut coronally according to the slant of these focal planes (Fig. 9-1). Although the lateral scans were useful to determine the anterior−posterior extent of these lesions, the coronal scans provided a measure of their depth. The anterior plane connected

THE FOCAL PLANE OF A.P. SCANS

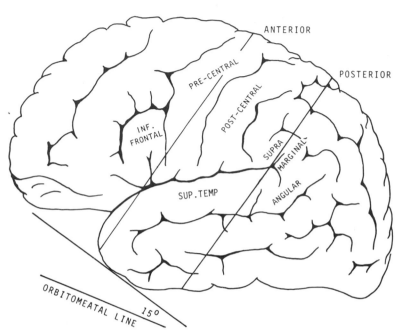

Fig. 9-1. Coronal cuts for anterior and posterior templates in focal planes of scans. (Reprinted from Arch Neurol 34:590−601, 1977. Copyright 1977, American Medical Association.)

the tip of the temporal lobe with the superior aspect of the precentral convolution, cutting across Broca's area (the posterior inferior third frontal convolution) and the posterior plane 4 cm behind the anterior template, which was cut across the posterior superior first temporal convolution (Wernicke's area) and the supramarginal gyrus.

Table 9-1 shows the number of aphasics, mean age, onset−test interval, test−scan interval, and the measure of severity (AQ) in each group. We divided aphasics into groups according to taxonomic criteria (see Table 4-2). Standard deviations and F ratios were calculated for the population. Analysis of variance shows that they are matched for age and test−scan and onset−test interval, but the groups differ significantly in their severity of aphasia.

The tracings of individual cases are presented in each group in the lateral and coronal (AP) views. The individual traces were overlapped on the lateral and coronal templates, and the overlap area for each group was selected on the basis of maximum density by the medical illustrator, who had no knowledge of the patients or the anatomic areas.

Table 9–1

Age, Scan–Test, and Onset–Test Interval, and Aphasia Quotient

Type of Aphasia	Age, year*		Scan–Test*		Onset–Test*		Aphasia Quotient‡	
	X	SD	X	SD	X	SD	X	SD
Global (N=12)	64.6	11.2	7.9	6.9	15.4	7.1	5.9	5.8
Broca's (N=14)	55.1	14.9	4.4	3.7	11.5	6.1	31.9	18.4
Wernicke's (N=13)	65.5	14.6	9.5	7.4	14.7	10.7	34.0	11.2
Conduction (N=11)	64.5	7.7	8.5	9.8	12.0	8.3	57.0	13.7
Anomic (N=7)	65.7	16.5	2.3	2.4	9.4	6.4	88.8	6.5

*F is not significant ($P \geqslant 0.01$).

‡F is significant ($P \leqslant 0.01$, df = 52.4).

(Reprinted from Arch Neurol 34:590−601, 1977. Copyright 1977, American Medical Association.)

Global Aphasics

This group ($N = 12$) had large scan uptakes, some involving most of the left hemisphere (Figs. 9-2−9-4). All cases without exception involved the inferior frontal and superior temporal convolution and the Sylvian fissure between them. The relatively limited, more anterior lesion occurred in a patient (case 5) who had the best comprehension (almost a Broca's aphasic). The coronal tracings similarly showed extensive lesions, practically all involving the basal ganglia as well as large areas of cortex and subcortical matter (Fig. 9-3). The large number of localizable global aphasics is not surprising, since the large infarcts producing these lesions will invariably produce an uptake.

Broca's Aphasics

These patients ($N = 14$) have a smaller and more anteriorly located lesion when compared with global aphasics (Figs. 9-5−9-7). Broca's aphasia is rather uniform in its clinical manifestation, with low fluency associated with relatively well-preserved comprehension. The common area is the third forntal convolution and this area is involved in all patients, except in one (case 25), where the uptake only touches the gyrus. In case 20, where the first temporal convolution is involved, the patient had relatively low comprehension scores and could be considered globally aphasic by some clinicians. His uptake was more like the smaller lesions in the global group. This is in a borderline area between the Broca's and global groups.

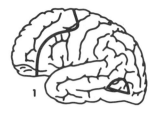
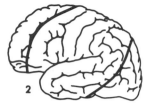
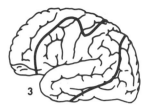

GLOBAL APHASIA

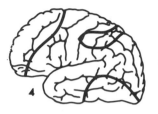
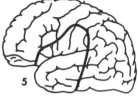
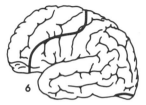

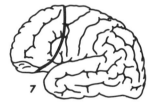
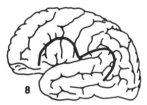
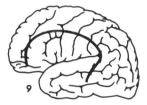

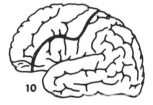
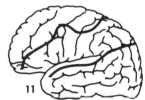
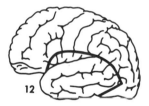

Fig. 9-2. Individual lesions of Global aphasics on lateral templates. (Reprinted from Arch Neurol 34:590–601, 1977. Copyright 1977, American Medical Association.)

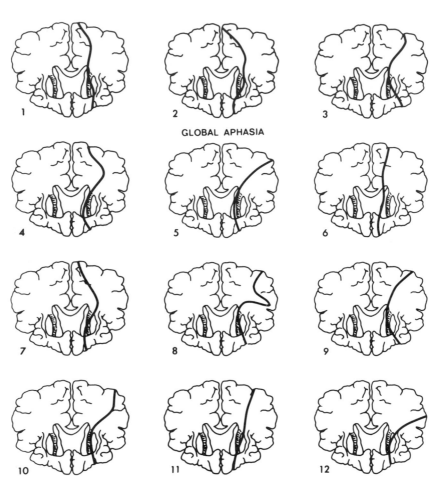

GLOBAL APHASIA

Fig. 9-3. Global aphasics. Anterior template. (Reprinted from Arch Neurol 35:590−601, 1977. Copyright 1977, American Medical Association.)

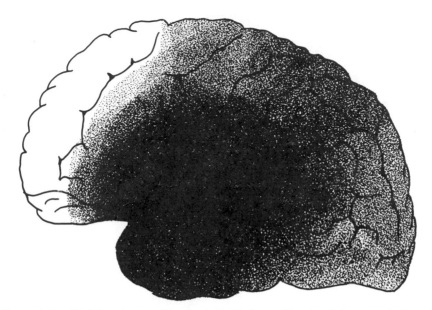

Figure 9-4.   Global aphasics. Composite of lesions. (Reprinted from Arch Neurol 34:590−601, 1977. Copyright 1977, American Medical Association.)

Conduction Aphasics

This group ($N = 11$) appeared to have lesions primarily between Broca's and Wernicke's areas, although some appeared right over these areas as well (Figs. 9-8−9-10). The common area appeared to be the superior lip of the sylvian fissure consisting of the inferior ends of the precentral, postcentral, inferior parietal, and supramarginal gyri. Some of these lesions were relatively small but quite deep, involving much of the insular tissue and connecting white matter between the frontal and temporal lobes. The less fluent patients (cases 47, 48, 49, and 50) in this group had more anterior lesions. Those with higher fluency scores (cases 40, 42, and 43) had uptakes situated more posteriorly. The most extensive lesions in this group occurred in the right hemispheres of two right-handed patients (cases 49 and 50). Bilateral speech representation may account for their relatively moderate aphasia. They are also examples of the rare "crossed" aphasia.

Wernicke's Aphasics

These patients ($N = 13$) have lesions involving the postrolandic areas (Figs. 9-11−9-13) Some are mostly parietal, others mostly temporal, but all involve the posterior third of the superior temporal gyrus to some extent. The patient

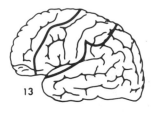
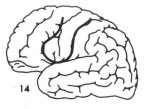
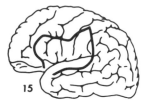

BROCA'S APHASIA

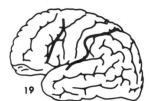
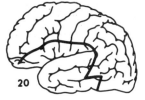
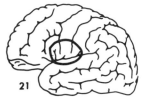

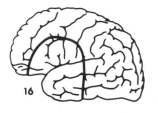
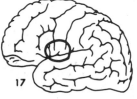
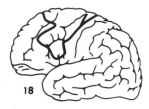

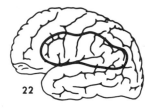
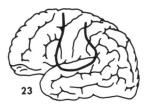
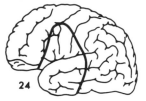

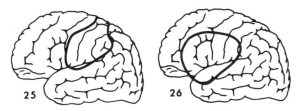

Fig. 9-5. Broca's aphasics. Lateral template. (Reprinted from Arch Neurol 34:590−601, 1977. Copyright 1977, American Medical Association.)

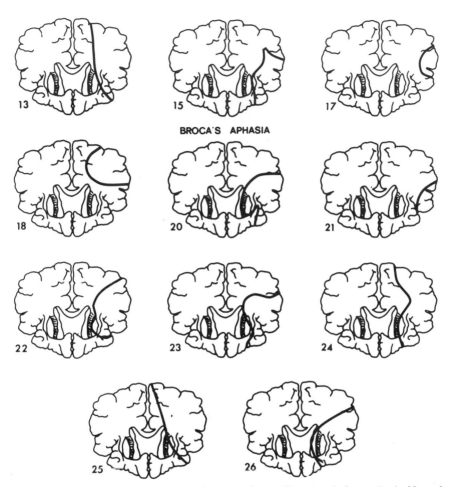

BROCA'S APHASIA

Fig. 9-6. Broca's aphasics. Anterior template. (Reprinted from Arch Neurol 34:590–601, 1977. Copyright 1977, American Medical Association.)

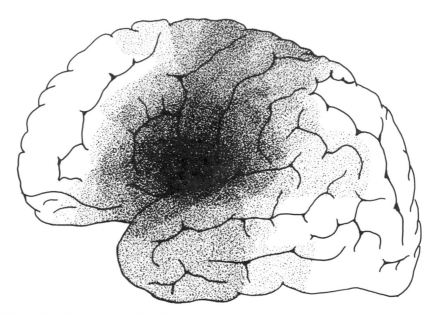

Fig. 9-7. Broca's aphasics. Composite of lesions. (Reprinted from Arch Neurol 34:590−601, 1977. Copyright 1977, American Medical Association.)

whose temporo-occipital lesion was only in the lower part of the superior temporal gyrus (case 36) had the highest comprehension and repetition scores of the Wernicke's group and, as such, represents a transitional stage between this group and anomic aphasia. The recovery pattern of Wernicke's aphasia is towards anomic aphasia in most cases and the extent of recovery seems to depend on the size of the lesion.

Anomic Aphasics

Anomic aphasia ($N = 7$) is notoriously difficult to localize in stroke patients in contrast to tumors (Figs. 9-14−9-16). Anomic patients are less disabled than others and less likely to have a large uptake on the scan after a stroke; the more stable patients with localizable lesions had posterior parietal and temporal lesions that tended to spare the superior temporal gyrus but not invariably. Broca's area was involved in one patient with transient anomia. We collected language data on a large number of anomics, but the majority of them recovered without localizing information. Often, anomic aphasia is the end-stage for various posterior or sensory aphasics, but it also appears *de novo* after mild strokes and often in tumors with larger lesions. Anomia as a linguistic phenomenon is common to almost all aphasics and therefore has little, if any, anatomical specificity.

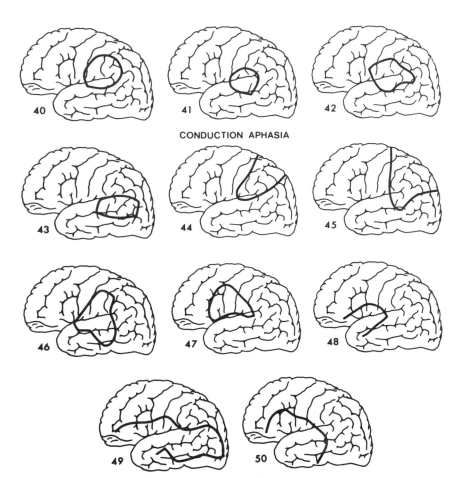

CONDUCTION APHASIA

Fig. 9-8. Conduction aphasics. Lateral template. (Reprinted from Arch Neurol 34:590–601, 1977. Copyright 1977, American Medical Association.)

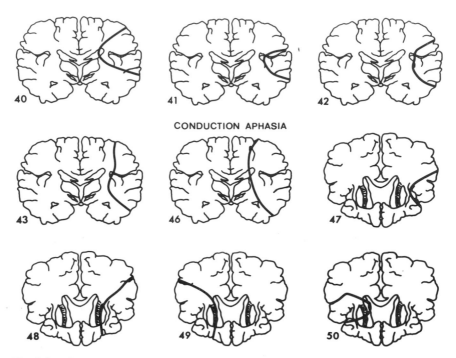

CONDUCTION APHASIA

Fig. 9-9. Conduction aphasics. Posterior template. Cases 47, 48, 49, and 50 are anterior templates. (Reprinted from Arch Neurol 34:590–601, 1977. Copyright 1977, American Medical Association.)

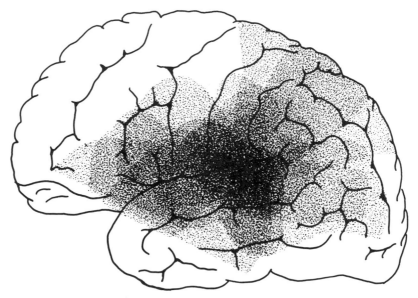

Fig. 9-10. Conduction aphasics. Composite of lesions. (Reprinted from Arch Neurol 34:590–601, 1977. Copyright 1977, American Medical Association.)

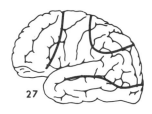 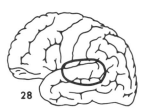 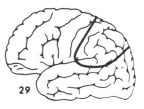

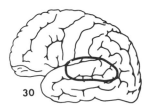 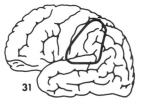 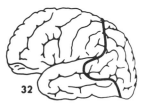

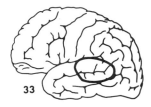 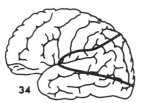 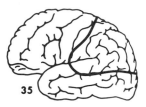

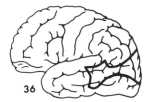 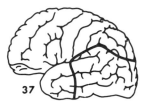 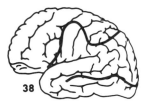

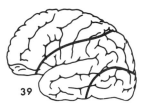

Fig. 9-11. Wernicke's aphasics. Lateral template. (Reprinted from Arch Neurol 34:590–601, 1977. Copyright 1977, American Medical Association.)

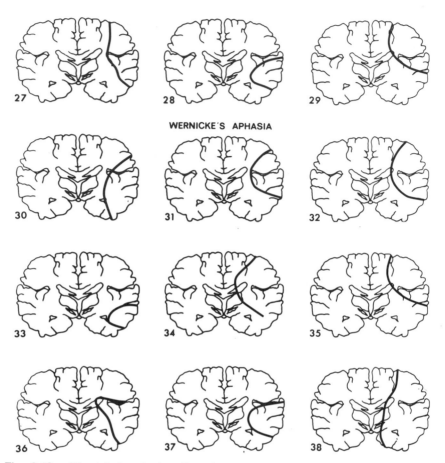

Fig. 9-12. Wernicke's aphasics. Posterior template. Cases 61, 63, 65 are anterior templates. (Reprinted from Arch Neurol 34:590–601, 1977. Copyright 1977, American Medical Association.)

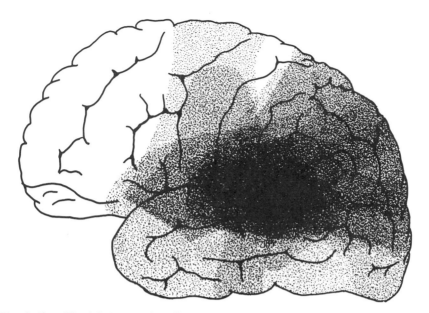

Fig. 9-13. Wernicke's aphasics. Composite of lesions. (Reprinted from Arch Neurol 34:590−601, 1977. Copyright 1977. American Medical Association.)

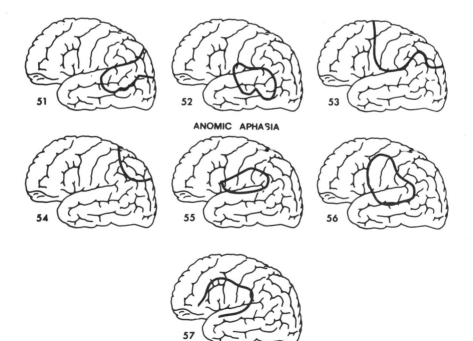

ANOMIC APHASIA

Fig. 9-14. Anomic aphasics. Lateral template. (Reprinted from Arch Neurol 34:590−601, 1977. Copyright 1977, American Medical Association.)

157

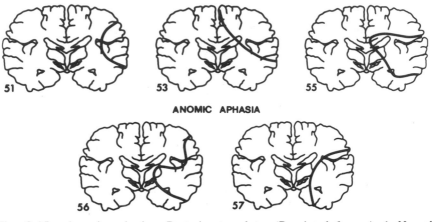

Fig. 9-15. Anomic aphasics. Posterior template. (Reprinted from Arch Neurol 34:590–601, 1977. Copyright 1977, American Medical Association.)

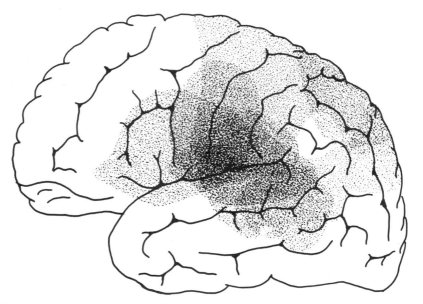

Fig. 9-16. Anomic aphasics. Composite of lesions. (Reprinted from Arch Neurol 34:590–601, 1977. Copyright 1977, American Medical Association.)

Transcortical Sensory Aphasics

Transcortical sensory aphasics ($N = 3$) characterized by fluent speech and comprehension difficulty but good repetition appear to have posterior parietal lesions (Figs. 9-17−9-19). Cases 58, 59, and 60 have predominantly subcortical infarcts.

Transcortical Motor Aphasics

Transcortical motor aphasia ($N = 3$) seems to involve the prerolandic portion of the speech area and in case 62, the distribution of the anterior cerebral artery (Figs. 9-17−19-19; cases 61, 62, and 63).

Isolation Syndrome

Isolation syndrome ($N = 2$), a recently described entity, was seen infrequently, but the lesions appear to be involving the watershed areas of cerebral circulation (Figs. 9-17−9-19, cases 64 and 65).

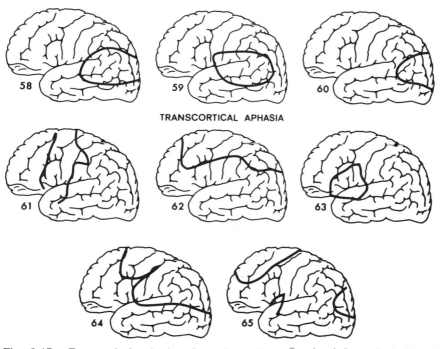

Fig. 9-17. Transcortical aphasics. Lateral template. (Reprinted from Arch Neurol 34:590−601, 1977, Copyright, 1977, American Medical Association.)

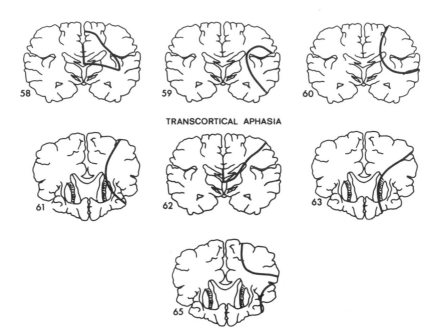

TRANSCORTICAL APHASIA

Fig. 9-18. Transcortical aphasics. Posterior template. Cases 61, 63, and 65 are anterior templates. (Reprinted from Arch Neurol 34:590–601, 1977. Copyright 1977, American Medical Association.)

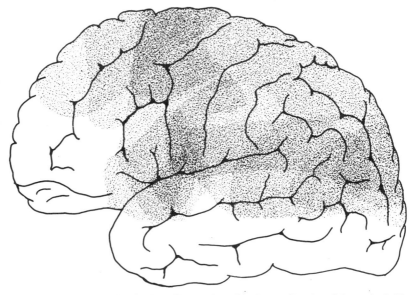

Fig. 9-19. Transcortical aphasics. Composite of lesions. (Reprinted from Arch Neurol 34:590–601, 1977. Copyright 1977, American Medical Association.)

THE OVERLAP OF AREAS PRODUCING APHASIA

The summary of the results on the lateral template illustrates the overlap areas for each group of aphasics (Fig. 9-20). The distribution of these along the anteroposterior parasylvian axis corresponds to the following order: Broca's, conduction, and Wernicke's aphasia. Transcortical lesions overlap outside the main "speech areas," except for a small portion that is adjacent to Broca's area. The anterior and posterior overlap areas in the coronal plane are less well separated for each group (Fig. 9-21). It is remarkable that the area for global aphasia is the only one deep enough to reach the basal ganglia. Transcortical overlap areas seem to be deep or superior to other "speech areas."

Finally, we calculated the number and percentage of the lesions in each group that covered Broca's and Wernicke's areas (Table 9-2) as defined by the overlap technique on the lateral template (Fig. 9-20). The criteria was defined as more than 75% of Broca's or Wernicke's overlap area being covered by the individual lesion. According to this criteria, 85% of the lesions among Broca's aphasics and 69% of the lesions of the Wernicke's group covered their respective

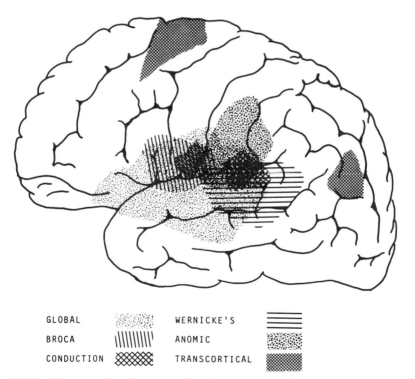

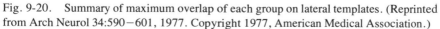

GLOBAL		WERNICKE'S	
BROCA		ANOMIC	
CONDUCTION		TRANSCORTICAL	

Fig. 9-20.   Summary of maximum overlap of each group on lateral templates. (Reprinted from Arch Neurol 34:590−601, 1977. Copyright 1977, American Medical Association.)

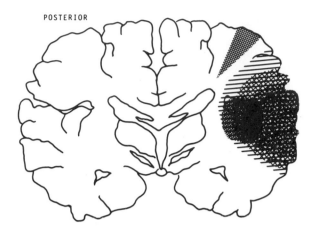

POSTERIOR

GLOBAL

BROCA

CONDUCTION

WERNICKE'S

ANOMIC

TRANSCORTICAL

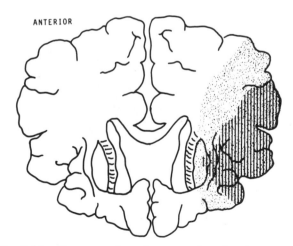

ANTERIOR

Fig. 9-21.   Summary of maximum overlap of each group on anterior and posterior templates. (Reprinted from Arch Neurol
34:590−601, 1977. Copyright 1977, American Medical Association.)

Table 9-2

Percentage of Lesions Covering Speech Areas

Groups	Percentage of Lesions Covering	
	Broca's Area	*Wernicke's Area*
Global (N=12)	100	83
Broca's (N=14)	85	7
Conduction (N=11)	36	36
Wernicke's (N=13)	24	69
Anomic (N=7)	14	28
Transcortical motor (N=3)	67	0
Transcortical sensory (N=3)	0	66
Isolation (N=2)	0	0

(Reprinted from Arch Neurol 34:590−601, 1977. Copyright 1977, American Medical Association.)

areas. Global aphasics cover both areas: 12 of 12 cover Broca's area, and 10 of 12 cover Wernicke's area. Conduction aphasics seem to have an anterior group (4 of 11 patients) covering Broca's area and a posterior group (4 of 11 patients) covering Wernicke's area. Only 1 of 7 anomics covered Broca's area and 2 of 7 covered Wernicke's area. Transcortical aphasics are few, but the transcortical sensory variety (2 of 3 patients) seem to have lesions near Wernicke's area and transcortical motor aphasics (2 of 3) near Broca's area. Isolation lesions lie outside of the speech areas.

LESION SIZE AND SEVERITY

In our preliminary survey of a somewhat larger population of aphasics, the correlation between the area as measured by a planimeter on the lateral uptake and the AQ was found to be significant (Pearson $r = -0.67$ at 55 df). This is in contrast to other studies (R. Karis et al., 1976 and M. Verhas, 1975) denying correlation between severity and lesion size. This is likely related to methodological differences. None of these other studies quantified aphasic impairment as we have. Outlining aphasia-producing lesions may help to predict recovery as well. Large lesions corresponded to poorer outcomes in a neuroradiological study using isotope and CT scans in strokes (P. Yarnell et al., 1976).

DISCUSSION

This study attempts to correlate systematic examination of aphasics with radioisotope scans, which provide the best available localizing information for recent infarcts at the time of testing. The variability of the technique and the difficulty in transferring the images of the isotope uptake to anatomical structures limit the localizing value of this procedure. The latter is a major problem since a centimeter difference may mean missing an important area. We hoped to overcome this by standardizing our templates and by transferring the lesions onto them by an unbiased observer. Head and brain sizes are variable; adjustments during the process of transfer are difficult to make. Even though the angulation of the anteroposterior tube was to be 15° to the orbitomeatal line, variations in this angle occur also. Notwithstanding these limitations, the results are rather gratifying in that we were able to demonstrate distinct areas for Broca's and Wernicke's aphasics and to show that lesions of global aphasics involve both these regions, while conduction aphasics have lesions in between. Conduction aphasia appeared less homogeneous clinically in our taxonomic study (see Chapter 6) and this may account for the bimodal clustering of the lesions as well. An example of a posterior lesion causing conduction aphasia is shown in Fig. 9-22. This right-handed 67-year-old woman had fluent spontaneous speech with frequent paraphasias, phonemic approximations, and word-finding difficulty, and a severe repetition disturbance in contrast to excellent comprehension. Her clinical picture was quite different from Wernicke's aphasia, even though the location of the lesion is in the posterior temporal parietal region, commonly associated with Wernicke's aphasia. Some transcortical motor aphasics and isolation syndromes have lesions surrounding speech areas. Transcortical sensory aphasics have lesions posterior and subcortical to the superior temporal gyrus. Anomic aphasia remains difficult to localize on the basis of these data. Lesions are seen anteriorly, as well as in the more usual posterior location.

Positive scan uptakes are usually obtained in the first month of the stroke, restricting our study to the early stages of aphasic impairment. This allowed us to look at some patients who were classified as Broca's aphasics from the first test. Mohr's patients were considered Broca's aphasics months later after recovering from "total" (global) aphasia (J.P. Mohr, 1976). We have documented this recovery process in another study, (A. Kertesz et al., 1977), but many global aphasics remain the same without significant recovery of comprehension. Recovery from Broca's aphasia can be considerable, but this should not obscure the common finding of a posterior inferior frontal lesion with the initial picture of Broca's aphasia. These clinical entities are distinct probably because of the variable involvement of structures concerned with comprehension. The size of the lesion is another obvious variable. The use of CT scans in conjunction with isotope scanning allows us to determine the lesion size and location in a more chronic state (see Chapter 10).

CORRELATION WITH CT SCANS

We had 54 cases with isotope and CT scans both available for correlation; 23 were within 35 days of each other. There were two cases where the CT scan was negative or too vague for localization in the acute state, and the isotope scan

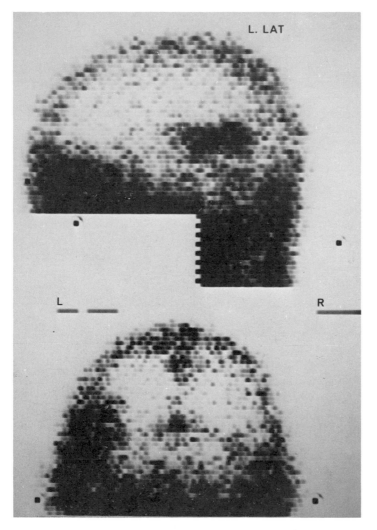

Fig. 9-22.   Conduction aphasia. Left lateral view on top; posterior view on bottom.

showed clear cut evidence of a lesion. Subsequently, the CT scans became more distinct. The opposite situation, that is, a negative isotope scan and early localization on the CT scan, occurred in three cases. In two of these, the isotope scans were done too early and were not repeated subsequently. We found only one case (Fig. 9-23), where the initial isotope scan showed a lesion but the subsequent CT scan was negative. This patient had a transcortical motor aphasia with a pre-rolandic posterior frontal, superficial uptake. He improved to a clinical picture of anomic aphasia with continuing word-finding difficulty and hesitancy.

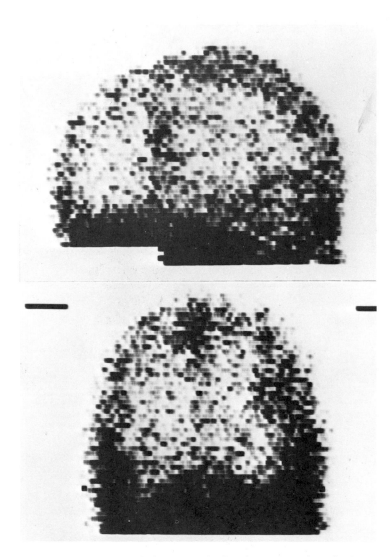

Fig. 9-23. A case of transcortical motor aphasic who recovered, and subsequent CT scan showed no lesion. Left lateral view is on top. Short dash is the left side of the anterior view (right on the photo).

166

SUMMARY

Cerebral infarcts causing aphasia were outlined on the isotope scans without the knowledge of the clinical features, and then overlapped in each clinically and taxonomically distinct group of aphasics. The maximum overlap area for Broca's aphasia was over Broca's area and at the foot of the Rolandic fissure. Wernicke's aphasia involved the posterior superior temporal fissure and the posterior perisylvian region; conduction aphasia involved a similar but somewhat anterior area. Lesions causing conduction aphasia appeared to cluster bimodally: anterior and posterior groups. Lesions of anomic aphasics were widely scattered and transcortical aphasics were outside of the speech area. The severity of aphasia (AQ) correlated inversely with lesion size on planimetry. These results suggest the usefulness of clinical examination and taxonomic diagnosis of aphasics with infarcts for localization. Occasionally, the isotope scan will be the only one to show a lesion.

10

Computerized Tomography in Aphasia

Mr. Hounsfield with great ingenuity coupled radiation physics with computer technology to provide a novel and practical method of direct imaging of the cranial contents.

Paul F. J. New (1975)

INTRODUCTION

Computerized tomography (CT) is the most important advancement in neurodiagnostic methods recently. Infarcts show decreased, and hemorrhages increased densities. The outline of lesions reflects the postmortem findings accurately (Kinkel et al., 1976). Early infarcts may be seen on the CT scan (Fig. 10-1) before they appear on isotope scans. Old infarcts, on the other hand, are quite distinct with sharp margins and lower density than the surrounding brain (Fig. 10-2). Hematomas are dramatic (Fig. 10-3) and even old ones correspond to the size measured at postmortem (Messina et al., 1975). Contrast enhancement of CT increases the diagnostic yield of infarcts especially in the acute stage (Fig. 10-1). In 11 percent of the cases, the infarct was detected only after injection of contrast material (Wing et al., 1976). A positive RN scan is related to a recent

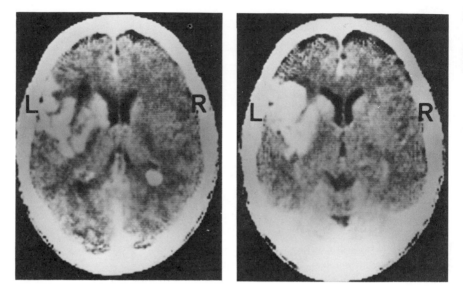

Fig. 10-1. Persisting Broca's aphasia with Broca's area infarct initially. The lesion is restricted to the inferior frontal and Rolandic area. The white area is contrast enhancement. (Reprinted with permission from Kertesz A, Harlock W, Coates R: Computer tomographic localization, lesion size, and prognosis in aphasia and nonverbal impairment. Brain Lang 8:34−50, 1979.)

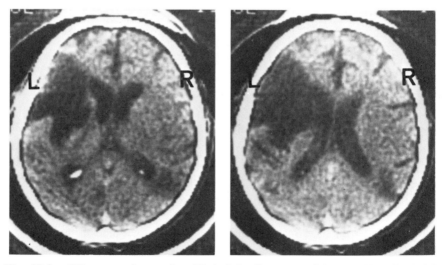

Fig. 10-2. CT a year after stroke. Clinical details presented in text. Note large left frontal and smaller right parietotemporal lesion. (Reprinted with permission from Kertesz A, Harlock W, Coates R: Computer tomographic localization, lesion size, and prognosis in aphasia and nonverbal impairment. Brain Lang 8:34−50, 1979.)

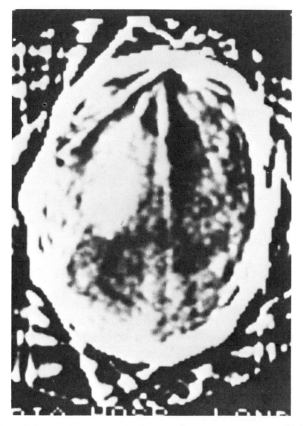

Fig. 10-3. A large putaminal hemorrhage causing initial Global
aphasia with eventual recovery to Broca's aphasia. The superior
temporal area is spared. (Reprinted with permission from Kertesz
A, Harlock W, Coates R: Computer tomographic localization,
lesion size, and prognosis in aphasia and nonverbal impairment.
Brain Lang 8:34—50, 1979.)

stroke, and in combination with a CT scan, may be used to differentiate between
recent and old infarcts, and may help to exclude previous lesions when the
history is unclear. A comparison of CT and RN scanning by Gado et al. (1976)
showed that slightly more (69%) of the recent infarcts showed abnormality on the
RN scan than on the CT scan (55%). On the other hand, infarcts more than 2
months old will rarely show on RN scans but will be seen on CT if they are larger
than 2 cm. This gives us the unique opportunity to examine stable neuropsychological deficits long after initial edema and cellular infiltration subsides and even
after second stage recovery, 3—6 months post onset, which is considered to be
variously related to axonal sprouting, functional compensation, or release from

"diaschisis." Thus, the minimal lesion size and location that will produce various cognitive, language, and behavior symptom complexes can be determined.

Our previous RN scan studies revealed a significant correlation between lesion location and type of aphasia, and lesion size and severity in recent stroke (Kertesz et al., 1977). Naeser and Hayward (1978), utilizing 19 CT scans, 2 months or older post stroke, and the Boston Diagnostic Aphasia Examination, suggested similar correlation. Mohr et al. (1978) outlined the large perisylvian lesions causing severe chronic Broca's aphasia evolving from total aphasia, and lesions affecting the third frontal convolution, associated with a milder, rapidly recovering, motor aphasia. Yarnell et al. (1976) correlated the size of chronic CT lesions with the outcome of aphasia in 16 cases.

CT LOCALIZATION OF INFARCTS ACCORDING TO TYPES OF APHASIA

We undertook a prospective study of aphasics with left hemisphere strokes and equivalent right hemisphere lesions without aphasia, in an effort to correlate the location and extent of the lesion as seen on CT, as soon as the scanner became available to us. We have obtained scans on all acute stroke patients in our unit and followed them for a year. In addition, we examined all stroke patients who had a scan from the other hospitals in London. We have also obtained scans on those chronic aphasics who were known to our laboratory and were able to return for retesting and scanning a year or more after their stroke. Most cases were infarcts but two cases of stable hemorrhage and one with an aneurysm were also included, as their clinical features were identical to the occlusive etiology. Of the 188 patients considered, 103 were excluded for various reasons such as multiple lesions, medical deterioration, confusion, hydrocephalus, atrophy, trauma, arteriovenous malformation, subarachnoid hemorrhage, and seizures. Four of these exclusions with deficit had no abnormality on the CT, and eight with CT lesions had no deficit by the time they were seen. Eighty-five scans have been included so far: 23 aphasics had CT scans within 5 weeks (acute), 39 after a year from their stroke (chronic), ten of these in both acute and chronic state. There were also ten acute and eight chronic, nonaphasic, right hemisphere lesions.

All subjects had CT, and some RN, scans as well within 35 days of neuropsychological testing. The CT 1010-S EMI Scanner, with a 160 × 160 matrix and 8-mm thickness slices, 8-mm apart, was used for the majority of cases but nine were done on a General Electric CTT 7800 Scanner, using 288 × 288 matrix and 10-mm cuts. A radiologist, who had no knowledge of symptoms or test scores, outlined the lesions on templates drawn for each of the six middle slices, 15° above the orbitomeatal line. The angle of CT scanning is different from the usual orientation of anatomical atlases and the templates are based on Gonzalez's atlas, the only one which indicates the cuts in relationship to the lateral landmarks (1976). The section which includes Broca's area only (the third frontal convolution) is B2 (the "smiling face" CT). This is our template 2. The section involving Broca's and just below Wernicke's area, in Gonzalez's atlas (1976) also involves the choroid plexuses (the "sad face" CT). This is our template 3. The cut through the posterior aspect of the superior temporal gyrus is represented by our template 4, which was drawn from cut 2a of Shipps' atlas (1975), as this corresponded more to our CT scans than Gonzalez's equivalent level. Template 5 cuts through the supramarginal gyrus. Cuts 2, 3, and 4 were chosen for representing the lesions. The outlines were overlapped in groups, defined *a priori* according to test scores as described above. The groups were further defined, according to the time of CT and neuropsychological testing, as acute (within 35 days of onset), or chronic (beyond one year from onset). For some of the chronically examined patients, acute test results were also available, and these were used to study the effect of lesion size on recovery. Where both CT scans were available, the tracings appear both in the acute and the chronic group.

Chronic Global Aphasia (Fig. 10-4)

Global aphasics had extensive lesions, involving both the posterior frontal and superior temporal, or Broca's and Wernicke's areas ($N = 6$). One of these was somewhat central, not quite reaching the periphery. There were two acute global aphasics but both of them evolved into Broca's aphasics on the long-term examination. Both had large frontal lesions and these were slightly more anterior, sparing postrolandic temporal structures. These are not displayed separately, but the same lesions appear in the chronic Broca's group (Fig. 10-3).

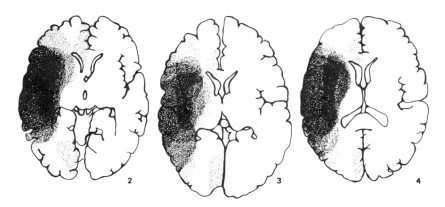

CHRONIC   GLOBALS

Fig. 10-4.   Chronic Global aphasia $N = 6$. (Reprinted with permission from Kertesz A, Harlock W, Coates R: Computer tomographic localization, lesion size, and prognosis in aphasia and nonverbal impairment. Brain Lang 8:34−50, 1979.)

Chronic Broca's Aphasia (Fig. 10-5)

Some of the patients who fell into Broca's category, in the chronic state, also had large lesions ($N = 4$). This group was distinguished from those global aphasics who remained global after a year by the location and size of their lesion, which did not extend quite as far back to involve Wernicke's area. They were clinically similar to global aphasics, especially in the acute state, except for their slightly better comprehension. However, two of the chronic Broca's aphasics had relatively small posterior frontal lesions (Broca's aphasia with Broca's area infarct) (Fig. 10-2).

Acute Broca's Aphasia (Fig. 10-6)

A tightly clustered identical group of lesions was found in six patients who had Broca's aphasia in the acute phase. These patients had relatively small posterior frontal lesions, underlying and restricted to Broca's area. When these patients were examined three months later, even though the lesions had not changed significantly, two of them had anomic aphasia, one transcortical motor aphasia, one recovered, and one remained unchanged.

Chronic Anomic Aphasia—Recovered from Initial Broca's Aphasia (Fig. 10-7)

Exactly the same localization was obtained from patients who were seen in the chronic phase as anomic aphasics, but who had fallen into Broca's category initially ($N = 7$). The only reason to separate this group from the acute Broca's group was that the scans were obtained only a year after the stroke. Two of these

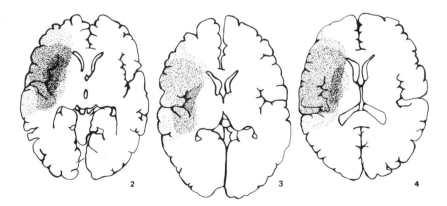

CHRONIC BROCA'S

Fig. 10-5.   Chronic Broca's aphasia $N = 4$. (Reprinted with permission from Kertesz A, Harlock W, Coates R: Computer tomographic localization, lesion size, and prognosis in aphasia and nonverbal impairment. Brain Lang 8:34–50, 1979.)

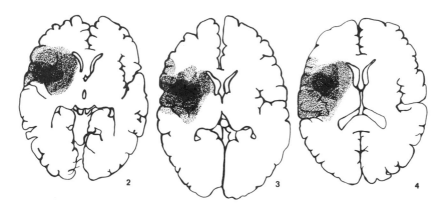

ACUTE BROCA'S

Fig. 10-6. Acute Broca's aphasia $N = 6$. (Reprinted with permission from Kertesz A, Harlock W, Coates R: Computer tomographic localization, lesion size, and prognosis in aphasia and nonverbal impairment. Brain Lang 8:34–50, 1979.)

patients had acute and chronic scans, both without any significant differences between them. This, then, is a common site for a lesion producing Broca's aphasia, which often recovers.

Acute Wernicke's Aphasia (Fig. 10-8)

Two cases of acute Wernicke's aphasia occupied the classical posterior temporal area. One of these patients had an anterior lesion as well, and during recovery resembled conduction aphasia, with improved fluency but continuing paraphasias.

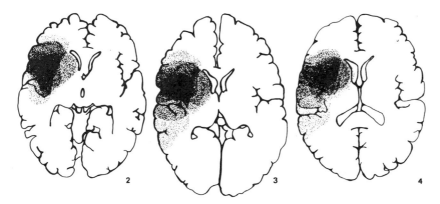

RECOVERED BROCA'S

Fig. 10-7. Chronic anomic aphasia—recovered aphasia $N = 7$. (Reprinted with permission from Kertesz A, Harlock W, Coates R: Computer tomographic localization, lesion size, and prognosis in aphasia and nonverbal impairment. Brain Lang 8:34–50, 1979.)

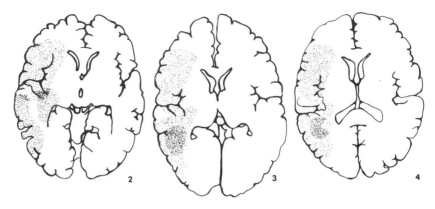

ACUTE WERNICKE'S

Fig. 10-8.   Acute Wernicke's aphasia $N = 2$. (Reprinted with permission from Kertesz A, Harlock W, Coates R: Computer tomographic localization, lesion size, and prognosis in aphasia and nonverbal impairment. Brain Lang 8:34–50, 1979.)

Chronic Wernicke's Aphasia (Fig. 10-9)

Persisting Wernicke's aphasia is exemplified by an infarct in association with an aneurysm with a large posterior lesion, but sparing the frontal operculum. This patient had persisting voluble jargon aphasia for years and remained essentially unchanged from the initial examination.

Acute Transcortical Sensory Aphasia (Fig. 10-10)

Transcortical lesions were rather posterior and deep to Wernicke's area ($N = 3$). The exception is a patient who had a lesion very similar to Wernicke's aphasia; in fact, his test scores were also similar, except for relatively well-

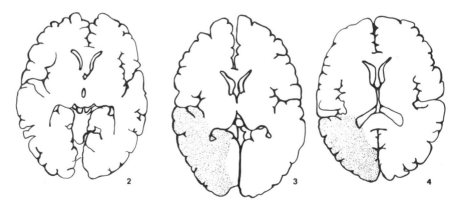

CHRONIC WERNICKE'S

Fig. 10-9.   Chronic Wernicke's aphasia $N = 1$. (Reprinted with permission from Kertesz A, Harlock W, Coates R: Computer tomographic localization, lesion size, and prognosis in aphasia and nonverbal impairment. Brain Lang 8:34–50, 1979.)

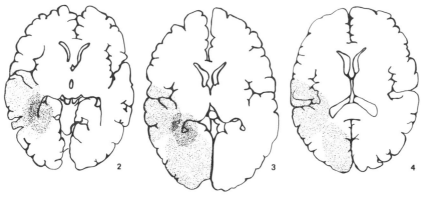

ACUTE TRANSCORTICAL
SENSORY

Fig. 10-10.   Acute transcortical sensory aphasia $N = 3$. (Reprinted with permission from Kertesz A, Harlock W, Coates R: Computer tomographic localization, lesion size, and prognosis in aphasia and nonverbal impairment. Brain Lang 8:34−50, 1979.)

preserved repetition as compared to his poor comprehension. His spontaneous speech was not very paraphasic, and initially he was considered to have pure word deafness. Subsequently, his repetition became so good that it was classified as transcortical sensory aphasia. This patient was unique in many respects, except that his lesion was really in Wernicke's area.

Chronic Conduction Aphasia (Fig. 10-11)

Chronic conduction aphasic patients had large lesions, one anterior, one posterior, and one both $(N = 3)$. One, with a clearly posterior lesion, as well as a

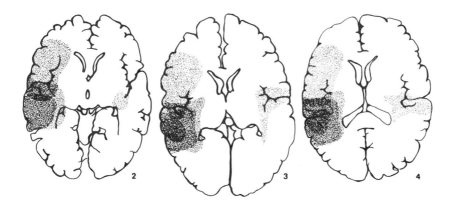

CHRONIC CONDUCTION

Fig. 10-11.   Chronic conduction aphasia $N = 3$. (Reprinted with permission from Kertesz A, Harlock W, Coates R: Computer tomographic localization, lesion size, and prognosis in aphasia and nonverbal impairment. Brain Lang 8:34−50, 1979.)

more anterior one, evolved from Wernicke's aphasia and is also included in Figure 10-8. The lesion on the right is from an acute conduction aphasic who was right-handed! This represents another case of crossed aphasia (See Chapter 9).

Acute Anomic Aphasia (Fig. 10-12) ($N = 8$)

Some patients with anomia initially had small lesions in Broca's area. Their fluency was low; e.g., one had a fluency score of six and another five. Because of their low fluency, some clinicians may consider them, rather, to be mild Broca's aphasics. They all had good prognosis, as they went on to complete recovery in a year. Three other acute anomics had smaller temporal lesions than Wernicke's aphasics, in a similar location. These patients had fluent paraphasic speech, with slightly lower comprehension than the others in this group, resembling mild Wernicke's aphasia. Mild anomic aphasics with subsequent recovery had large lesions, just touching the speech area (Fig. 10-12).

Chronic Anomic Aphasia (Fig. 10-13)

Chronic anomic aphasia was common and the lesions occupied anterior and posterior locations, depending on their initial associated linguistic features. In other words, mild Broca's aphasics, conduction aphasics and Wernicke's aphasics all ended up in a similar chronic anomic state, indistinguishable by our test results, a year or more after their stroke ($N = 13$).

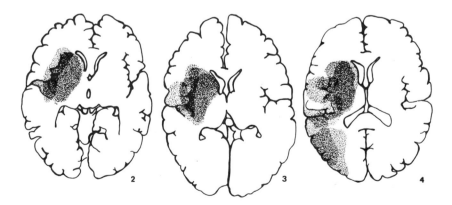

ACUTE ANOMIC

Fig. 10-12.   Acute anomic aphasia $N = 8$. (Reprinted with permission from Kertesz A, Harlock W, Coates R: Computer tomographic localization, lesion size, and prognosis in aphasia and nonverbal impairment. Brain Lang 8:34−50, 1979.)

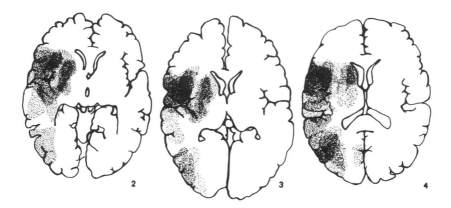

CHRONIC ANOMIC

Fig. 10-13.   Chronic anomic aphasia $N = 13$. (Reprinted with permission from Kertesz A, Harlock W, Coates R: Computer tomographic localization, lesion size, and prognosis in aphasia and nonverbal impairment. Brain Lang 8:34−50, 1979.)

Nondominant Lesions with Constructional Apraxia (Fig. 10-14)

Among the 15 nondominant cases, there was a group of 6 clearly distinguished by severe constructional apraxia, as defined by the scores on the block design and drawing tasks. Most of these patients also had neglect and other visuospatial difficulties. There was another unexpected finding of significant reading difficulty in three acute nondominant hemisphere cases admitted to this study. These patients had a similar, rather central lesion, like the rest of the group and all had constructional apraxia.

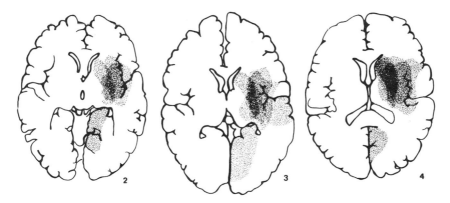

NON-DOMINANT WITH
CONSTRUCTIONAL   APRAXIA

Fig. 10-14.   Nondominant with constructional apraxia $N = 6$. (Reprinted with permission from Kertesz A, Harlock W, Coates R: Computer tomographic localization, lesion size, and prognosis in aphasia and nonverbal impairment. Brain Lang 8:34−50, 1979.)

Nondominant Lesions without Constructional Apraxia (Fig. 10-15)

The acute and chronic cases were combined as in the previous group. There was no essential anatomical difference between this and the other group with constructional apraxia.

OVERLAPPING OF LESIONS

Acute Aphasia (Fig. 10-16)

The overlaps of each type are summarized in Fig. 10-16, except when there were too few to be meaningful. At least 80 percent of the lesions in each group are included in the area of overlap selected by the medical illustrator as the optically densest region.

Chronic Aphasia (Fig. 10-17)

These were overlapped separately from acute cases, using the same method as in the previous group. We did not include the single chronic Wernicke's aphasic (see Fig. 10-9), as the lesion was disproportionately larger than the other areas, and obviously not comparable to the composite overlaps obtained from several cases.

We have discussed some of the deficiencies of the overlap technique in our previous chapter on isotope scan localization. The more cases included, the smaller is the overlap. Therefore, the size of the composite areas is also a

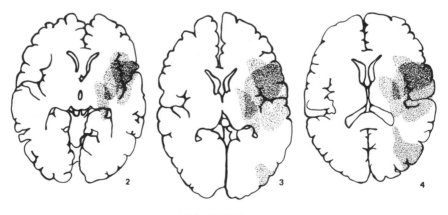

NON-DOMINANT NO
CONSTRUCTIONAL
APRAXIA

Fig. 10-15.   Nondominant without constructional apraxia $N = 5$. (Reprinted with permission from Kertesz A, Harlock W, Coates R: Computer tomographic localization, lesion size, and prognosis in aphasia and nonverbal impairment. Brain Lang 8:34−50, 1979.)

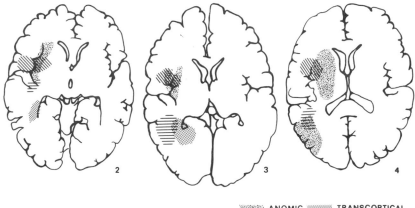

ACUTE   APHASIA

▓▓▓ ANOMIC ▓▓▓ TRANSCORTICAL
\\\\\\\ BROCA ═══ WERNICKE'S

Fig. 10-16.   Composite of overlaps—acute aphasics $N = 19$. (Reprinted with permission from Kertesz A, Harlock W, Coates R: Computer tomographic localization, lesion size, and prognosis in aphasia and nonverbal impairment. Brain Lang 8:34−50, 1979.)

reflection on the number of cases in that group, as well as the size of the lesions necessary to produce the deficit. We did not include in the composite pictures chronic Wernicke's (only one), acute globals (two), acute transcortical motor (one), isolation (one), and acute conduction (one), in order to avoid discrepancy between the size of the composites.

One of the constraining factors in the study of localization of lesions by syndromes is the limitation imposed by any classification system. There are patients in different groups who resemble each other more than their group mates, and our study suggests that their lesions may be more similar to each other

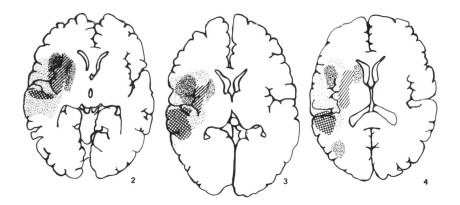

CHRONIC APHASIA

░░░ GLOBAL ▓▓▓ CONDUCTION
\\\\\\\ BROCA ▒▒▒ ANOMIC

Fig. 10-17.   Composite of overlaps—chronic aphasics $N = 33$. (Reprinted with permission from Kertesz A, Harlock W, Coates R: Computer tomographic localization, lesion size, and prognosis in aphasia and nonverbal impairment. Brain Lang 8:34−50, 1979.)

also! This decreases the extent of overlapping within each group and increases the overlap between groups. At times, mild Broca's aphasics resemble some anomic aphasics more than severe Broca's aphasics in some respects, and the globally affected patients may be quite close to severe Broca's aphasics, except for one important parameter: comprehension. Some anomic aphasics who evolve from Broca's area lesions retain characteristics of mild Broca's aphasia (relatively low fluency), and those with damage in Wernicke's area resemble mild Wernicke's aphasia (higher fluency and lower comprehension). Nevertheless, the validity of our clinical classifications has been supported by objective numerical taxonomy indicating a highly significant clustering of patients (see Chapter 6). The extent of the overlap results also justifies the separation of groups according to limits defined by scores rather than treating them as a continuum. We could conceivably increase discrimination by using more tests in the formation of groups. However, the resulting increase in the number of groups could be to the detriment of practicality, and may not be valid clinically either. We could divide anomics and possibly the conduction group when more cases become available.

SEVERITY AND LESION SIZE

The size of the lesions traced was determined by the digitizer program on a Hewlett–Packard computer. This allowed us to outline the lesions and calculate the area. Coefficients of correlation (Pearson r) were calculated to determine the relationship between the lesion size and severity of aphasia, as measured by the aphasia quotient (AQ) (see Table 10-1). The AQ is the summary score of the WAB and it has face validity for severity. A component analysis showed that various subtests contribute evenly to this severity factor (see Chapters 4 and 6). The correlation coefficient (Pearson r) between the largest area traced in each aphasic; their AQ was -0.60, significant at $P \leq 0.01$ (df = 61). The negative correlation means that the larger the lesion, the lower the AQ (the more severe the aphasia).

A similar, highly significant, negative correlation was obtained between the lesion size and the performance quotient (PQ) (the sum of nonverbal test scores): Pearson $r = 0.54, P \leq 0.01$ (df = 61). Among the various groups of aphasics, the anomics had the highest degree of correlation between AQ and area: $r = -0.81$. This underscores the clinical experience, that in anomic aphasia, the size of the lesion is more significant in determining the degree of aphasia than its location. This is in contrast to other types, such as Wernicke's aphasia, where a small but strategically placed lesion in Wernicke's area may produce severe Wernicke's aphasia. Other aphasic groups had less than significant correlation between severity and lesion size.

Nondominant lesion size did not correlate with language tasks, as these

Table 10–1
Correlation between Area and Severity

Groups	N	Pearson r	Significance
All aphasics language	62	−0.60	$p \leq 0.01$
Nondominant language	18	−0.02	NS*
Anomic language	13	−0.81	$p \leq 0.01$
All aphasics performance	62	−0.54	$p \leq 0.01$
Nondominant performance	18	−0.22	NS*

*Not significant.

The correlation between the area and severity of language deficit of all aphasics and the anomic group, and between the area and the performance total of nondominant hemisphere lesions was estimated by the Pearson r. (Reprinted with permission from Kertesz A, Harlock W, Coates R: Computer tomographic localization, lesion size, and prognosis in aphasia and nonverbal impairment. Brain Lang 8:34−50, 1979.)

patients were not aphasic. There was a negative trend, even though statistically not significant, between lesion size and nonverbal performance.

Our findings in the nondominant group can only be considered preliminary. The lesions were generally smaller than those involving the speech hemispheres. This may be due to sampling, as we had more opportunity to examine stable dominant hemisphere lesions known to our aphasia laboratory, than chronic left hemiplegias. Further sophistication and improvement in the clinical description and categorization of nondominant lesions and deficits are needed to study localization of abnormalities in the right hemisphere.

LANGUAGE PARAMETERS, RECOVERY, AND LESION SIZE

Among acute aphasics, the larger the lesion, the poorer is the comprehension (a significant negative correlation). Similar trends (negative correlations) were seen for naming, repetition, and overall severity, but they reached statistical significance only in the chronic group. On the other hand, fluency did not correlate with lesion size, due to the large lesions of some of the very fluent Wernicke's and transcortical sensory aphasics and the relatively smaller lesions of the nonfluent Broca's aphasics. Some of the very fluent anomic aphasics also had small lesions (Table 10-2).

Chronic aphasics showed significant negative correlation across the board between lesion size and all language parameters, related to the larger lesions of the severely affected Global aphasics.

The extent of language recovery was calculated as the difference in scores between the initial and one year follow-up examination in 32 patients. The positive correlation between recovery of comprehension and lesion size was the only one reaching statistical significance. A trend of negative correlation was

Table 10–2

Language and Performance Parameters and Lesion Size

Group	N	Fluency	Comprehension	Repetition	Naming Total	AQ
Acute aphasics	23	−0.1437	−0.595**	−0.328	−0.357	−0.367
Chronic aphasics	33	−0.666**	−0.740**	−0.679**	−0.702**	−0.725**

		Drawing		Block Design	
Acute nondominant	10		−0.503		−0.375
Chronic nondominant	8		−0.514		−0.127

**p ≤ 0.01.

Various language parameters were correlated in both the chronic and acute groups of aphasics, and drawing and block design for the nondominant lesions. (Reprinted with permission from Kertesz A, Harlock W, Coates R: Computer tomographic localization, lesion size, and prognosis in aphasia and nonverbal impairment. Brain Lang 8:34−50, 1979.)

observed for the other parameters (Table 10-3). This can be easily understood if one considers that the comprehension deficit caused by large lesions often recovers considerably more than other parameters (Lomas and Kertesz, 1978). The more severe the deficit initially, the more room there is for recovery. Smaller lesions, on the other hand, often result in aphasia with little, if any, comprehension deficit; the extent of recovery is small with the higher scores to begin with. The negative correlations between the recovery rates of fluency, repetition, naming, AQ, and lesion size indicate that the larger the lesion, the less overall recovery occurs in the total language deficit (AQ) and in the parameters other than comprehension.

Table 10–3

Language Recovery and Lesion Size

Parameters	Pearson r	Significance
AQ (severity)	−0.253	NS
Fluency	−0.348	NS
Comprehension	+0.350	p ≤ 0.05
Repetition	−0.300	NS
Naming	−0.255	NS

Recovery rates of language parameters are correlated with lesion size using Pearson r. (Reprinted with permission from Kertesz A, Harlock W, Coates R: Computer tomographic localization, lesion size, and prognosis in aphasia and nonverbal impairment. Brain Lang 8:34−50, 1979.)

ACUTE AND CHRONIC LESIONS

The lesion sizes in acute and chronic scans in the same patients were compared with the t tests for paired samples. The difference was not significant ($t = 0.02$, df $= 9$). A slight decrease in the lesion size was noted in the few cases of hemorrhage, but there was no change between the acute and chronic lesions as a rule.

The constancy of the lesion size in our study suggested that a CT image obtained in a chronic stable state is a good indication of the extent of the structural damage in the acute state, although effects of edema or other pathochemical or histological changes in the acute state may not be evident on the scans. Not testing patients in the acute state, as done by Naeser and Hayward (1978), eliminates some of the variability, but it also misses the interesting variations in the acute syndromes which change subsequently.

The lesions of chronic aphasic groups are most important because they represent stable deficits. Even though the lesion may be larger than the portion necessary to produce this deficit, the essential structure can be determined, to some extent, by overlapping several larger lesions. The major problem with chronic lesions on the CT scan is that recovery often alters the clinical picture considerably, while the lesion changes little, if any. It is evident from this study that a great deal of functional compensation and restructuring of speech mechanisms must take place to achieve the degree of recovery observed, with relatively large areas of the brain remaining destroyed.

Acute aphasics have lesions, on the other hand, that are related to uncompensated and, therefore, greater deficit than is seen in the chronic cases. The overlapping reveals generally the same structures involved in the acute and chronic groups and confirms our findings with isotope scans.

The timing of the localizing tests has to be carefully planned and coordinated with the time course of evolution of aphasic and neurological deficit. Three weeks postonset is probably optimal to obtain localizing information and clinical tests in the acute patients. For chronic assessment, we chose a year as a period of stabilization based on our previous study of recovery (Kertesz and McCabe, 1977). Although we only used CT scans obtained within a month from the neuropsychological tests, for the chronic scans this restriction may not be necessary, since our data indicate that the lesions do not change to any significant extent.

The evolution of aphasic syndromes can be correlated with lesion size and location. Large perisylvian infarcts produced persisting global aphasia. Similarly large infarcts, but somewhat more anterior in location, showed evolution toward Broca's aphasia in the chronic state, mainly with improved comprehension. This is essentially in agreement with Mohr's (1978) finding that larger lesions involving the superior division of the middle cerebral artery territory will produce lasting Broca's aphasia. Nevertheless, there are global aphasics whose deficit remains the same and whose comprehension does not recover. These patients are distinguishable clinically, as well as on the CT scan, by their more extensive and posterior spread of lesions.

Results indicate that the CT scan is best for localizing chronic, and as shown by our previous study, the RN scan acute infarcts (see Chapter 9). In some of the acute cases the CT was negative, while RN scan showed an uptake. CT scans that are normal initially, may change to abnormal in 48 hrs. The early infarction appears as a speckled area of ill-defined, decreased density, and 14−30 days later, the borders become more clearly defined and decreased density is more homogenous (Kinkel and Jacobs, 1976). RN scans, on the other hand, show maximum uptake in 7−21 days (Gado et al., 1976), but cannot be used beyond 6−8 weeks for reliable localization. It is in this chronic state where CT scans provide a real advantage over RN scans. Another advantage is seen shortly after a stroke, in the first few days, when the RN scan is still negative: the CT scan may already show a lesion. Few infarcts have been scanned serially, due to the large demand for CT time, but in one study, 19 percent of CT scans were negative, 31 percent equivocal, and 50 percent only were positive in the first week; in the second week, this changes to 12 percent, 12 percent, and 76 percent; and after four weeks to 2 percent, 13 percent, and 85 percent, respectively (Davis et al., 1975). RN abnormalities are often less distinct than chronic CT images, although rectilinear images are better suited for isotope localization than the gamma scan.

A CASE WITH UNUSUAL LOCALIZATION

It is important to present exceptions which defy our system of classification and have unusual localizing features. A case which was not included in the previous study because of another lesion on the right side may serve as an example. E H, a 67-year-old, right-handed man had a sudden onset of right hemiplegia and global aphasia, on July 10, 1977, as a result of a left internal carorid artery occlusion. Ten days after his stroke, he was nonfluent, said mainly "yes" and "no," and his comprehension was poor. His subsequent recovery was unusual and well documented. Three months after his stroke, his spontaneous speech became considerably more fluent, with paraphasias and word-finding difficulty. His comprehension continued to be mildly but significantly impaired and his repetition was less affected, even though striking phonemic paraphasias were produced. He was considered a Wernicke's aphasic by a speech pathologist, Dr. C Shewan, but his repetition score placed him in the transcortical sensory group. Several others who saw him agreed that it was difficult to put him in any category. His spontaneous speech reminded us of recovered Broca's aphasia, but his comprehension remained poor enough to consider his clinical picture among the sensory aphasics. Although his comprehension and fluency improved slightly, his category and AQ remained quite similar a year after his stroke, when a CT scan was done (Fig. 10-2). This showed a left frontal lesion with inferior Rolandic and parietal operculum involvement and sparing of Wernicke's or posterior areas. On the other hand, the opposite supramarginal and parietal region was clearly involved in another infarct, for which no history could be obtained.

Various possibilities can be considered to correlate the frontal localization by CT with the fluent paraphasic speech and impaired comprehension. One of the most plausible explanations is that he had a right-sided infarct before the left-sided one and this made the initial insult much more severe, causing global aphasia. The left frontal lesion, by itself, would have resulted only in Broca's aphasia, possibly a rapidly recovering one. Some of his speech recovery was compatible with this, except his comprehension which remained impaired, possibly because the right parietotemporal area could not contribute to recovery as fully as in others. The right parietotemporal lesion may block transcallosal access of the intact left Wernicke's area to the substituting right hemisphere.

This case illustrates the contribution of the CT scan to the analysis of unusual cases, as well as the difficulty in trying to localize certain infarcts which deviate a great deal from others in their location or association with other lesions. This is similar to the unique location and distance effects of tumors, which make it so difficult to rely on their localization.

DISCUSSION

An interesting finding was the nearly identical location of lesions of Broca's aphasia and some anomic aphasia in the frontal operculum and third frontal convolution (Broca's area). The essential center producing chronic Broca's aphasia (as defined by our methods) is the same as in those anomic patients who recovered from acute Broca's aphasia to a milder deficit. The important difference is the size of the lesion. A larger lesion will produce a more lasting deficit. There is a spectrum of syndromes produced by Broca's area infarct. More than just initial mutism and verbal apraxia, the larger lesions produce the full-blown symptom complex of Broca's aphasia with decreased fluency, effortful speech production, and relatively good comprehension. This syndrome persists for a variable length of time, and one's view is influenced by the time one looks at the deficit.

It came as no surprise that acute Wernicke's aphasics had postrolandic lesions, and that those of conduction aphasics were just slightly forward to this, but nearly in the same area in the chronic state. We had only one example of a Wernicke's aphasia with jargon in the chronic state, although such cases have been published previously in a clinicopathological correlation of jargon aphasics (Kertesz and Benson, 1970). Our acute Wernicke's cases recover most often as

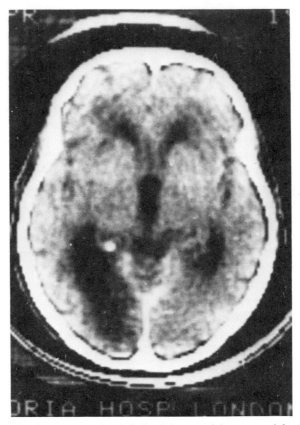

Fig. 10-18. A posterior inferior infarct and large ventricles in case of Transcortical Sensory aphasia. Note intact Wernicke's and Broca's area. (Reprinted with permission from Kertesz A, Harlock W, Coates R: Computer tomographic localization, lesion size, and prognosis in aphasia and nonverbal impairment. Brain Lang 8:34−50, 1979.)

anomic and occasionally emerge in the conduction category. Relatively large posteriorly placed lesions, with transcortical sensory or anomic aphasia, are compatible with complete recovery. Anomic aphasics have posterior lesions when the condition appears *de novo*, but anterior lesions with initial nonfluent aphasia (Broca's or transcortical motor types) often become anomic, with their lesions unchanged.

CT cuts provide accurate information about the anteroposterior (AP) extent and the depth of the lesion in two dimensions, while RN scans image the lesions in vertical, anteroposterior, and coronal planes. It is likely that future technology will integrate the horizontal slices to obtain a vertical projection as well as to

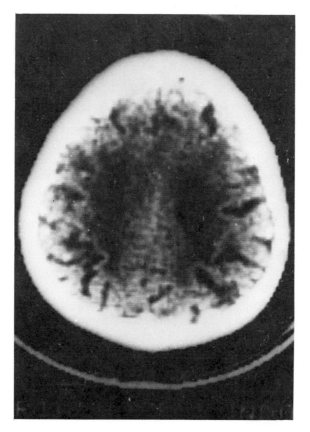

Fig. 10-19. Significant cerebral atrophy added to a cerebral infarct in a 78-year-old female patient without history of dementia (same as Fig. 10-18 but higher cut). (Reprinted with permission from Kertesz A, Harlock W, Coates R: Computer tomographic localization, lesion size, and prognosis in aphasia and nonverbal impairment. Brain Lang 8:34−50, 1979.)

achieve a three-dimensional CT image. A reasonably accurate estimate of the vertical and lateral dimension can be achieved by connecting the edges of the horizontal cuts (Mazzocchi and Vignolo, 1978).

CT scans have another substantial contribution to neuropsychological investigation—they are excellent in showing cerebral atropy (Figs. 10-18 and 10-19). The extent of atrophy and dementia has been correlated on CT scans, although some atrophy is, at times, related to aging without dementia. Atrophic cases can be excluded from a series, or the presence or absence of atrophy can be considered in the interpretation. This 78-year-old female patient whose chronic CT scan is illustrated in Figs. 10-18 and 10-19 had a transcortical sensory aphasia, which has recovered despite the large posterior lesion (Fig. 10-18) in the lower cut. She was not demented despite either the large ventricles and sulci indicating age-related atrophy (Fig. 10-19). One should be cautious not to equate the presence of atrophy to dementia. Further data are needed to clarify the significance of atrophy.

SUMMARY

CT is a powerful tool to correlate structural abnormality in the nervous system with neuropsychological impairment. Relatively small changes in the infarcted area are compatible with considerable recovery, accounting for some of the discrepancies between structures and function reported in the literature.

Chronic global aphasics have lesions that are more extensive posteriorly than patients with persisting Broca's aphasia. The area of persisting Broca's aphasia is similarly anterior but larger than recovered motor aphasia. Anomic aphasics evolve from Broca's and Wernicke's types with differing localization. Lesion size correlates with severity and impairment of comprehension, repetition, and naming. Positive correlation between lesion size and recovery of comprehension corresponded to the observation that comprehension recovers more in large lesions than other parameters.

11

Alexia

Reading maketh a full man, conference a ready man, and writing an exact man.

Francis Bacon (1625)

INTRODUCTION

Alexia, by definition, is the failure of comprehension of written material. It often accompanies aphasia and agraphia but can be independent from them; the reverse is true also. Reading involves visual attention, optokinetic functions, perception of forms, spatial relations, and symbolic significance. These multiple functions are not always clearly separable. Early descriptions of alexia have been reviewed by Benton (1964). Broadbent (1872) recorded a case of severe alexia, with only mild aphasic disturbance and minimal disturbance of writing. Kussmaul (1877) applied the term ''word blindness'' and considered alexia a form of aphasia. Dejerine (1892) published two cases of alexia, one with agraphia and the other one without agraphia, at the outset. The case of alexia and agraphia had an infarct in the angular gyrus. The patient with alexia without agraphia and a right homonymous hemianopsia had a second stroke producing agraphia as well. A postmortem examination revealed an infarct of the left angular gyrus in addition to involvement of the medial and inferior aspects of the left occipital lobe, and the splenium of the corpus callosum. Dejerine (1892) concluded that the combination of these lesions produced alexia by disconnecting the visual from the verbal system. Hinshelwood (1900) collected 28 cases of word blindness. Recent reviews summarized the extensive literature on the subject of alexia by Leischner (1957), Benson and Geschwind (1969), and Hecaen and Kremin (1976). Table 11-1 represents an overview of classification which attempts to list equivalent terminology in the same row. Most authors agree on the following classifications: (1) alexia without agraphia, (2) alexia with agraphia, (3) aphasic alexia.

ALEXIA WITHOUT AGRAPHIA

Pure alexia, pure word blindness, optic alexia, subcortical visual aphasia, or agnosic alexia in modern terminology are known simply as alexia without agraphia. Other speech functions and writing to dictation and spontaneously remains intact; however, the patient may not be able to read his own writing after an interval! The term "word blindness" refers to the often observed phenomenon discussed below that the patient may recognize individual letters but not words (verbal alexia). Some alexic patients can read words better than letters; this is often called "letter blindness" or "literal alexia." "Global alexia" is used for patients who cannot read either letters or words.

Some patients are able to read letters but unable to join them together (asyllabia). Simply patterned letters, such as "i" and "o" are recognized more readily than complex ones. Sometimes, this reading disability is considered to be similar to simultanagnosia. Kinsbourne and Warrington (1962) described such patients and called it "spelling dyslexia," because these patients could read laboriously by spelling each letter individually. According to many authors the difference between literal and verbal alexia results only from differences in the severity of the lesion and, perhaps, also from the different educational levels of the patients. Others consider this distinction useful clinically (Benson et al., 1971).

Hecaen (1967) described 14 cases of pure alexia, which were further subdivided. *Verbal alexia* (seven cases), was characterized by preservation of the ability to read letters but inability to read words, other than by a process of spelling (spelling dyslexia). Items, whether meaningful or not, could be read, except when they were too long. Simple commands could be understood; but when they were more complex, the breakdown seemed to be related to a failure to memorize various elements. Copying was erratic but could be carried out from block to cursive script. Spelling was good, but verbal naming was poor, and

Table 11-1

Classification of Alexia

Author	Year				
Kussmaul	1877	Word blindness	Word blindness with agraphia		
Wernicke	1885	Subcortical (Literal, Verbal)	Cortical	Transcortical	
Dejerine	1892	Pure word blindness (Pure alexia)	Word blindness with agraphia		
Pick	1931	Word form blindness			
Kleist	1934	Subcortical, corticocomissural	Word meaning blindness (Cortical)	Sentence alexia	
Nielsen	1939	Verbal–visual agnosia	Word meaning blindness		
Quesnel	1931	Occipital	Parietal	Temporal	Aphasic
Alajouanine	1960	Agnosic (optic)			
Brain	1961	Agnosic	Visual asymbolia	Aphasic	
Kinsbourne, Warrington	1962	Spelling dyslexia	Paralexia		
Benson, Geschwind	1969	Alexia without agraphia (Literal, Verbal, Global)	Alexia with agraphia	Aphasic (Paralexia, Pseudoalexia)	
Marshall, Newcombe	1973	Visual dyslexia (grapheme confusion)	Surface dyslexia (grapheme phoneme conversion)	Deep dyslexia (syntactosemantic)	
Hecaen, Kremin	1976	Alexia without agraphia (Literal, Verbal, Global)	Alexia with agraphia	Aphasic (Sentence)	
Benson	1977	Posterior (sensory)	Central (associative)	Sensory Motor	Frontal

color naming appeared to be frequently affected. Digits and numbers could be read easily but arithmetical operations were often erroneous. In *literal alexia* (five cases), the reading of letters resulted in more errors than the reading of words, and both visual and semantic types of paralexias were produced during reading. The length of the word was not a major factor. Function words and nonsense syllables were read with difficulty. Although one or two words might be understood, complex commands could not be read and there were numerous paralexias. Digits and numbers could not be read. Copying was impossible or resembled copying meaningless designs; writing often showed paragraphias. *Global alexia* (two cases) indicated the total inability to read letters and words. This condition is often associated with a more global agnosia. A further study by Dubois-Charlier (1970), on 11 patients, indicated the presence of yet another form of alexia, called *sentence alexia*. In these cases, grammatical endings were misread and the meaning of a sentence or a text was not understood.

In cases of verbal alexia, the grammatical category or word frequency or even word length did not exert a systematic influence; the paralexias seemed to be the result of "oversights." In literal alexia, a global strategy or guessing was observed. Words in context were read better than those in isolation; semantic paralexias were common. The failure of literal alexia was considered to be at a phonographemic level, and verbal alexia at the morphographemic level (that is, the inability to apply the rules of written morphemes correctly), and finally, sentence alexia at syntactic level, with an incorrect application of syntactic rules for written language.

Color identification defect is common in pure alexia, occurring in 70 percent of the series of Gloning et al. (1968). The combination of word blindness and color naming defect is also called Pötzl's syndrome, and two further cases with anatomical verification were published by Hoff et al. (1962). The patient usually preserves the ability to sort colors and they can usually point to colors on verbal request much better than they can name them. The nature of the color-naming defect has been clarified by Geschwind and Fusillo (1966), who thought that the exclusive visual—verbal associations are affected in the recognition of both colors and printed material, in contrast to object recognition, which can be mediated through tactile associations that remain intact.

Lissauer (1889) suggested a close association between agnostic disorders and alexia without agraphia. Goldstein (1948) considered pure alexia a disturbance of figure—ground relationship, resulting in the loss of "simultaneity," leaving only "successivity." He considered "primary alexia" a loss of the abstract attitude. Although most cases of alexia without agraphia are not associated with visual agnosia, it should be noted that in most cases of visual agnosia, there is alexia without agraphia. The recently presented cases of Albert et al. (1978) and Mack and Boller (1977) are rare but important exceptions to this rule.

A right homonymous hemianopia is usually present, although there have been exceptions described. Greenblatt's (1973) case without hemianopia had a left occipital tumor invading the splenium but sparing the calcarine fissure. As the majority of patients with hemianopsia are not alexic, pure word blindness is not caused by lesions responsible for hemianopsia alone. There has to be an interruption of connections from the intact right visual area.

The ability to read numbers may be lost in alexia, although at times number reading is better preserved than letter reading. There is less agreement about musical notation. This is related to the low rate of musical literacy. The reading of musical notes, while not recorded in most cases, may be impaired also. Dejerine's original case showed retention of number reading (1892) which was explained by Alajouanine (1960) by the smaller vocabulary for numbers and the more thorough overlearning, as well as the less complex phonemic qualities of numbers, when compared to letters, and, thirdly, that numbers are learned by counting on fingers, thus producing bilateral somasthetic associations and, perhaps, alternate association pathways for number reading (Geschwind, 1962). Acalculia, itself, is not usually a part of alexia and its presence may indicate a severe number reading disturbance.

Although writing is preserved in pure alexia, it shows certain features which are similar to the writing of blind persons. These patients have difficulty moving from one line to the next and often, the writing is slanted and extra loops are observed. The patient has difficulty copying and the ability to transfer printed to cursive script is absent. At times, the patient cannot copy at all; other times, copying is slavish, as if for a meaningless design. It has been observed in some cases of alexia without agraphia that the patients could improve their recognition of letters by tracing them or palpating cardboard letters with their fingers. Also, these patients readily comprehend words spelled aloud to them and can also spell aloud correctly. On the other hand, patients with alexia with agraphia usually cannot do this task. Identifying printed words after hearing them, called auditory word recognition or phonetic association, is easier for patients with pure alexia, in contrast to aphasic alexia, where the deficit is more bidirectional.

Benson and Geschwind (1969) collected 15 cases from the literature, where pathology was available for the syndrome of alexia without agraphia. Nine of these had involvement of the splenium of the corpus callosum and all but two involved the occipital lobe on the left; one had a bilateral infarct and one a right-sided infarct. It was suggested that a deep white matter lesion in the left medial occipital region could produce the same effect as actual involvement of the splenium. There have been a number of postoperative cases of alexia without agraphia, when only a lateral parieto-occipital lesion was present, but often, the exact depth of occipital involvement was unknown. The pathology supports the disconnection theory that when the left occipital lobe or primary visual area is destroyed, the right side cannot convey the stimulus to the intact left angular gyrus. More anterior portions of the corpus callosum remain available to transmit other visual stimuli, such as objects or numbers, because these have more tactile associations and can utilize parietal systems to get across the corpus callosum. The possible interhemispheric dissociation of reading ability from spoken language was presented by Erkulvrawatr (1978) in a patient who had alexia without agraphia from a right occipital infarction but had speech dominance on the left, according to a sodium Amytal test. Although most of the documented instances of alexia without agraphia are related to posterior cerebral artery thrombosis, which supplies the dominant occipital lobe and the splenium of the corpus callosum, the syndrome has been produced by dominant occipital lobectomy (David et al., 1955). The author also had a personal case, associated with visual agnosia due to closed head injury (Kertesz, 1979). In addition to the usual splenio-occipital lesion due to infarct, the "subangular" pathology has been described with A−V malformation (Greenblatt, 1976).

ALEXIA WITH AGRAPHIA

This disorder used to be called visual asymbolia or cortical visual aphasia, since both reading and writing are affected. Aphasia more often accompanies it and there are often other signs, such as acalculia, right and left disorientation, finger agnosia, construction apraxia, and naming difficulty. The term should be used only when the reading and writing disturbances are distinctly more prominent than the other associated features. Right homonymous hemianopsia is a less constant defect than it is in pure alexia. The recognition of letters is impaired even in tactile presentation, and also, when the letters are spelled ("auditory reading"). The preservation of word reading over letters can be marked, with words read without phonemic errors, even though semantic paralexias are common. Context seems to improve word recognition. Isolated letters such as B, P, and U may not be recognized, but the words "Bee," "Pea," and "You" are read well (literal alexia). The writing defect is variable. In severe cases, the patient only scrawls on the paper. Copying is more successful than writing spontaneously or on dictation. This is just the opposite of alexia without agraphia. Writing is often parallel with the reading disturbance; it is often paragraphic, that is, incorrect forms are produced, although at times, some letters, and even words, are preserved. The associated aphasia is often a mild anomic type, but at times paraphasias and comprehension difficulty are seen. Paraphasic responses while reading are often called paralexia and may be more commonly seen for pictureable words. According to Benson and Geschwind's review, most cases of alexia with agraphia also have features of Gerstmann's syndrome. However, Gerstmann's original description did not include alexia as an integral part of the syndrome. In alexia with agraphia, the dominant angular gyrus is involved as a rule. Tumors and trauma also play a larger role in the cause of this symptom than in alexia without agraphia, which is usually caused by vascular occlusion of the posterior cerebral artery. The importance of the angular gyrus in cross modal associations has been emphasized by Geschwind (1965). That the complex au-ditory—visual functions of reading are impaired by lesions in between the impor-tant speech and visual perceptual areas is not surprising.

APHASIC ALEXIA

Aphasic alexia refers to the alexia which accompanies aphasia in most cases. Patients with Wernicke's aphasia have alexia with agraphia and often, have very copious, paragraphic output of writing, and defects in reading similar to that of speaking. In these cases, usually the posterior superior temporal lobe, as well as the angular gyrus, is destroyed together, although some authors do not consider angular gyrus involvement essential (Nielsen, 1939). Since language is acquired through auditory pathways, the subsequent acquisition of visual lan-guage depends on this initial mechanism. Visual language may be disturbed in isolation, by disconnecting visual—auditory associations, but lesions in the corti-cal areas of speech will affect all modalities of language (Benson and Ges-chwind, 1969). Exceptions to this rule are the cases of pure word deafness, when the patient can read but has difficulty understanding spoken language. At the same time, these patients have only mild difficulty in spontaneous speech and writing! Heilman et al. (1978) presented an initially global aphasic, who, in the course of recovery, read better than he understood spoken language. A second right hemisphere stroke deprived him of this residual ability. In another patient with fluent aphasia, better reading than auditory comprehension was observed by Hier and Mohr (1977). Although the authors make a point of dissociation of auditory and visual mechanisms of comprehension, their findings of better semantic than phonetic association in the synonym—homophone reading task in fact suggested that the errors of visual identification were related to the auditory disturbance.

Alexia with Broca's aphasia is less frequently documented. It is often con-fused with the patient's inability to read aloud. Slowness and dislike of reading is often observed in Broca's aphasia, even though reading comprehension may be quite good. Benson (1977) considered alexia with frontal lobe pathology distinc-tive enough to call it "the third alexia." In Broca's aphasia, the reading com-prehension of meaningful content words is better than the relational or syntactic structures, similar to auditory comprehension. Other features characteristic of this variety of alexia were: scanning difficulty (gaze paresis), inability to main-tain verbal sequences, and literal alexia. Transcortical aphasia or isolation syn-drome have been described with severe alexia and agraphia. On the other hand, conduction aphasics seem to have normal reading comprehension, but writing is often paragraphic to the same extent that their speech is paraphasic. Those with more severe alexia usually have a more posterior lesion. Letter (literal) alexia is seen frequently in aphasics; patients with anomic aphasia who have difficulty naming letters may be able to read words quite well. Benson and Geschwind (1969) thought that some cases of letter alexia were, in fact, letter naming difficulty. There is less dissociation, however, between letter and word reading than in the other two forms of alexia (Brown, 1972). At times, questions or commands read aloud normally may lead to incorrect response. This may represent impaired comprehension or impaired praxis, depending on the nature of the response. Also, paralexic reading may still result in correct response. Reading aloud without comprehension was called transcortical alexia by Dejerine (1880), and word-meaning blindness by Nielsen (1939). This seemingly paradoxical phenomenon is easier to understand if one considers that some sensory aphasics do not comprehend even their own fluent speech, and that even normals can read foreign text without understanding it. A nearly opposite clinical state is the loss of phonemic reading ability but the retention of semantic reading ability, which was described by Albert et al. (1973). Their patient, who only had Anomic aphasia, could not read letters, words or sentences, but could identify them by auditory stimuli from a multiple choice, select a written word on the basis of their semantic category, or match it to pictures. This is different from pseudoalexia, in that reading comprehension was impaired, even though recognition through other modalities appeared to be facilitated. According to Brain (1961), and in our personal observations also, alexia with agraphia can be the residual disturbance after aphasia involving spoken speech resolves.

SURVEYS, LINGUISTIC FEATURES, ANATOMY, AND RECOVERY

Alajouanine (1960) reviewed 22 cases with alexia and found eight with agnosic alexia or optic alexia and considered that the dissociation between the overall reading loss and relative preservation of analytical reading was characteristic of this variety. On the other hand, in aphasic alexia, a frequent dissociation is observed between verbalization and comprehension. The reading is global and not analytical. Hecaen and Kremin (1976) studied 41 cases with left hemisphere lesions with a reading battery. Three of these patients had pure alexia and five other patients came close to the alexic patients in performance; these had paraphasias, verbal comprehension problems, writing, copying and spelling disturbances, acalculia, and visual field defects, and three of these patients had color naming defects, as well as constructional apraxia. He did not find any significant correlation with the apraxias and agnosias. A principle component analysis to study the relationship between the clustered variables of the tests was performed; there seemed to be a dichotomy between recognition and reading, and between recognition of meaningful and nonmeaningful material. There appears to be a trichotomy between reading of meaningful material and nonsense syllables and letters. One patient had selective deficit at the sentence level, one at the level of letters, and another for words. Anatomical studies of 14 alexic patients by Hecaen, showed that verbal alexia may exist with occipital lesion, without any involvement of the splenium (Hecaen and Kremin, 1976). In a case of literal alexia, a double lesion involving the occipital lobe and the temporoparietal lobe seemed to be necessary. The frequency of reading impairment was higher with isolated temporal lesions than with occipital and parietal lesions in a large number of left hemisphere lesions (Hecaen and Angelergues, 1964). Recovery from occipital lobectomy, with initial global alexia, subsequently revealed that after 10−12 days, individual letters could be read again, and shortly afterwards, syllables and short words. After a month, a text could be read slowly. Some words were deciphered by spelling. Writing disorders were absent or slight, with the exception of inability to copy. Eventually, considerable recovery was observed, but the patients continued to be slow and they disliked reading.

Gardner, Denes, and Zurif (1975) suggested that aphasics with anterior lesions tend to read "for meaning," focusing on substantive, pictureable elements and encountering difficulty with lexical elements that bear a contiguous, "syntagmatic" relationship to one another. Patients with posterior lesions have more difficulty with substantives than with interstitial words and benefit from lengthier, redundant messages. Gardner and Zurif (1976) found significant correlation between the severity of comprehension deficit and the reading of words and phrases. Patients with significant comprehension deficit were good at recognizing misspelled words, poor at matching nouns with depicted referents, better at recognizing the syntactical than the semantic value of words, and better at matching words that belonged together than choosing the odd word out. Mild aphasics benefited from the addition of lengthier phrases while severe aphasics did not. The severely aphasic patient approaches a text using strategies more morphologically than semantically. Reading comprehension seems to be better preserved in comparison to auditory comprehension in posterior lesions, while the reverse obtains in anterior ones.

A quantitative and qualitative analysis of the paralexias was done by Marshall and Newcombe (1966). The patient had a traumatic left temporoparietal lesion. Errors were more frequent for adjectives and verbs than for nouns. Functional words were omitted frequently. Semantic paralexias occurred with nouns and visual paralexias occurred with adjectives and verbs. In a subsequent paper, Marshall and Newcombe (1973) distinguished three types of alexias:

1. a *visual alexia,* in which paralexias consist of confusion of letters or words that are graphically similar
2. a *surface dyslexia,* in which the paralexias result from a partial failure in the application of the grapheme−phoneme conversion rules, producing a large number of neologisms
3. a *deep dyslexia,* or syntactic or semantic dyslexia, in which the paralexias are of a semantic type

Weigl and Bierwisch (1970) postulated two stages in reading; first, the identification of the graphemic structure and then, the actualization of the meaning. Newcombe and Marshall (1973) described stages of recovery of reading, following removal of a left occipital abscess. Reading errors consisted of a breakdown in grapheme to phoneme recording and in late stages, errors of visual analysis were predominant. Central deficits of lexical access manifested in word finding difficulty and syntactical problems may persist and not respond to treatment.

HEMIALEXIA AND THE ROLE OF THE CALLOSUM

Trescher and Ford (1937) and Maspes (1948) presented cases of alexia following sectioning of the splenium of the corpus callosum, involving only the left visual field. Benson and Geschwind classify this as hemialexia. As a result of sectioning of the splenium of the corpus callosum, some patients have difficulty reading in the left visual field. However, there are some patients who can comprehend words with the right hemisphere and can choose the correct objects with their left hand, flashed to the left visual field, on a tachistoscope (Sperry and Gazzaniga, 1967). It is possible that patients who can do this had some damage in childhood or infancy, allowing the right hemisphere to develop certain perceptual functions, otherwise dominated by the left hemisphere. Geschwind (1962) revived the importance of the callosal lesions in pure alexia. Visual input from the right hemisphere relating to objects is spared in pure alexia because it evokes other sensory associations. Another hypothesis considers that since the callosal lesion is incomplete, it has resulted in a reduction of capacity of transferring information and only the less sophisticated or advanced forms of visual information are transferred (Oxbury et al., 1969). Hecaen (1975) presented a case of alexia, unchanged for four years, and, on autopsy, the splenium appeared to be intact. He felt that the presence of lesion in the white matter of the occipital lobe may have given the same effect of interrupting the callosal fibers from the other hemisphere.

PSEUDOALEXIA AND PARALEXIA

Under "pseudoalexia," Benson and Geschwind included difficulty reading aloud by some Broca's aphasics and Conduction aphasics, while reading comprehension is preserved. Kinsbourne and Warrington (1962) distinguished unilateral paralexia, which was incorrect reading of part of a word of part of a sentence, such as seen with right posterior hemisphere damage and neglect of the left visual field. These patients continue to read correctly in their good visual field with vertical presentation. Paralexia then is used also in the sense of a reading difficulty due to a perceptual problem, such as hemianopia, visual neglect, or scanning difficulty. "Paralexia of the visual completion" refers to errors at the end of the words. This is attributed to hemianopia with macular involvement, impairing the left to right scanning movements. The opposite side is impaired in Hebrew readers with alexia (Sroka et al., 1973). Tachistoscopic perception of words in the right visual field was superior to the left (Mishkin and Forgays, 1952). This was attributed initially to the attentional habit of English readers, as contrasted to Hebrew readers, who showed left visual field superiority. This was not confirmed subsequently and the right field superiority for words is attributed to cerebral asymmetry (Kimura, 1966). The left field, on the other hand, has been found to be superior for letters; this has been suggested as a mechanism whereby patients with alexia without agraphia were better in letter reading than word reading (they were using their right hemisphere) (Woods and Poppel, 1974). Howes (1962) noticed that alexic patients needed higher luminance and longer exposure duration for three-letter words, and that they did much worse with seven-letter words. There was a lack of influence of word frequency for three-letter words, but the presence of this influence for longer words and the elevation of perceptual threshold in alexic patients compared to normals. Difference for object perception, however, was much less than for lexical items.

SPECIAL READING DISORDERS, ORIENTAL SCRIPT, AND BRAILLE

Special reading disorders were described in Japanese patients, with two systems of reading affected separately. The Kana system of phonetic, syllabic script is more often involved and its disturbance is equivalent to alexia related to angular gyrus and aphasic alexia. On the other hand, the Kanji system of ideographic writing is more susceptible to more posterior, occipital involvement. An article by Kotani (1935) describes a case of alexia with agraphia, in which the reading of Kana was more affected than Kanji. The opposite situation, that is retaining Kana symbols better than Kanji, was seen in "mixed" forms of transcortical aphasia (Sasanuma, 1975). Apparently, reading words in Kanji involves direct graphic strategy or a direct access to the semantic representation of lexical items, while reading words in Kana involves an indirect phonetic strategy, since reading requires an intermediate phonological process to arrive at the meaning. Sasanuma et al. found right hemisphere superiority for Kanji words and left hemisphere superiority for Kana words presented tachistoscopically. Alexia in a patient with acquired blindness who could read Braille was observed by Gloning et al. (1955). They demonstrated the loss of Braille from biparietal cerebral metastases. The patient had more trouble with words than letters and could not type. They considered that the lesion near the right-hand kinaesthetic association area in the left parietal lobe was crucial to produce verbal alexia in the blind.

Another case of tactile alexia for Braille, due to a stroke, was described by Simonyi and Palotas (1959). They considered the type "aphasic alexia" and described a method of retraining the patient. Another patient with alexia and agraphia in Braille recovered faster than the therapist could learn Braille (Parker, 1970)! Various degrees of alexia for different languages in a polyglot were described by Hinshelwood (1917). Interestingly, the impairment was greatest in English and the least in Greek, the reverse of what was expected from the patient's use of these languages.

ALEXIA AND APHASIA: A STUDY OF OUR POPULATION

We decided to explore the relationship of alexia and aphasia further, and determine the extent of reading disability in various aphasic groups. This information is lacking in the literature. We examined 225 aphasics on a reading task, consisting of nine subtests. It includes the shortened version of the reading comprehension of sentences task of the Boston Diagnostic Aphasia Examination, using a multiple choice response requiring no verbal output (Read Sent). Another task involves reading commands aloud and performing them (Read Comm). The others are word−object choice matching (word−obj), picture stimulus−word choice matching (pict−word), word stimulus−picture choice matching (word−pict), phonetic association (phon assn), letter reading (letter read), recognition of spelled words (spell recog), and spelling (spell)—see Chapter 3 for detailed description of these tasks. The requirements for inclusion in this study

Table 11–2

Reading Subtests Means and Standard Deviation

| Group | N | Subtests and maximum score | | | | | |
		Read Sent 40	Read Comm 20	Word Obj 6	Pict Word 6	Word Pict 6	Phon Assoc 4
Global	29	2.68±6.3	1.62±4.2	1.06±1.5	1.17±1.9	1.10±1.6	0.55±0.8
Broca	37	13.6±11.4	6.12±7.5	4.42±2.1	4.91±1.8	4.62±1.8	2.40±1.3
Isolation	4	5.0±8.7	5.50±9.7	4.25±2.8	2.50±2.6	2.50±2.5	2.50±1.9
Transcortical Motor	9	19.7±16.5	15.8±4.0	4.50±2.3	3.66±2.8	3.66±2.3	3.33±1.6
Transcortical Sensory	20	7.0±10.6	4.57±7.2	1.89±2.4	2.10±2.2	2.52±2.3	1.89±1.6
Conduction	23	20.9±11.3	13.8±7.0	5.68±0.8	5.68±0.5	5.78±0.5	3.05±1.2
Wernicke	17	5.29±7.5	4.00±6.5	3.35±2.5	3.17±2.5	3.82±2.5	1.64±1.3
Anomic	86	25.1±11.5	17.7±4.1	5.74±0.9	5.62±1.2	5.70±1.2	3.52±0.8
N.A.A.R.	18	34.7±5.4	19.8±0.4	6.00±0	6.00±0	6.00±0	4.00±0
Nondominant	69	33.2±7.7	19.1±2.8	5.50±1.4	5.61±1.0	5.72±1.1	3.66±0.8
Normal	22	36.0±6.8	19.6±1.1	6.00±0	6.00±0	6.00±0	4.00±0

were that the patients attempted the tasks and scores were recorded: 69 nondominant hemisphere lesion patients and 22 normal controls were also examined on the reading tasks, as well as on written and spoken subtests of the WAB. The patients were classified taxonomically, according to the spoken language tasks (see Table 4-2).

The means and standard deviations on the reading subtests are displayed in Table 11-2. Nonfluent aphasics are in the top half of the table, the fluent ones in the bottom. They are ranked according to severity (the AQs are displayed on the right side). Globals, of course, achieve low scores, but Broca's aphasics indeed comprehend written material much better than isolation, transcortical sensory, and Wernicke's aphasics with higher AQs. The best reading comprehension scores are achieved by conduction and anomic aphasics. Transcortical motor aphasics are better in reading and performing commands than conduction aphasics, even though the results of reading comprehension are the reverse. This may be related to the poor praxis of conduction aphasics. Even though transcortical sensory and isolation aphasics have low reading comprehension, they are considerably better in recognition of spelled words than Broca's and transcortical motor aphasics. The total reading scores follow reading comprehension closely, the lowest being global, then Wernicke's, isolation, and transcortical sensory aphasics. Relatively good reading totals are achieved by Broca's, transcortical motor, conduction, and anomic aphasics. Nondominant hemisphere controls achieve significantly better total reading scores than anomics, the best aphasic group.

The correlation coefficients of reading tasks with other language subtests for

Table 11-2 (continued)

Letter Read 6	Spell Recog 6	Spell 6	Reading Total 100	Writing 100	Compre-hension 100	AQ 100
0.58±1.2	0.17±0.53	0.17±0.60	9.13±13.8	2.7±9.5	2.38±1.0	11.7±8.9
3.48±2.5	0.68±1.2	0.34±1.1	41.2±23.4	20.1±20.4	6.58±1.5	30.9±17.3
2.25±2.8	3.25±1.7	1.50±1.0	29.2±30.3	12.0±23.3	4.67±2.9	48.7±15.9
4.66±2.4	2.66±2.3	1.83±1.9	64.2±29.1	34.4±29.7	6.82±1.7	62.7±8.4
3.47±2.2	3.05±2.3	3.52±2.1	30.9±26.1	27.5±22.6	5.63±1.5	64.6±11.3
5.52±0.84	1.89±1.9	1.94±1.9	65.4±20.5	40.5±26.7	8.31±0.92	65.2±12.3
3.52±2.6	0.88±1.7	1.29±1.7	28.1±20.7	16.5±18.1	4.20±2.0	44.5±17.2
5.70±1.0	4.62±1.4	4.30±1.5	77.7±17.0	57.3±23.3	8.87±1.1	83.9±10.4
6.00±0	5.40±0.8	5.40±0.8	91.6±7.0	85.8±21.5	9.82±0.2	97.1±1.4
5.57±1.3	4.90±1.4	4.55±1.3	88.1±13.2	69.6±22.1	9.65±0.45	94.9±5.3
6.00±0	5.42±0.5	5.14±0.6	95.9±8.2	85.5±14.7	9.94±0.13	98.8±1.3

all aphasics ($N = 225$) revealed that the reading total correlated best with the naming score, then with the aphasia quotient (overall severity of aphasia), and these were closely followed by writing and calculation (Table 11-3). RCPM, repetition, fluency, and comprehension have somewhat lower correlations with reading but they are all significant. Correlation coefficients for the reading subtests revealed similar trends, except that reading comprehension correlates best with auditory comprehension, then with naming, calculation, writing, and the aphasia quotient.

The correlation of reading total with other language subtests in each aphasic group (Table 11-4) revealed a high correlation with AQ in all groups. Low values in the control groups reflect little or no variability. Comprehension total, naming, calculation, and writing seemed to have high correlations for all groups.

In conclusion, these results show that reading is impaired in all aphasic groups but the variation between aphasic groups is significant. Reading comprehension is better in Broca's and transcortical motor (or nonfluent) aphasics,

Table 11–3
Reading Tasks/Group Correlation with Language Subtests

	SSFL	Comp	Rep	Nam	AQ	Calc	RCPM	Writ T
Read Sent	0.41**	0.70	0.45	0.66	0.62	0.64	0.61	0.64
Read Comm	0.52	0.76	0.59	0.78	0.73	0.64	0.55	0.71
Word Obj	0.34	0.34	0.37	0.63	0.57	0.61	0.51	0.54
Pict Word	0.30	0.30	0.29	0.55	0.50	0.57	0.53	0.55
Word Pict	0.39	0.39	0.36	0.60	0.57	0.57	0.51	0.55
Phon Assoc	0.41	0.41	0.49	0.65	0.63	0.59	0.55	0.61
Letter Read	0.50	0.50	0.51	0.65	0.68	0.59	0.56	0.62
Spell Recog	0.60	0.60	0.75	0.77	0.77	0.54	0.37	0.61
Spell	0.65	0.65	0.70	0.69	0.73	0.50	0.27	0.64
Read Total	0.55	0.55	0.61	0.81	0.78	0.73	0.66	0.75**

**$p \leq 0.01$ in all cases.
Aphasic N: 225

Table 11-4
Reading Total/Group Correlation with Language Subtests, AQ Writing

Group	N	AQ	SSFL	Comt	Rep	Nam	Calc	Writ T	RCPM	Prax	Draw
Global	29	0.406*	0.073	0.388*	0.383*	0.608**	0.237	0.044	-0.110	-0.031	0.233
Broca	37	0.571**	0.102	0.737**	0.398**	0.663**	0.587**	0.679**	0.497**	0.595**	0.622**
Isolation	4	0.968*	0.576	0.950*	-0.892	0.997**	0.975	0.963*	1.000**	0.895	0.975
Transcortical Motor	9	0.394	-0.228	0.612*	-0.154	0.018	0.724*	0.555	0.894**	0.768**	0.873*
Transcortical Sensory	20	0.491*	-0.080	0.537**	-0.184	0.699**	0.454*	0.498*	0.405	0.377	0.276
Conduction	23	0.513**	0.270	0.309	0.395*	0.516**	0.651**	0.673**	0.618**	0.337	0.597**
Wernicke	17	0.651**	0.422*	0.816**	0.312	0.440*	0.665**	0.692**	0.395	0.598**	0.118
Anomic	86	0.632**	0.158	0.629**	0.568**	0.625**	0.435**	0.430**	0.504**	0.431**	0.442**
N.A.A.R.	18	0.193	-0.087	0.186	-0.044	0.159	0.072	-0.226	0.190	-0.478*	0.036
Nondominant	69	0.314**	0.079	0.439**	0.323**	0.285**	0.514**	0.415**	0.457**	0.219*	0.444**
Normal	22	0.835**	—	0.565**	0.664**	0.752**	0.623**	0.587**	0.758**	0.225	0.602**

even though their aphasia quotient is worse than some of the fluent aphasics with poorer reading. The one exception to this seems to be the recognition of orally spelled words, which is more impaired in nonfluent aphasics. This is not strictly a reading task and it is spared in pure alexia. Reading scores correlated best with naming, severity (AQ), writing, and calculation.

READING ALOUD VERSUS READING COMPREHENSION

In an attempt to determine if there was any difference in the aphasics' ability to read aloud and to perform commands, 56 patients were given six commands of increasing complexity printed one to a card. The patient was asked to read it aloud and then to follow the command. Each section was worth ten points and a difference of more than two points was considered significant. The patient was penalized for paraphasias and only partial performance. Of the 14 patients with Broca's aphasia, six patients or 43 percent were able to perform the commands better than they could read them aloud. Only one severely apractic patient was able to read aloud better than he could follow commands. Two patients with conduction aphasia were tested. One of these read aloud and performed the commands easily. The other patient made abundant paraphasic errors in reading the commands but performed them well. Twenty anomics were examined and 20 percent of these were significantly alexic. However, only one of these patients had significantly better reading aloud than performing the commands and he was also apractic. Wernicke's and global aphasics had difficulty reading aloud or performing the commands, although it has been reported that a few patients with Wernicke's or transcortical sensory aphasia will read aloud, some without comprehending it.

VARIETIES OF ALEXIA

The incidence of the varieties of alexia, such as literal, verbal, global, and sentence alexia, was determined in our population of aphasics who had the reading task completed. Those who achieved better than 50 on the combined score of sentence comprehension (maximum 40), reading of commands aloud (maximum 10), and performing same commands (maximum 10) were considered not alexic (normal reading) for the purpose of this study. The rest were divided into the various groups of alexias taxonomically, according to their sentence reading comprehension (maximum 40), word reading (maximum 12)—actually a matching task—and letter reading (maximum six)—also visual matching of a sample stimulus to a choice of six. A synoptic table was constructed to define the alexic syndromes unequivocally (Table 11-5).

Literal alexia was defined as poor letter reading ($\leqslant 3/6$) and good word

Table 11–5
Classification of Alexia

	Sentence (40)	Word (12)	Letter (6)
Literal	0–40	7–12	0–3
Verbal	0–40	0–6	4–6
Sentence	0–20	7–12	4–6
Global	0–20	0–6	0–3
Diffuse	21–40	7–12	4–6

Normal: Achieved better than 50 on the combined score of sentence comprehension (maximum 40) and reading of commands aloud (maximum 10) and performing same commands (maximum 10).

reading ($\geqslant 7/12$). Verbal alexia was defined as poor word reading ($\leqslant 6/12$) and good letter reading ($\geqslant 4/6$). Sentence alexia was poor sentence reading comprehension ($\leqslant 20/40$) with good word and letter reading. When all aspects of reading were severely affected, we used the term global alexia, and when all aspects were moderately affected, diffuse alexia.

The incidence of each variety was determined in each aphasic group (Fig. 11-1), and the percentages in each group and the subtotals of the varieties are displayed in Table 11-6. These results indicate that literal alexia ($N = 22$) occurs most frequently with Broca's aphasia, a point made by Benson (1977). Literal and sentence alexia are often seen together when word reading is spared and one is tempted to establish a separate category. However, in this study, the more severely affected individuals with literal and sentence alexia fall in the category of literal alexia and the less severely affected ones into the diffuse group. The high incidence of sentence alexia in Broca's aphasia is noteworthy although it is seen with equal frequency in anomic aphasia. Verbal alexia is the least common variety ($N = 16$), but it is seen relatively frequently in transcortical sensory, Wernicke's, and Broca's aphasia. Global aphasics commonly have global alexia but the spared word reading in a few provides a relatively high incidence of literal alexia. Broca's aphasics predominantly have literal and sentence alexia, while Wernicke's aphasics suffer from sentence and global alexia. Conduction aphasics show sentence and diffuse alexia.

In conclusion, this study attempts to assess and analyze the varieties of alexias in aphasia, in a quantitative and objective fashion. The taxonomic analysis of alexia in aphasia indicates that most aphasics are alexic as well, with the exception of 53 percent of anomic aphasics, many of them mild, 30 percent of transcortical motor aphasics, and 20 percent of conduction aphasics who were not alexic. Only one Broca's aphasic had normal reading. We also found one Wernicke's aphasic without alexia, small percentages in this large and representative aphasic population. The Wernicke's aphasic was atypical with borderline auditory comprehension scores. Apart from a few paraphasias, these resembled "pure word deafness." There was also a case of global aphasia who

THE VARIETIES OF ALEXIA IN APHASICS

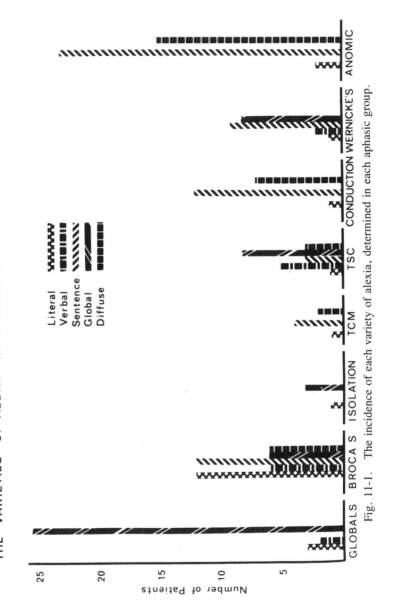

Fig. 11-1. The incidence of each variety of alexia, determined in each aphasic group.

Table 11-6

The Percentages of the Varieties of Alexia in Aphasics

Type of Alexia	Globals (34) %	Broca's (43) %	Isolation (4) %	Transcortical motor (10) %	Transcortical sensory (20) %	Conduction (25) %	Wernicke's (21) %	Anomic (87) %
Litera (22)	9	28	25	10	5	4	5	2
Verbal (16)	6	14	0	0	25	0	9	1
Sentence (63)	0	28	0	40	15	48	43	27
Global (54)	85	14	75	0	40	0	38	0
Diffuse-A (33)	0	14	0	20	15	28	0	17
Normal (56)	0	2	0	30	0	20	5	53

did significantly better on sentence comprehension than on word or letter reading. He did not fit into any of the taxonomically defined varieties. His better
sentence reading performance may be related to random pointing to the multiple
choice answers, rather than to true reading comprehension.

The variability of reading skills will tend to increase the levels of breakdown
in alexia due to brain damage. Much speculation has been made about the
relationships of the linguistic processes involved. The error patterns of *literal
alexia* suggest a disturbance of grapheme to phoneme strategy, which is prominent in some cases of Broca's or other motor aphasias. In these cases, a direct
route between visual images and semantic analysis without an acoustic element is
likely. Pattern recognition of words is retained, but some lexical elements can not
be "sounded out."

On the other hand in *verbal alexia,* the semantic interpretation of written
words (word finding) appears to be impaired selectively. A failure of pattern
recognition or a disconnection from auditory associations could both result in this
deficit. It is the least common variety but more likely to be encountered with
alexia without agraphia.

In most cases of aphasic alexia, the error types are multiple and the distinction is blurred as to which strategy of reading is impaired. The semantic
phonological and orthographic factors of reading are often affected together,
although most of the above mentioned varieties can be distinguished in patients.

SUMMARY

Alexia is defined and classified with a review of the pertinent literature. The
main varieties of pure alexia, alexia with agraphia, and aphasic alexia are described in detail. Anatomic, linguistic, and epidemiological studies, as well as
special varieties of alexia and closely related disorders are reviewed. Our study
of the reading performance of 225 aphasics is briefly presented, indicating good
reading comprehension in nonfluent aphasics, and high correlation between reading, naming, severity of aphasia, writing, and calculation.

Another study compared reading aloud and reading comprehension. Only
one anomic patient read aloud better than his comprehension, but the reverse
dissociation was more common, especially in Broca's aphasics.

A third study of the incidence and distribution of the taxonomically defined
varieties of alexia is presented. Literal alexia was common in Broca's aphasia,
while verbal alexia, which is the least frequent variety, was seen in Wernicke's
and transcortical sensory aphasia. Sentence alexia was seen in Broca's, conduction, and anomic aphasia.

12

Agraphia, Acalculia, and the Gerstmann Syndrome

The Moving Finger writes; and, having writ, moves on.

Omar Khayyam

THE LITERATURE ON AGRAPHIA

Writing has developed relatively late in man's history, and also in his individual development. Writing was regarded as the symbol of symbols by Hughlings Jackson (1864). Written speech is usually more premeditated, precise, and terse than the spoken word. The vocabulary used is more extensive and stylistic, and grammatical constraints are more rigorous. The differences between the spoken "vernacular" and written forms of language can be considerable, as pointed out by MacDonald Critchley (1970). Benedikt (1865) used the term "agraphia" for the first time in the literature, and Ogle (1867) classified agraphia as ataxic when the letters cannot be written, and amnemonic when the letters are used incorrectly. Subsequently, many classifications for agraphia were attempted; Table 12-1 summarizes these. It became evident that agraphia differs when it is associated with a reading disorder alone, or with sensory aphasia or motor aphasia. Pitres, in 1873, classified agraphia as: (1) occurring with word blindness, (2) with word deafness, or as (3) motor agraphia (graphoplegia). Wernicke (1886) divided agraphias along the lines of his classification of

Table 12-1

The Classification of Agraphias

Ogle	1867	Ataxic			Amnemonic			
Pitres	1873	Graphoplegia	With word deafness		With word blindness			
Wernicke	1886			Cortical Form	Subcortical	Transcortical	Conduction	
Monakow	1914	Cheiro-kinesthetic	Sound					
Henschen	1920	Frontal	Temporal	Parietal	Angular	Occipital		
Pick	1931	Secondary to motor defect	Paragraphic		With Alexia	Without alexia	Ideational	
Kleist	1934			Constructional	Ideokinetic			
Nielsen	1946	Frontal apraxic	Formulation	Constructional	Angular gyrus	Parieto-occipital	Ideokinetic apraxic (callosal)	External capsule
Goldstein	1948	Motor (pure)		Innervatory (cortical)	Amnestic apraxic		Ideational apraxic (callosal)	
Leonhard	1952				Ideokinetic	Optokinetic	Conduction (callosal)	
Critchley	1953	Frontal	Temporal	Parietal	Dyslexic	With Gerstmann		
Leischner	1957	Linguistic motor	Linguistic sensory	Constructional	Amnestic	Apraxic		
Hecaen	1963	Expressive	Sensory	Spatial	Parietal			Developmental

aphasias: (1) cortical, (2) subcortical, (3) transcortical, and (4) conduction. He also distinguished between literal and verbal agraphia. Wernicke did not think a separate writing center likely, as he considered writing to be very closely associated with language and with visual copying. Henschen (1922) promoted Exner's writing center in the second frontal convolution, opposite to the hand area (Exner, 1881). Since then, this has been debated vigorously. The localization of agraphia producing lesions has been reviewed recently by Leischner (1969). Most authors will agree that pure agraphia probably cannot be produced by a localized lesion at F2, but that one can come close to it in a Gerstmann syndrome, with an angular gyrus lesion, associated with very little, if any, aphasia or alexia.

Arnold Pick (1931) considered the mechanism of agraphia to be dependent upon the availability of the image of a script and its evocation, which is related to the activity of the angular gyrus region; this, in turn, activates automatized motor sequences in the F2 region. Pick observed that copying may be preserved, in contrast to dictation, but that they are often affected together. He contrasted the act of volition and automatism and found that copying one's name may be more affected than the signature. He considered writing a more difficult task than speaking, but occasionally, it is better performed, and although paragraphia often corresponds to paraphasia, the two sometimes diverge. Discussing the relationship of agraphia to aphasia, Pick concluded that although writing from dictation is influenced by disorders of the acoustic component, word deafness may not be accompanied by agraphia, indicating that the motor patterns of writing can be activated apart from the auditory system. Goldstein (1948) distinguished primary agraphia without aphasia, which could be:

1. Ideational apraxic agraphia, in which the concept of the letter shape is impaired
2. Amnestic apraxic agraphia, when the patient cannot write names
3. Motor or pure agraphia, when the use of the hand is preserved for everything else
4. Innervatory or cortical agraphia
   Secondary agraphia occurred with aphasia

Nielsen (1946) believed in:

1. Angular agraphia
2. Ideokinetic–apraxic parieto-occipital agraphia
3. Ideokinetic–apraxic corpus callosum agraphia
4. Formulation agraphia
5. Frontal apraxic agraphia
6. Capsula externa agraphia.

Callosal agraphia in the left hand has been called conduction agraphia by Leonhard (1952). He also believed that bilaterality of writing occurs more often than bilaterality of language. He thought that, in cases of agraphia with right-sided lesions, reading may be dissociated from writing, and that writing may be located on the right and reading on the left side.

Leischner (1957) reviewed 23 cases of agraphia. The first group consisted of linguistic agraphias, which were closely related to aphasias. The second group was called constructional agraphias, associated with parieto-occipital symptoms. The third group consisted of apraxic agraphias, and the fourth group was developmental agraphia, related to parietal lobe damage before the age of learning to write. He observed that agraphia was obligatory in total aphasia, except for a few automated words, such as name and address. A paragraphic style of writing, with nouns and verbs, but without connecting words, is seen with motor aphasia. Paragraphias of the literal or verbal type usually accompany motor agrammatisms; as motor aphasia recovers, mistakes of spelling and syntax are seen. Sensory aphasia produces more frequent paragraphias, and, at times, the amount of writing is similar to the jargonlike speech output; the patient may show an overproduction. Cases of copious jargon agraphia (graphorrhea) have been published by various authors: Moutier (1908), Hecaen et al. (1963), and Kertesz and Benson (1970). Figure 12-1 is an example from a jargon aphasic whose writing approached quantity and quality of his spoken speech. In amnesic aphasia, the patient has word-finding difficulty in writing as well as in speech. Goldstein (1948) describes the agraphia associated with conduction aphasia and transcortical aphasia as similar to the spoken deficit. The association of agraphia with acalculia, right–left confusion and finger agnosia, has been described by

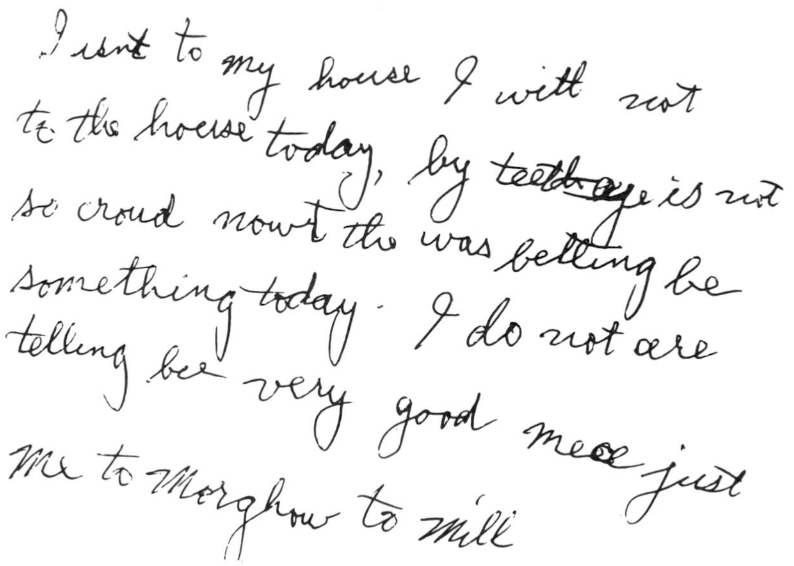

Fig. 12-1.   Jargon agraphia or graphorrhea.

Gerstmann (1924) (see below). The agraphia in this syndrome is more marked in spontaneous writing and dictation than in copying. It differs from the parietal syndrome associated with constructional apraxia, in that copying is not as much affected. In the more extensive parietal syndrome, copying may be more difficult than spontaneous writing. Abnormalities occur in letter formation, separation of words, and direction of words. Lineation becomes defective and the lines run into each other (Critchley, 1953). In moderate cases, semantic disturbances, omissions, misspelling, paragraphias, and neologisms may be observed, and in severe cases, the writing becomes illegible and amorphic. De Ajuriaguerra and Hecaen (1960) also emphasized the specificity of the spatial type of dysgraphia. This could be identified by a sudden steplike change in the line in the middle of a word, and the writing of single letters and small groups of letters in isolation. Similar symptoms can be found in posterior lesions of the right hemisphere. These are often characterized by writing only on the right side of the page, perseveration of the basic strokes of a letter, especially m, n, i, and v, and inability to keep to a line. In copying, only the right side is reproduced and the left is neglected.

Hecaen et al. (1963) delineated various types of agraphia.

1. Agraphia with expressive aphasia, with frontal and rolandic lesions, characterized by literal paragraphias and paragrammatisms. The patient can write common words, names, and addresses, but cannot describe his own profession or case history; copying is usually not affected. A direct parallel exists between verbal and written expression. Motor aphasia without writing disturbance is observed in purely cortical dysarthria. The paragrammatism is characterized by the use of nouns and the infinitive form of verbs.
2. Sensory aphasia due to temporal lesions often produces garbled and senseless, written speech.
3. In parietal agraphia, literal paraphasias, paragrammatisms, and word-finding difficulties are seen. The language disturbance, however, may be mild and the agraphia severe. Severe perseveration is often seen. Disturbance of copying points to the associated constructional apraxia.
4. Agraphia with conduction aphasia is characterized by better writing on dictation than spontaneously.

Special attention was paid, in the study, to the problem of agraphia in left-handers. They considered writing in left-handers to be more sensitive to brain damage than other linguistic functions. It did not seem to matter whether they wrote with the left or right hand. In right-sided lesions, agraphia was found to be more frequent among left-handers than right-handers. Alexia, sensory, and mixed aphasia occurred as much in the left-handed as in the right-handed patients. Motor aphasia was more often observed in the left-handers without agraphia, indicating a further dissociation of speech from writing between the hemispheres. Dubois et al. (1969) further pointed out the relative increase of pure agraphia in left-handers. It is considered possible that left-handers handle writing differently, on the basis of alternative functional organization of the brain. Heilman et al. (1973) presented a case of a left-hander who developed left hemiplegia without aphasia, but who had agraphia and apraxia of the right hand, attributed to a right hemisphere lesion. This case suggested to them that the patient's language dominance was in the left hemisphere and that dominance for handedness, writing, and praxis was in the right hemisphere. They found another case, this time a right-hander, with presumed right hemisphere dominance for language (a rare event in itself), but with left hemisphere dominance for praxis and writing (Heilman et al., 1974).

Chedru and Geschwind (1972) examined agraphia occurring in acute confusional states. They found writing frequently impaired in motor, linguistic, and spatial aspects, even without oral language disorder. Reiterated curves and loops, which are often seen in "pure agraphia" were not seen but the spatial aspects of writing were more impaired. They thought that isolated agraphia occurs primarily in the presence of diffuse brain damage. Basso et al. (1978) examined the dissociation between oral and written expression and found two cases of pure agraphia with lesions in the upper left parietal lobule. The occurrence of fluent anomic aphasia without agraphia is another interesting finding by the same authors. It is similar to the interesting case report of better written than oral naming by Hier and Mohr (1977). This patient could not write on dictation or read words, and the authors concluded that this case represents a component or a subdivision of Wernicke's aphasia. Agraphia to dictation was considered a transcoding process by Weigl and Fradis (1977). They found it selectively blocked, that is, without associated disturbances of comprehension, repetition, reading, and audiovisual matching in five out of 15 cases. More defective written than oral spelling was observed in a patient with Gerstmann syndrome (Kinsbourne and Rosenfield, 1974). They made a point that perseverative repetition of letters suggests a frontal lobe lesion, order errors indicate posterior inferior parietal location, characteristic of the Gerstmann syndrome, and letter substitutions are more characteristic of aphasic agraphia.

A different form of agraphia—"efferent motor agraphia"—was postulated by Ferguson and Boller (1977) in three cases with nonaphasic motor disorders. They hypothesized that this may be produced by the disturbed feedback from hand and speech movements, just like artificial writing impairment can be induced in normal subjects by having them write while looking at their work under delayed visual feedback. Sasanuma and Fujimura (1972) investigated 50 aphasics and 30 controls on a writing task in Japanese. Graphical confusions were seen in aphasics and nonaphasics in the Kanji transcriptions (ideograms). Phonological confusions were most of the errors in Kana letters (syllabic script). Aphasics with "apraxia of speech" showed larger numbers of Kana errors than the rest of the aphasic group. They concluded that "Kana" is processed through a phonological mechanism, and "Kanji" may have direct access to the lexical items bypassing this "phonological process."

WRITING STUDY WITH THE WAB

We examined agraphia in the context of aphasia, with a standardized test of writing, in 225 aphasics and 109 controls. The test is a part of the WAB; a detailed description can be found in Chapter 3. It includes examination of writing on request, on dictation, and copying, the written output on describing a picture, and recalling written symbols. The means and standard deviations of the scores achieved by various aphasic and control groups on the writing subtests, as well as calculation, reading, comprehension and aphasia quotient (AQ), are compared in Table 12-2. The control groups consist of 18 patients who had recovered by the time of their first examination, 69 nondominant hemisphere damaged, nonaphasic patients, and 22 normal, age matched controls. Aphasics are grouped according to the taxonomic criteria described in Chapter 4 (Table 4-2).

Global aphasics have very low writing scores, although copying is better than all other subtests. The total writing scores of Broca's aphasics are considerably higher than those of isolation, Transcortical Sensory, and Wernicke's aphasics, even though these all have higher AQ or severity ratings. The low comprehension groups seem to have the low total writing scores! This relationship seemed to apply to all other writing subtests including copying. All aphasics had higher scores on copying, but Wernicke's improved the most, when compared to dictation. Writing scores discriminated all groups from normal controls (Table 12-2). Writing is a very sensitive measure of aphasic impairment and, at times, right hemisphere damage.

Correlation of writing with other language and nonverbal subtests (Table 12-3) revealed the most significant values for calculation, reading, Raven's matrices (RCPM), drawing, and comprehension, with a less impressive relationship to praxis, naming, and AQ. Fluency and repetition correlated the least with writing total.

ACALCULIA

Calculation involves a multiplicity of mental processes. First of all, there is the notion that quantities are bigger or smaller, and, also, that they are part of a whole. After dividing the whole, parts of the whole can be counted as units, and replaced by numerical symbols. Manipulation of these symbols requires spatial concepts and the special syntax of calculation; including addition, subtraction, division, and multiplication. The degree of acquired calculation skill is very much education dependent.

Table 12–2

Writing subtests, reading, AQ, and Calculation Means and Standard
Deviations

Tests and maximum scores	Global N=29	Broca's N=37	Isolation N=4	Transcortical motor N=9	Transcortical sensory N=20
Name, address (/6)	0.12±0.45	1.94±1.85	1.12±2.25	2.66±2.56	2.30±2.11
Picture description (/34)	0±0	2.40±5.81	1.50±3.00	2.72±4.91	2.07±4.00
Dictated sentences (/10)	0.34±1.8	1.22±2.67	0.25±0.50	3.05±3.43	2.60±3.02
Dictated words (/10)	0.32±1.7	1.34±2.33	1.12±2.25	3.88±3.65	3.35±2.82
Alphabet (/12.5)	0.34±1.50	2.01±3.04	1.50±3.00	4.55±4.60	4.75±4.76
Numbers (/10)	0.20±1.11	3.65±4.32	2.50±5.00	6.33±4.77	4.52±4.70
Dictated letters (/2.5)	0.12±0.49	0.87±0.98	0.75±1.19	1.61±1.21	1.37±0.97
Dictated numbers (/5)	0.17±0.92	1.12±1.69	1.00±2.00	2.77±2.16	2.75±1.97
Copy sentence (/10)	1.01±2.45	4.60±4.22	2.12±4.25	4.94±4.51	3.57±3.56
Writing total (/100)	2.75±9.54	20.18±20.48	12.00±23.33	34.44±27.71	27.50±22.67
Reading total (/100)	9.13±13.80	41.21±23.44	29.25±30.33	64.22±29.17	30.90±26.18
Calculation (/24)	1.46±3.60	12.62±8.32	5.33±9.23	12.88±7.55	11.35±6.65
Comprehension (/10)	2.38±1.07	6.58±1.54	4.67±2.94	6.82±1.75	5.63±1.56
Aphasia quotient (/100)	11.71±8.95	30.97±17.35	48.75±15.90	62.75±8.49	64.67±11.30

Table 12-2 (continued)

Conduction N=23	Wernicke's N=17	Anomic N=86	Recovered N=18	Nondominant N=69	Normal N=22
3.21±2.09	1.82±1.90	3.98±1.71	5.30±1.29	5.08±1.31	5.63±0.58
7.17±7.74	0.52±1.08	11.30±10.37	24.80±9.18	18.59±10.61	26.95±7.99
3.06±2.88	1.50±2.88	5.71±3.54	8.82±1.71	8.20±2.29	9.56±1.10
4.54±3.89	1.70±2.86	6.21±3.16	7.91±2.61	6.82±3.13	9.00±0.70
4.81±4.57	2.55±3.93	8.72±3.87	11.33±1.69	9.26±3.60	10.50±0.10
6.27±4.36	2.88±3.74	8.13±2.86	9.75±0.61	9.08±2.47	10.00±0.10
1.56±1.02	0.55±0.84	2.05±0.0	2.50±0.76	2.20±0.61	2.00±0.70
2.68±1.88	0.70±1.31	3.80±1.61	4.83±0.40	3.96±1.48	5.00±0
7.15±3.63	4.11±4.40	7.44±2.99	8.58±2.15	7.31±3.35	10.00±0.10
40.52±26.76	16.58±18.13	57.32±23.36	82.39±17.01	69.62±22.16	85.54±14.75
65.47±20.50	28.11±20.73	77.71±17.04	91.66±7.02	88.13±13.23	95.95±8.26
14.00±8.00	7.37±8.63	18.71±5.84	22.77±1.70	21.82±4.16	23.27±1.45
8.31±0.92	4.20±2.06	8.87±1.17	9.82±0.26	9.65±0.45	9.94±0.13
65.22±12.30	44.52±17.25	83.96±10.44	97.17±1.46	94.90±5.34	98.84±1.38

Table 12–3

Correlation of Writing with Language and Reading Subtests/Groups

Groups	N	AQ	Fluency	Comprehension	Repetition	Naming	Calculation	Reading	RCPM	Praxis	Drawing
Global	29	0.10	−0.02	0.26	0.17	0.01	0.83**	0.04	0.38*	0.31	0.37*
Broca's	37	0.37*	0.06	0.54**	0.20	0.41**	0.59**	0.67**	0.49**	0.47**	0.68**
Isolation	4	0.92*	0.34	0.94*	−0.73	0.97*	0.99**	0.96*	0.96*	0.78	0.99**
Transcortical motor	9	0.30	−0.25	0.40	0.03	−0.08	0.83**	0.55	0.45	0.62*	0.40
Transcortical sensory	20	0.39*	0.16	0.46*	−0.29	0.35	0.21	0.49*	0.45*	0.53*	0.57**
Conduction	23	0.44*	0.15	0.29	0.36*	0.40*	0.83**	0.67**	0.60**	0.56**	0.72**
Wernicke's	17	0.40	0.11	0.53*	0.38	0.19	0.71**	0.69**	0.32	0.63*	0.40
Anomic	86	0.39**	0.22*	0.43**	0.30**	0.25**	0.46**	0.43**	0.49**	0.38**	0.70**
Nondominant	69	0.51**	0.29**	0.43**	0.31**	0.49**	0.36**	0.41**	0.50**	0.42**	0.45**
Normals	22	0.83**	—	0.60**	0.35	0.43*	0.30	0.58**	0.58**	0.34	0.66**

*-$\leq$0.05. **$p\leq$0.01.

The Pearson r is used to calculate the correlation coefficients between writing and other parameters.

Lewandowsky and Stadelmann (1908) described a case of calculation disorder with agraphia and alexia in detail. Poppelreuter (1917) said that calculation is always involved in aphasia because of the auditory language factor in calculation. Peritz (1918) published a study of acalculias, and distinguished between visual, acoustical, and ideational forms. Henschen (1920) described the disorders of calculation after surveying the literature and named it acalculia; he differentiated cypher and number deafness, number blindness, and errors in the naming and writing of numbers, without actual disorders of calculation. He found that number reading difficulties may occur with occipital lesions, associated with an inability to copy. He observed acalculia in occipital, frontal, parietal, and temporal lesions, and drew the conclusion that calculation can be impaired from many different regions. He felt that the arithmetical system was independent of general intelligence, and also from the systems of language and music. Sittig (1921) described agnosia for operation symbols, such as a minus sign, multiplication sign, etc. The association of acalculia with Gerstmann syndrome (Gerstmann, 1924) and constructional apraxia (Kleist, 1934) is a well-recognized and important feature. Often, the nature of acalculia is considered a constructive one in parietal syndromes. This is characterized by the inability to manipulate parts of numbers or relate them to each other horizontally or vertically. Perseveration and memory disturbance also interfere with calculation. This makes the evaluation of acalculia exceedingly difficult.

Hecaen et al. (1961) found 183 cases of calculation disorders in postrolandic lesions. They differentiated between the groups.

1. Patients with predominantly number alexia and agraphia (aphasic acalculia)
2. Acalculia with spatial disorganization
3. True arithmetical difficulty

The second group occurred with right-sided lesions, and the first and third groups with aphasia and alexia in dominant hemisphere lesions. Grewel (1969), in his review of the acalculias, divided primary acalculia into asymbolic acalculia and asyntactic acalculia. Secondary acalculia occurs with aphasia and with the Gerstmann syndrome (see below). A complicating factor in aphasics is the interference of expressive difficulties with calculation. Paraphasic responses may create the impression of acalculia. Benson and Denckla (1969) reported two patients with Gerstmann syndrome who appeared to have calculation disturbance, one caused by paraphasic substitution of numbers, which improved when a multiple choice response was used. They warned against accepting acalculia with a single mode of presentation and response. The second patient was considered to have more of a primary computational disorder, as he had no obvious aphasia. Benson and Weir (1972) presented a case with accidentally discovered difficulty with complex computation, who actually complained of reading problems and also had a right inferior quadrantanopsia and agraphia. They felt that in the absence of language or spatial disturbance, the patient had true "anarithmetia" (Hecaen's third variety). It seems that the process of calculation can be disturbed in a multiple and complex fashion. The isolation and analysis of various factors involving acalculia remains difficult and unstandardized.

CALCULATION STUDY WITH THE WAB

The calculation subtest of the WAB was deliberately designed to be simple, to avoid intellectual and educational influences. Only two-digit additions, subtractions, multiplications, and divisions are included, and the task is given verbally; at the same time, the patient is allowed to look at a card showing the task in print (to eliminate perceptual or input difficulties), and the correct answer out of a choice of four. The patient is allowed to respond verbally or by pointing, thus minimizing the output problems as well. Responses are accepted also by pointing to the multiple choice of four, out of which one is correct, and another, incorrect choice is correct for the opposite maneuver (addition instead of subtraction, etc.). The response choices are placed one under another to exclude hemianopic problems which may interfere with the test.

We analyzed the calculation scores according to various taxonomic groups of aphasics. The grouping is the same as it is for writing (see Table 4-2). The mean values and standard deviations of calculation scores for each group is displayed, along with the writing subtests, in Table 12-2. The variation within the various aphasic groups is most similar to the writing scores. Globals do poorly, but Broca's aphasics are much better than would be expected on the basis of the aphasia quotient or severity rating alone. Among the rest of the aphasics, low comprehension groups had poor calculation scores also.

Calculation correlated best with writing in all groups (Table 12-4). Reading, drawing, RCPM, and praxis were next, followed by naming, comprehension, and AQ, with a lesser degree of correlation.

THE GERSTMANN SYNDROME

Finger agnosia, right and left disorientation, agraphia, and acalculia was described by Gerstmann as a clinical syndrome, in 1924. In a subsequent paper, Gerstmann (1940) described the acalculia as involving either complex arithmetical operations or even simple numbers. The patient is disoriented regarding the sequence and the decimal values of the digits. Gerstmann explained the relationship between finger agnosia, agraphia, acalculia, and right and left disorientation, by the important part played by individual fingers and the right and left laterality in acquisition of the functions of writing and calculating. He argued that fingers supply the first aid in learning to calculate and they are important in the development of writing. The word "digit" means both finger and numeral. In

Table 12-4

Correlation of Calculation with Reading, Writing, and Language Subtests

Type	N	Fluency	Comprehension	Repetition	Naming	AQ	Praxis	Drawing	RCPM	Reading	Writing
Global	29	0.04	0.19	0.28	0.43*	0.27	0.00	0.30	−0.01	0.23	0.83**
Broca's	37	0.02	0.57**	0.23	0.47**	0.39**	0.45**	0.48**	0.45**	0.58**	0.59**
Isolation	4	0.50	0.99*	−0.84	0.98*	0.99*	0.77	1.00**	0.97	0.97	0.99**
Transcortical motor	9	−0.36	0.62*	0.15	−0.11	0.31	0.87**	0.51	0.61*	0.72*	0.83**
Transcortical sensory	20	−0.45*	0.17	0.21	0.38*	0.00	0.19	0.12	0.55*	0.45*	0.21
Conduction	23	0.17	0.23	0.16	0.28	0.29	0.51**	0.71**	0.56**	0.65**	0.83**
Wernicke's	17	0.04	0.49*	0.12	0.34	0.31	0.55*	0.07	0.18	0.66**	0.71**
Anomic	86	0.04	0.62**	0.33**	0.54**	0.54**	0.50**	0.50**	0.51**	0.43**	0.46**
Nondominant	69	0.11	0.22*	0.36**	0.21*	0.26*	0.04	0.24*	0.33**	0.51**	0.36**
Normal	22	—	0.17	0.64**	0.52**	0.61**	0.00	0.23	0.54**	0.62**	0.30

$*p \le 0.05.$ $**p \le 0.01.$

The Pearson r is used to calculate the correlation coefficients between calculation and other parameters.

this later paper, he also acknowledged that constructive apraxia, word-finding difficulty and mild reading difficulty, impairment of color perception, and absence of optokinetic nystagmus may be associated with this syndrome. He interpreted this as involvement of the neighborhood structures. He also mentioned four cases himself; two with glioma and two with infarct, with localization to the parieto-occipital region, particularly the angular gyus and the area of transition to the second occipital convolution. He went on to distinguish between a primary and a secondary syndrome. In the secondary syndrome, the clinical picture is dominated first by a more extensive complex of signs, and only after regression of these symptoms does the syndrome of finger agnosia and its related disturbance emerge. The development of this syndrome depends on the nature of the underlying lesion. More extensive lesions will include other symptoms. He emphasized the practical use of the syndrome in the local diagnosis of space-taking lesions in the lower part of the parietal lobe, or in the transitional zone of the parieto-occipital region. The Gerstmann syndrome was further detailed by Schilder (1931), who spoke about finger aphasia, optic finger agnosia, and constructive finger apraxia. Most clinicians consider these further divisions superfluous and clinically not contributory. Subsequently, Critchley (1953) discussed the syndrome in detail in his monograph on the parietal lobes. Kinsbourne and Warrington (1962) characterized the problem as a finger sense defect, and emphasized the frequent occurrence of constructional apraxia and other supernumerary symptoms.

Recently, several articles attacked this syndrome as a fiction and an artifact of biased observation. Benton (1961) felt that the four components occurred together only in a case of a large lesion; and that the isolation of the syndrome occurred only when other symptoms were ignored. Heimburger et al. (1964) claimed that the individual components are more likely to appear separately. Poeck et al. (1966) said that the bond between the symptoms in Gerstmann's syndrome is no closer than the association between these symptoms and others outside of them. They also suggested that acalculia is an aphasic symptom. Critchley (1966) summarized the controversy about Gerstmann's syndrome, and withdrew his support of the developmental variety he himself described in 1942. Cases of developmental Gerstmann syndrome continue to be published, such as the two cases of Benson and Geschwind's (1970), who had constructional apraxia but were both good readers. Strub and Geschwind (1974) described a case of Gerstmann syndrome without aphasia, and in their reply to Poeck's (1975) criticism they stated that it did not matter whether the intercorrelation is low between the symptoms; it was important that the syndrome had a predictive value of a left parietal lesion. They agreed that Gerstmann's syndrome was typically associated with other deficits, but that this did not invalidate its usefulness. Benton (1977) had the last word recently. After reviewing both sides of the issue, he felt that the localizing significance appears to be related to the components of agraphia and acalculia. Finger agnosia appears to be carrying only the implication of either aphasic disorder or mental impairment. To most neurologists and neurosurgeons, the syndrome remains synonymous with a left parieto-occipital lesion. Whether its components are arbitrarily selected or not, the traditional use of the syndrome will likely continue in the future.

GERSTMANN SYNDROME IN OUR POPULATION

Although the criteria as to what is an acceptable Gerstmann syndrome vary considerably, we have labeled nine patients clinically in our population of 556 aphasics and controls examined on the WAB (see Table 12-5). There were others called Gerstmann syndrome casually, by a resident or a staff neurologist, but they were either not examined in detail for some reason or, on examination, they turned out to be frankly aphasic or demented. The ones under this label had agraphia, acalculia, right and left disturbance, and finger agnosia outstanding from other deficits. One with a large parietal meningioma and another with traumatic hemorrhage had mild Wernicke's aphasia, and a third with metastatic tumor fell in the transcortical sensory category. Six patients were not considered significantly aphasic, although every one of them had mild word-finding difficulty and some had naming difficulty. In one patient, both finger agnosia and agraphia were very mild but definite enough for this diagnosis. None of them were "pure" examples of the tetrad. Cases 3, 5, and 7 had significant naming difficulty, and 3, 6, and 7 significant constructional apraxia (see drawing, block design, and RCPM scores). Cases 1, 3, and 6 were the most typical, in that they had the severe tetrad (with constructional apraxia) but no significant language impairment. A left parieto-occipital lesion was discovered in seven out of nine cases. (Figs. 12-2 and 12-3). One patient had bilateral lesions, and one with trauma, a negative scan. This is a representative example of the clinically diagnosed syndrome in our unit. If we exclude the three cases with definite aphasia and the mild one with near normal scores, we are left with five cases (1,3,5,6,7) which would be acceptable to most clinicians. We then established a control group of patients with significant agraphia (<57), acalculia (<14), but without significant aphasia (AQ>74.2, word discrimination>50), based on the limits set by the test scores of this clinical group.

We found 23 other patients within the above criteria but only five of these would fit "Gerstmann syndrome" as the rest of them either did not have finger agnosia or right−left disorientation, or either of these two components. These five patients did not receive the clinical label of Gerstmann syndrome because two of them had transcortical motor aphasia, two of them presented with severe alexia, and one was seen for bilateral subdural hematomas. Localization of lesions in this control group, when it was available (13 cases), still yielded a high number of left parietal lesions (six). There were also three frontal, two bilateral, one temporal, and one right parietal abnormalities. This suggests that agraphia

Table 12–5
Clinical Features—Gerstmann's Syndrome

Patient	Sex	Age	Etiology	Aphasia	Scan	Writing	Calculation	Finger recognition	Right-left discrimination	AQ	Information	Fluency	Comprehension	Repetition	Naming	Reading	Praxis	Drawing	Block Design	RCPM
1	M	64	Infarct	—	Left parietal	24	14	2	6	83.4	9	8	7.4	9.4	7.9	61	83	18	6	17
2	F	70	Infarct	—	Left parietal	70	18	4	7	91.9	9	9	9.5	9.4	9.0	84	—	11	9	20
3	F	63	Aneurysm	—	Left pareital	7	12	4	3	86.2	9	9	8.1	10.0	7.0	74	—	9	3	—
4	F	42	Hemorrhage Trauma	Wernicke's	Left parietal	16	0	2	5	68.6	7	9	6.3	7.8	4.2	3	84	9	1	12
5	M	39	Trauma	—	Normal	57	12	3	6	79.2	8	8	8.4	8.0	7.2	68	—	24	9	27
6	M	59	Neoplasm	—	Left pareital	14	10	3	4	93.4	10	10	7.9	10.0	8.8	78	—	13	5	15
7	M	76	Neoplasm	—	Left parietal	45	12	4	4	74.2	7	8	7.1	8.2	6.8	76	65	9	4	19
8	M	75	Neoplasm	Wernicke's	Left parietal	4	0	0	3	62.6	6	5	6.2	7.5	6.6	22	42	13	3	15
9	M	76	Neoplasm	Transcortical sensory	Bilateral	21	10	2	0	52.8	4	6	6.2	9.2	1.0	21	63	17	0	7
Maximum Scores						100	24	5	7	100	10	10	10	10	10	100	90	30	9	36

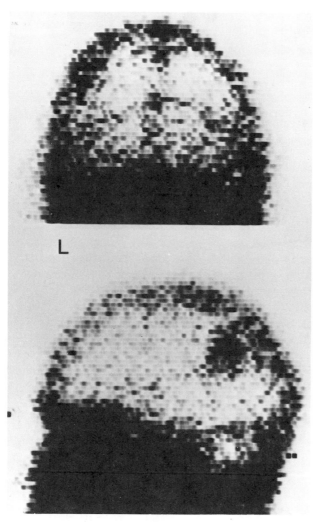

L

Fig. 12-2.   Case 1—Gerstmann syndrome.

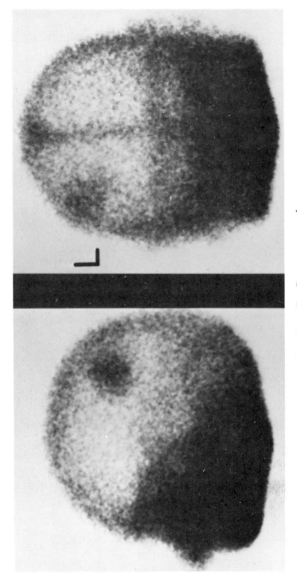

Fig. 12-3. Case 7—Gerstmann syndrome.

and acalculia without significant aphasia are also significant determinants of a left parietal lesion, even in the absence of finger agnosia and right−left disorientation.

SUMMARY

Writing is a late learned system of symbols, secondary to speech. Disturbances of writing, and of calculation, are closely associated with aphasia. The categories of parietal, angular gyrus, constructional, apractic, amnestic, ideokinetic, etc., agraphia more or less overlap, and there is little justification to separate them. Some agraphias appear to have more constructional than linguistic components. Agraphias are mostly distinguished by the symptoms they are accompanying (aphasia, alexia, acalculia, etc.). The severity of agraphia and acalculia seemed to correlate with comprehension deficit more than the severity of aphasia. Right-sided lesions can cause agraphia and acalculia but these are quantitatively different and usually relate to spatial, constructional difficulties.

Relatively isolated agraphia and acalculia are rare, and they often occur together or with alexia and constructional apraxia in left parietal lesions. The addition of finger agnosia and right−left disorientation to agraphia and acalculia constitutes the Gerstmann syndrome, which often signifies a left parietal tumor when it appears *de novo*. Although the specificity of this tetrad is questioned, in our experience it may be more predictive of a left parietal lesion than agraphia and acalculia alone.

13

Apraxia

Shape without form, shade without color
Paralyzed force, gesture without motion.

T. S. Eliot (1927)

DEFINITION

Liepmann defined apraxia as a "disturbance of purposeful movement" despite retained mobility, assuming that it was not due to lack of comprehension. He credited Steinthal with the first use of the word "apraxia." Hughlings Jackson (1866) called attention to the frequency of motor disturbances in aphasics, especially the difficulty protruding the tongue. He said that voluntary actions were lost before automatic ones because of the hierarchial dissolution of the nervous system in disease. Nothnagel (1887) wrote about "paralysis of intent," a motor disturbance which would be distinct from paralysis or ataxia, but rather an impairment of the memories for motor patterns. Meynert, in 1890, compared this motor disturbance to motor aphasia and called it a lack of motor symbols. Wernicke (1900) considered apraxia as a transcortical disconnection of the substrate of intellectual activity from the motor region. The general idea of attributing these clinically common motor disturbances to a failure of intellectual function or lack of comprehension or agnosia was prevalent before Liepmann. In a series of articles, from 1900—1920, Hugo Liepmann described three kinds of apraxia: (1) limb kinetic (2) ideomotor (3) ideational (Liepmann, 1920). Actually, he accepted Pick's (1905) addition of ideational apraxia.

This classification, although often quoted, has not gained universal acceptance and, to some extent, it has confused the issue because it is difficult to apply to clinical cases. It seems that the majority of authors now doubt the separate existence of limb-kinetic apraxia and consider ideational apraxia as either apraxia of complex movements or as a severe form of ideomotor apraxia in which even the use of objects is impaired. Yet this classification continues to be the base of discussion in modern work, and cannot be disregarded. In Table 13-1, the equivalent terms are aligned.

VARIETIES OF APRAXIA

Ideomotor (ideokinetic) apraxia (IMA)

This is the common variety, seen with many aphasic syndromes, often with the anterior or motor (Broca's) type. It is equivalent to Heilbronner's (1907) transcortical apraxia. The patient has difficulty performing simple voluntary acts with his nonparalyzed hand, whether he has to pretend or use actual objects, although the use of the latter usually improves the performance, as does imitation. There is no paralysis in the limb and the patient comprehends the command (these are implied conditions). The performance of "automatic" or "emotional" acts with the same set of muscles is not impaired. An example is the patient with "motor aphasia" and right hemiplegia, who cannot wave goodbye with his left hand on command, but will do so in response to the departure of the examiner. Liepmann interpreted this kind of apraxia as a "gap" between the normal kinetic engrams and the rest of cerebral functioning. Liepmann found apraxia of the left hand in 14 of 18 patients with right hemiplegia and severe aphasia and six of 23 right hemiplegics without severe aphasia and termed it "sympathetic dyspraxia." It did not occur in the right hand of left hemiplegics (Liepmann, 1905). He thought the lesions were subcortical in the left frontal lobe, producing, in addition to the right hemiplegia, a disconnection of the callosal transmission of motor patterns to the right frontal lobe. Geschwind (1963) considers this syndrome a subset of ideomotor apraxia, in addition to the other forms associated with callosal and supramarginal region lesions.

Liepmann's first case, the "Regierungsrat," who had right-hand apraxia, was found later to have left supramarginal as well as a callosal lesion (Liepmann, 1900). He thought that the posterior aspects and the motor regions of the left

Table 13-1
Classification of Apraxia

Liepmann 1900–1920	Pick 1905	Heilbronner 1905	Kleist 1907	Monakow 1914	Morlaas 1928	Sittig 1931	Denny-Brown 1958	Geschwind 1965
Limb kinetic		Cortical	Innervatory		Spatiodyskinetic		Kinetic	
Ideomotor		Transcortical	Ideomotor			Aphasic		Sympathetic Callosal
Ideational	Ideational		Amnestic	Ideogenic Amnestic	Object use	Agnostic	Kinesthetic	Ideational
Pseudopraxia				Parapraxia				
Parapraxia	Parapraxia							

Shilder and Gerstmann, 1926—gait apraxia.
Kleist, 1934—constructional apraxia.
Brain, 1941—dressing apraxia.
Goodglass and Kaplan, 1963 (modern descriptive)—buccofacial, transitive, intransitive, complex, truncal, upper limb, lower limb, performance on command, imitation, with object use.

233

hemisphere were disconnected and handling of objects, learned visually, was impaired, but buttoning, which required only tactile control, was not. He then originated the formulation that the left hemisphere was not only dominant for language but also for skilled movements. His second famous case, "Ochs," had extensive callosal disconnection (Liepmann and Maas, 1907). Monakow, although critical of Liepmann, seemed to agree with some of his ideas. "Bilateral ideomotor apraxia" was associated with left supramarginal gyrus lesions in 13 cases out of 41 with anatomical verifications (Monakow, 1914).

Limb-Kinetic Apraxia

Liepmann (1905) did not report a case of *limb-kinetic* (melokinetic) *apraxia* but he described it as: "The virtuosity which practice lends to movements is lost. Therefore the movements are. . .clumsy, without precision." He thought that this related to the destruction of kinetic engrams. Kleist (1907) called this cortical or innervatory apraxia. The existence of this type, however, is seriously doubted or denied by many authors. The relationship of manual dexterity to apraxia has been a subject of controversy. Although Pieczuro and Vignolo (1967) found ideomotor apraxia independent of manual dexterity, Heilman (1975) showed that apractic patients were slower on a finger tapping task than nonapractic aphasics.

Ideational Apraxia (IA)

This is a third form, representing a defect of purposeful movements, where the ideational project or plan appeared to be disordered, although engrams for individual movements were considered to be intact. Instead of accomplishing the desired objective, a false one is realized. The patient puts the match into his mouth in trying to light a cigarette; tries to drink from a cup by leaning over or under it, etc. Here, the whole series of action is impaired due to the conceptual disturbance. This failure of performing a series of complex movements was interpreted as a loss of goal concept by Pick (1905) and Marcuse (1904). Liepmann (1908) reported 6 cases of ideational apraxia in a series with 24 cases of ideomotor apraxia. More recently, Hecaen and Gimeno (1960) collected 8 cases of ideational apraxia with 47 cases of ideomotor apraxia.

Sittig (1931) felt that ideational apraxia was only a severe form of ideomotor apraxia, and refuted the concept of IA being a loss of serial, complex actions on the basis that even simple gestures may be disturbed at an ideational level. Pick (1905) showed that in diffuse brain diseases such as general paresis, degenerative diseases, etc., marked apractic disturbances occur. He differentiated this from that of Liepmann's ideomotor apraxia by its bilateral appearance and called it ideational apraxia. He explained it on the basis of a dissociation of a higher order caused by a loss of original intention. Monakow (1914) divided apraxia into six categories of which the description of "agnostic apraxia" or "parapraxia" seems to conform to the concept of ideational apraxia best; he felt that ideational apraxia had little or no localizing value as the lesions were diffuse or very large. Nathan (1947), Zangwill (1960), and Ajuriaguerra (1960) felt that ideomotor and ideational apraxia coincide and that the independence of ideational apraxia has not been reliably demonstrated.

Exceptions were cases with visuoperceptual deficits, suggesting bilateral damage. Ideational apraxia seems to be characterized by disturbance with or without the actual objects present, according to Denny-Brown (1958). He emphasized the loss of conceptual process in IA. DeRenzi et al. (1968) adopted Morlaas' (1928) definition of IA as the inability to demonstrate the use of actual objects. They defined IMA, on the other hand, as the inability to perform intransitive gestures on imitation (to wave "goodbye"). According to these definitions, IA was found in 33 percent of the aphasic group. They also found 11 patients with IA, who did not have IMA and 11 who showed the opposite dissociation. IA was closely tied to left hemisphere damage and aphasia, and it occurred mainly in patients with Global and severe Broca's and Wernicke's aphasia, all with poor comprehension, although the tests used did not require auditory comprehension. Clinical observations on the ward suggested that these patients could still eat, wash, brush their hair, etc., in real life situations. These observations point to the essential difference between their definition of IA (demonstrating the use of actual objects) and the much less common "true IA" when complex movements are disturbed outside the test situations also.

More common is the patient who does poorly on verbal command and imitation, but does better in the presence of the normal stimuli or objects. Geschwind (1965) made the point that he has not seen patients who fail with objects but succeed in carrying out the task on imitation or verbal command. He implicated the visuomotor connections of the dominant hemisphere and the corpus callosum, both being necessary for bilateral imitation of the examiner's movement. He also postulated that there are some people who can make use of the right visuomotor connection, however. These patients with left hemisphere lesions could still carry on movements, on imitation, with the left hand. In the case of Geschwind and Kaplan (1962), the patient showed difficulty only with the left hand, when the information had to be transferred from the left hemisphere, such as in performing verbal commands, drawing, or identifying objects with the left hand. However, he could imitate with his left hand. Apractic difficulties could be induced in the right hand when the stimulus came from the right hemisphere, such as drawing objects held in the left hand. Their patient had a massive involvement of the left frontal lobe by tumor and the corpus callosum was markedly thinned in its anterior portion. Infarct was seen in the anterior cerebral artery distribution.

Another simplification of the concept of ideational apraxia is that it means the loss of ability to "pretend," Heilman (1973) presented three cases of what he considered ideational apraxia. In contrast to the cases of DeRenzi (1968), his patients had no difficulty handling objects or imitating movements, but demonstrated a disorder of intransitive, as well as transitive movements on command. He felt that the distinction between ideomotor apraxia and what he considered ideational apraxia was that his patients improved on imitation, while the patients with IMA frequently failed to do so. Many would doubt that this distinction is sufficient to define ideational apraxia.

The controversy, then, continues in the interpretation of ideational apraxia. Most clinicians feel that the defect in the actual use of objects represents a severe form of ideomotor apraxia. The definition of ideational apraxia as a defect in the performance of a series of movements, or, on the other hand, as a defective use of objects, has not been fully satisfactory. Patients who have trouble using objects in common, natural situations usually have bilateral or diffuse lesions and may also be described as having ideational apraxia. It is recognized that there is an apraxic defect, which is usually related to a dominant parietal lobe lesion, in which, although the commands are understood, the idea of the movement seems to be lost, in contrast to the more frontal type of apraxia associated with Broca's aphasia. This type of apraxia is perceived as a deficit of symbolic function, similar to the loss of abstract attitude of Goldstein (1948). This is the recurring theme of "asymbolia" which originated with Finkelnburg (1876), and has been popular with subsequent authors. A recent opponent of this concept is Kimura (1976). She found that right-handers gesticulated with the right hand, while left-handers tended to use both hands during speaking. This asymmetry in hand movements appeared as early as the evidence of functional asymmetry for speech in children. Kimura and Archibald (1974) pointed out that unfamiliar and less verbalizable movements are also impaired in apraxia, in support of the notion that impairment of gesture may be independent from that of language.

Their study with left hemisphere lesion patients showed impairment in the performance of meaningless manual sequences, but not of finger flexion or copying static hand postures, indicating that the impairment was more salient when a series of movements was required. Kimura has put forth the theory that symbolic language functions of the left hemisphere are secondary to the specialization of motor function. She also cited the case of Leischner (1957) in support of this theory. This patient, who was congenitally deaf, had impairment in manual signing, and his lesion was in the angular and supramarginal gyrus and the underlying white matter, on the left side. One could argue the opposite view, also, that this is exactly the area where symbolic functions are processed, regardless of the output modalities, such as speaking, writing, or signing.

LOCALIZATION

There is general agreement that lesions causing apraxia are in the left hemisphere when it is dominant for speech. Only occasionally will apraxia in the left hand be the result of a right hemispheric lesion. Hecaen et al. (1960) found

13 cases in the literature and added three of their own. Some of these were left-handers and some had left hemisphere lesions also. It is at times difficult, but nevertheless, important to differentiate apractic disturbances from motor neglect, impersistence and perseveration which are features of nondominant hemisphere lesions. The magnetic and repulsive types of kinetic response described by Denny Brown (1958) are also in this realm.

Ajuriaguerra et al. (1960) had 58 cases of apraxia, 11 ideational, and 47 ideomotor: 48 occurred with left hemisphere damage and ten had bilateral lesions. There were none with right-sided lesions. The callosal localization has been discussed above in the cases of Liepmann and Geschwind. Zaidel and Sperry (1977) observed the persistence of mild left-handed apraxia and right-handed copying difficulty 6 to 8 years after callosal section. Bimanual coordination was also impaired.

Foix (1916) believed that ideomotor apraxia occurred with occlusion of the parietal branch of the artery to the angular gyrus and ideational apraxia with the temporal branch. Ajuriaguerra et al. (1960) found ideomotor apraxia with parietal and temporal lesions, and ideational apraxia with large posterior parietal lesions.

According to Luria (1966), damage to the premotor area leads to disruption of movements requiring sequencing responses with preservation of movements requiring unique parts of the same response. Lesions of the postcentral regions forming part of the "proprioceptive analyses" leads to an "afferent" apraxia, in which the accurate direction and fine control of movements is lost. Parieto-occipital lesions cause impairment of the spatial organization of action.

DESCRIPTIVE CLASSIFICATION

Classification by the region involved or by the actual movement tested is gradually taking the place of the ideomotor-ideational dichotomy.

Facial Apraxia

Facial apraxia was considered to be the most common variety (Nathan, 1947). DeRenzi et al. (1966) found it in 90 percent of Broca's aphasics and in 33 percent of conduction aphasics. It may be seen in isolation, without significant limb apraxia. Geschwind (1965) thought it represented only a special form of sympathetic dyspraxia, in which those parts of the pathways involving the limbs are relatively spared, but not those involving the face, which are lower lying and closer to Broca's area.

Trunkal Apraxia

Trunkal apraxia or complex whole body movements may be retained, while limb and face movements fail. Geschwind considered axial movements to be mediated by the temporopontine bundle of Turck, from Wernicke's area to the pontine nuclei. Later on, however, he modified this idea by considering that there is an outflow from Wernicke's area to some brain stem motor system, although this is not by way of the pontine nuclei (Geschwind, 1979). There are other explanations such as those by Brown (1972), that the right hemisphere comprehends and carries out body movements, as opposed to limb movements, directed by the left hemisphere. Sittig (1931), in his monograph on apraxia, felt that more automatic functions, such as body movements, have lower and more generalized localization and may be preserved in local hemispheric damage.

Gait Apraxia

Gait apraxia was described by Gerstmann and Shilder (1926) as a disorder of walking in the absence of limb weakness, ataxia, or sensory impairment. Various other terms have been in use, such as frontal disequilibrium and frontal apraxia. Some of these phenomena are closer to extrapyramidal akinesia or paresis than true apraxia.

Dressing Apraxia

Dressing apraxia has been described as a specific inability to put garments on (Brain, 1941). Hecaen (1962) found dressing apraxia in 22 percent of right and 4 percent of left hemisphere cases. It is probably not a true apraxia but more related to the visuospatial difficulties of the nondominant hemisphere, such as "constructional apraxia." Denny-Brown (1958) considered it with the framework of neglect and "amorphosynthesis."

APRAXIA AND APHASIA

Goodglass and Kaplan (1972) preferred to use descriptive terminology to study apraxia. They assessed buccofacial, intransitive limb, transitive limb, whole body, and serial actions. In their previous study (Goodglass and Kaplan, 1963), natural expressive gestures, conventional gestures, and pantomime were also studied. Gestural enhancement, vocal overflow—when a patient verbalized the action instead of doing it—and the use of body parts for objects were special features noted.

The coexistence of apraxia with aphasia is well accepted. More controversial is their interdependence. Goodglass and Kaplan did not find significant correlation between the severity of aphasia and gestural ability in their study of 20 patients (1963). We have studied the gestural disturbances in a large population of aphasics, with special reference to the severity of their aphasia and language parameters.

APRAXIA STUDY WITH THE WAB

We employed a comprehensive apraxia test, to include most aspects of gestural expression, similar to that used by Goodglass and Kaplan (1972). Rather than dividing apraxia into ideomotor or ideational apraxia, we used descriptive terms, pertaining to the actual movements. Such categories were:

1. "Upper limb praxis," such as making a fist or waving goodbye.
2. "Buccofacial praxis," such as sticking out the tongue, sniffing, or closing the eyes.
3. "Instrumental," which involved the use of a comb, a hammer, or a spoon.
4. "Complex," such as asking the patient to pretend to drive a car, play the piano, or fold a paper. These tasks were bimanual.

Initially, we included movements involving legs, as well as trunkal movements, but because of the difficulty employing these with most hemiplegic patients, we had to delete this part of the testing in some of the subjects; these data are not used here. The results were calculated by transforming the raw scores to percentages of the total maximum allowable score. Scoring was specifically tailored to the quality of performance: "acceptable or standard" performance, as judged by the examiner on the basis of clinical experience, was scored 3; "approximate" performance or performance on imitation only scored 2; and approximate performance on imitation or if only performed with an actual object scored one. The maximum score for the 20 item task was 60. The sequence of testing was suggested by Goodglass and Kaplan (1972). First, the command was given and if the patient did not understand it, it was repeated, again asking the patient to pretend the movement or to use a certain instrument. Approximate performance on verbal stimulation was accepted, but if the patient did not perform, the next step was requested, by asking the patient to imitate the examiner. If this was not performed either, finally the instrument or object was given to the patient for actual use.

We included 387 patients—262 aphasics and 125 controls—in the study. Some of these patients had a series of tests and when they changed from one aphasic category to another, the new tests were included in that particular category, as well as the original one. Altogether, 473 tests were done, where both the aphasia and apraxia tasks were completed, but only the first one for each patient was included in the study, if they remained in the same category.

The aphasic types were defined by our usual taxonomic criteria (see Table 4-2). There were three groups of control patients for comparison. The first were recovered aphasics, N-32, in whom the total score or Aphasia Quotient (AQ) on the Western Aphasia Battery reached 93.8, which is the cutoff point for the WAB, for aphasia, obtained from the mean of a previous control group of nonaphasic, brain damaged patients (Kertesz and Poole, 1974). The other groups were 72 cases of nondominant hemisphere lesions and 21 normal, age-matched patients, from the hospital, who were admitted for other than intracranial disease. The population consisted of stroke cases mainly, but a proportion of tumor and trauma were also tested (Table 13-2). The male−female ratio was 2.7:1 and the left-handed and ambidextrous patients were excluded. To reduce the effect of severe comprehension deficit, those patients whose comprehension was 2 standard deviations below the mean for the total aphasic group were excluded. This left 216 aphasics for analysis from the original total of 262.

THE EXTENT OF APRAXIA IN VARIOUS TYPES OF APHASIA

Mean scores for various categories of apraxia are tabulated in each group, including the total praxis score in addition to comprehension and the AQ (Table 13-3). Global aphasics, as expected, performed poorly on all gestural subtests and their apraxia score is low, like their AQ. Excluding those with the most severe comprehension deficit reduced the number of this group significantly. Broca's aphasics did much better than global aphasics, and, interestingly, also surpassed isolation aphasics, even though their mean AQ is lower than that group. However, their comprehension scores are much better also. Transcortical motor, transcortical sensory, and conduction aphasics have similar praxis scores and comparatively better AQ, indicating a milder from of aphasia. They are undistinguishable from each other, on the basis of their apraxia scores, although their comprehension is significantly different. Wernicke's aphasics, on the other hand, had relatively poor scores on praxis, along with a lower AQ and lower comprehension. Anomic aphasics approach normals in their performance on the praxis tests, but there is a significant difference between anomics and the control patients, especially in complex movements, where anomics seem to have

Table 13–2
The Etiology of Aphasics and Controls in the Praxis Study

| | APHASICS | | CONTROLS | | | |
| | | | | Recovered | | Nondominant |
Etiology	N	Percentage	N	Percentage	N	Percentage
CVA	151	69.9%	21	65.6%	60	83.3%
Hemorrhage	16	7.4%			3	4.2%
Aneurysms	14	6.5%	2	6.25%		
Neoplasms	21	9.7%	2	6.25%	8	11.1%
Trauma	14	6.5%	7	21.9%	1	1.4%
TOTAL	216		32		72	120

Table 13–3

Mean Scores for Subtests and Total Praxis, Comprehension, and
Aphasia Quotient

Type	N	Upper limb	Bucco-facial	Instru-mental	Complex	Praxis Total	AQ	Compre-hension
Maximum Score		*15*	*15*	*15*	*15*	*60*	*100*	*10*
1. Global	(18)	4.7	5.8	3.5	2.5	16.6	12.3	2.9
2. Broca's	(48)	11.9	9.8	8.9	7.7	38.4	33.4	6.3
3. Isolation	(6)	8.6	8.5	4.8	3.8	25.8	41.7	3.3
4. Transcortical motor	(7)	13.7	12.8	11.8	10.0	48.4	66.7	7.8
5. Transcortical sensory	(17)	12.8	13.5	11.1	10.2	47.2	62.5	5.3
6. Conduction	(24)	13.3	12.7	12.7	11.5	50.4	60.9	7.9
7. Wernicke's	(21)	11.8	12.0	9.3	8.3	41.6	48.1	4.8
8. Anomic	(75)	14.6	14.3	13.9	13.0	56.0	84.9	8.9
Total Aphasic	(216)							
9. Recovered	(32)	14.9	14.8	14.7	14.3	58.9	97.3	9.8
10. Nondominant	(72)	14.8	14.7	14.4	14.0	58.0	94.5	9.5
11. Normal	(21)	14.2	14.1	14.1	14.2	56.8	94.1	9.4
Total Control	(125)							

more difficulty than either normal aged controls or nondominant or recovered
patients. However, the total praxis score is comparable, even though the AQ of
anomics is significantly below that of the recovered group. The relatively
superior performance of the recovered aphasic group may be related to their
lower mean age, when compared to the ages of normal and nondominant hemisphere injured populations.

Analysis of variance and *t* tests showed the praxis means to be significantly
different from the rest of the aphasic population in global, Broca's, isolation,
and anomic groups. The significance of the differences between those aphasic
groups which were closet in their scores was also determined (Table 13-4).
Globals were different from Broca's in all respects, and Broca's from isolation
aphasics in limb, instrumental apraxia, and in total praxis. No significant difference was found between transcortical sensory or motor aphasics. The only
significant difference between Broca's and Wernicke's group was the poorer
facial praxis, even though total praxis scores are the same. This is in support of
the idea that Broca's aphasics have more facial apraxia. Recovered aphasics,
dominant hemisphere lesions, and normal controls were significantly different

Table 13–4

The Difference of Praxis between Groups

Comparisons	Upper limb	Bucco-facial	Instru-mental	Complex bimanual	Praxis Total	AQ
Global–Broca's	≤0.01	≤0.01	≤0.01	≤0.01	≤0.01	≤0.01
Broca's–Isolation	NS	NS	≤0.05	NS	≤0.05	NS
Broca's–Wernicke's	NS	≤0.01	NS	NS	≤0.01	≤0.01
Transcortical sensory–Motor	NS	NS	NS	NS	NS	NS
Transcortical sensory–Conduction	NS	NS	NS	NS	NS	≤0.01
Anomic-recovered	NS	≤0.05	≤0.01	≤0.01	≤0.01	≤0.01

The difference is calculated using student t test. For the n's of various groups, see Table 13–3.

from aphasics, even from anomics, underlining that even anomic aphasics may have significant apraxia.

COMPARISON OF PRAXIS SUBTESTS

It appears, that for each group, the complex movements are most difficult (See Table 13-3). This is invariably the case, even for the control groups. In transcortical motor and Broca's aphasia, buccofacial praxis seemed to be more difficult than upper limb praxis. In Transcortical Sensory aphasia, the relationship appeared to be reversed. In the rest of the groups, there was no significant difference between praxis subtests.

CORRELATION OF APRAXIA WITH LANGUAGE AND NONVERBAL TESTS/GROUPS

Each apraxia subtest was correlated with the language and nonverbal subtests of the WAB. In Table 13-5, only the total praxis score correlations are shown. We were specifically interested in spontaneous speech, fluency, comprehension of "yes" and "no" questions, word discrimination, sequential command comprehension, repetition, naming, and among the performance subtests, drawing, block design, Raven's Colored Progressive Matrices, and writing. In most aphasic subgroups, the correlation was significant with comprehension and naming and to a lesser extent, with writing, repetition, AQ, drawing and the Raven's Colored Progressive Matrices (RCPM). An exception to this was the conduction–Wernicke's group, where none of the language subtests seemed to correlate with praxis. Fluency and block design did not correlate significantly with praxis in any of the aphasic groups.

Table 13-5
Correlation of Praxis with Language and Nonverbal Tests/Groups

Group	N	Fluency	Yes-No	Comprehension Word	Sentence	Total	Repetition	Naming	AQ	Writing	Drawing	Block design	Raven's
Global	18	−0.10	−0.17	−0.12	0.81**	0.64**	−0.29	−0.21	−0.10	−0.36	−0.36	−0.06	0.32
Broca's	48	0.12	0.26*	0.45**	0.44**	0.47**	0.15	0.27*	0.28*	0.47**	0.47**	0.04	0.30*
Isolation	6	0.52	−0.25	0.22	0.11	0.17	−0.73	−0.23	−0.32	0.29	0.57	0.77	0.83
Transcortical motor	7	0.00	0.56	0.53	0.77*	85**	0.51	0.85**	0.75	0.18	0.18	−0.73	−0.07
Transcortical sensory	17	−0.02	−0.18	0.62**	0.13	0.27	−0.00	0.62**	0.36	0.39	−0.01	−0.36	−0.37
Conduction	24	−0.14	0.29	−0.03	−0.10	0.02	0.15	0.22	0.20	0.46*	0.57**	0.25	0.61**
Wernicke's	21	0.00	0.25	0.59	0.57	0.72	0.37	0.61	0.67	0.53	0.51	0.09	0.36
Anomic	75	0.02	0.56**	0.24*	0.17	0.37**	0.39**	0.55**	0.50**	0.19	0.07	0.10	0.05

**$p \leq 0.01$. *$p \leq 0.05$.

CORRELATION OF PRAXIS SUBTESTS WITH OTHER
WAB SUBTESTS/TOTAL POPULATION

In a previous section, the correlation between total praxis and the subtests of the WAB in each group was explored. In this study, we attempted to correlate various elements of the praxis test separately with other language and nonverbal parameters for the whole aphasic group. All correlations were statistically significant but the actual coefficients reveal interesting trends (Table 13-6). Comprehension again is the most important language subtotal to correlate with the praxis subtotal, followed closely by the aphasia quotient (AQ), word recognition, and sentence comprehension, with naming and writing next. For upper limb praxis, the comprehension total again is the most significant, followed by the comprehension subtests and AQ. The same pattern is valid for the other subtests, such as instrumental or complex movement, the exception being buccofacial praxis, which correlates best with the AQ and the naming subtest, but seems not as highly correlated with comprehension. We looked at Broca's aphasics for the explanation, and found that they had poor buccofacial praxis with good comprehension. The scores were lower for buccofacial than other praxis subtests in Broca's, transcortical motor, isolation, and conduction aphasics. Broca's and transcortical motor aphasics in the series had slightly more buccofacial apraxia than the other groups. Writing correlated best with complex and with instrumental or transitive movements and total praxis.

MOVEMENTS ON COMMAND VERSUS IMITATION AND
REAL USE OF OBJECTS

Another method to eliminate the effect of comprehension is to use imitation when the patient failed to perform on command. The effect of the mode of stimulation to elicit gestural responses was studied for 230 aphasics and 125 nonaphasic controls. A full description of the administration of the praxis task is given earlier. There are three modes of presentation.

1. The patient is asked to pretend a movement or action—performance on command (PC).
2. If the PC is failed, the patient is asked to imitate the movement or action performed by the examiner (IM).
3. If still not correctly performed (IM), the patient is asked to show the use of the actual object (OU) if the action is transitive (e.g., combing one's hair).

There were eight out of the 20 items in praxis, which involved the use of an instrument; five were unilateral, two buccofacial, and one bilateral complex movements. The performance of each aphasic and control group has been converted to a mean percentage of correct responses for each mode of presentation.

Table 13-6

Correlation of Praxis and Other Subtests for all Aphasics*

	AQ	Fluency	Comprehension				Repetition	Drawing	Block Design	Raven's	Writing	Naming
			Yes–No	Word	Sentence	Total						
Upper limb	0.66	0.50	0.54	0.70	0.65	0.71	0.50	0.56	0.29	0.46	0.56	0.62
Buccofacial	0.72	0.63	0.48	0.60	0.55	0.60	0.62	0.48	0.18	0.33	0.54	0.66
Instrumental	0.68	0.54	0.54	0.71	0.67	0.73	0.50	0.60	0.26	0.47	0.65	0.64
Complex	0.68	0.53	0.55	0.67	0.68	0.71	0.49	0.59	0.24	0.46	0.66	0.64
Total	0.74	0.60	0.56	0.73	0.70	0.75	0.57	0.60	0.26	0.47	0.60	0.70

*All correlations are significant @ $p \leq 0.01$.

Figures 13-1 and 13-2 show the number of patients who improved on imitation, and the number which required the actual object for certain transitive movements, after failing on imitation, and, finally, the number not performed in either mode (NP).

Globals (*N* = 32)

Globals generally showed poor performance, with no real difference displayed across modes of presentation. A mean of 67 percent of the items were not performed, (Fig. 13-1).

Broca's (*N* = 48)

Broca's aphasics performed 50 percent of the items PC, a further 25 percent IM, but only another 6 percent improved on OU. This group displayed a fair degree of apraxia; 19 percent of the items were NP, (Fig. 13-1).

Wernicke's (*N* = 21)

The performance rates for the Wernicke's group are similar to those of the Broca's aphasics (though slightly higher IM), but the parallel performances are

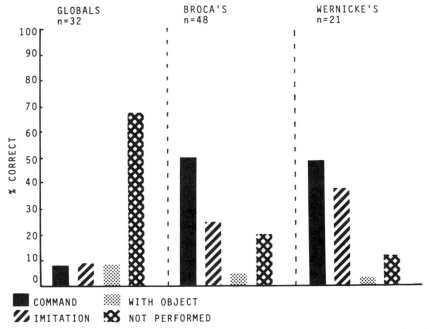

Fig. 13-1. The percentage of correct performance in each mode of presentation is represented by the height of the columns.

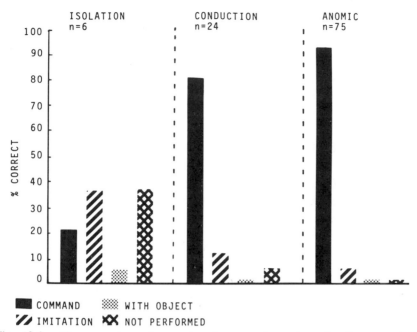

COMMAND   WITH OBJECT
IMITATION   NOT PERFORMED

Fig. 13-2. The percentage of correct performance in each mode of presentation is represented by the height of the columns.

attributable to different causes. The Wernicke's aphasics seem to be less apractic as a group, but performance on command is hampered by their auditory comprehension deficit. This may explain why they do so much better than other groups on IM: The stimulus is now visual rather than auditory. Performance PC plus IM yields a total of 86 percent of the items correctly performed, (Fig. 13-1).

Transcortical Motor (*N* = 7), Transcortical Sensory (*N* = 17), and Conduction (*N* = 24)

These three groups show very little variation from one another with PC = 76 percent, 75 percent, and 80 percent, respectively. Mode IM raises their total performance levels to 92 percent, 90 percent, and 92 percent, respectively. Only 6 percent, 8 percent, and 6 percent respectively, of the items were not performed at all, (Fig. 13-2).

Isolation (*N* = 6)

The isolation aphasics displayed generally poor performance: only 21 percent PC, 36 percent IM, 6 percent OU, and 37 percent NP. The improvement seen with the imitation mode of presentation may indicate that the same mechanism which underlies their speech output operates here also. Isolation aphasics repeat well—i.e., imitate speech well—in isolation from other cerebral functions, especially comprehension, (Fig. 13-2).

Anomic (N = 75), Naar (N = 32), Nondom (N = 72), and Normal (= 21)

The Anomics' performance approaches the levels achieved by the three control groups (not aphasic and recovered, nondominant lesions, and normals), which are not significantly different from each other with 98 percent, 97 percent, and 99.7 percent, respectively, on PC. Patients in these groups generally show very little if any difficulty with praxis, (Fig. 13-2).

We have presented all the items of the praxis test in all three modes (P.C.), (I.M.), and (O.U.) in 23 aphasics and 5 nondominant controls. The scores of object use were scaled so it could be compared to intransitive and buccofacial performance. In none of these patients did the performance on command surpass imitation or object use and similarly, in no instance was imitation better than actual object use. These results support the clinical impressions of Geschwind and the rationale of administrating the praxis test in the sequence of command, imitation and with object, as recommended by Goodglass and Kaplan.

DISCUSSION

The results indicate that different aphasic groups have different degrees of apraxia. Although apraxia is more severe in the severely affected aphasics, there seems to be more correlation with comprehension than with AQ (severity) in our study. The two groups of aphasics who showed more gestural failure than expected from their AQ were Wernicke's and isolation aphasics. This may be related to their low comprehension. In other groups with low scores on praxis, the comprehension deficit was also severe. Comprehension is clearly the most important factor when praxis is primarily tested with verbal commands. At times, it is difficult to tell whether the patient will not carry out a request because of comprehension difficulty, or true apraxia. Other times, it is obvious that the patient understands, from the verbal replies, and even from actual repetition of commands or from the satisfactory performance on other comprehension tasks. Should one examine apraxia then, by excluding those with auditory comprehension deficit? This would restrict the examination of higher motor functions to a limited portion of aphasics, usually those close to recovery or having only anomia. It seemed to us much more fruitful to survey all aphasics except those who did not seem to comprehend the task. We thought a great deal of information would be lost by eliminating the examination of praxis on command, as done by DeRenzi et al. (1968), but we reduced the effect of comprehension by having the patient imitate immediately after a failure of performance on verbal request.

DeRenzi et al. disregarded gestures on command being too dependent on comprehension and examined ten intransitive movements on imitation. They called these movements ideomotor apraxia (IM). They also examined the use of seven objects, which they called ideational apraxia (IA). Their 127 aphasics were divided into six groups; IA appeared in the global and severe Broca's and Wernicke's groups. The severity of aphasia was measured by their comprehension score, which correlated with their object use task significantly. The percentage of aphasics with ideational (object use) and ideomotor (imitation) apraxia was about the same. Twenty-one percent of the left brain damaged patients had both, indicating that the two, in fact, were closely related. The two tests may have measured the same form of praxis. An interesting finding was that 11 patients who had IA did not have IM. This is contrary to the common belief and to our results which show that movement on imitation is more difficult than movement with actual objects. The opposite association, which was also observed in their study, makes their findings difficult to interpret. Their tasks for object use were different from their imitation items (intransitive movements) and, therefore, the two categories are not as easily comparable as in our study. Their definition of ideational apraxia is quite different from the usual definition other authors use, accounting for the discrepancy between the rarity of the syndrome, as reported elsewhere, and the high frequency found in their study.

We examined only two patients who would fit the consensus of the description of ideational apraxia in the literature. Both had a great deal of difficulty using utensils and dressing apraxia, in addition to having apraxia of pretended and imitated movements and object use. One had bilateral vascular lesions and the other one was assumed to have early degenerative disease, with cortical atrophy, on the CT scan. These individuals had relatively less difficulty with simple, common, overlearned gestures but a great deal more trouble with complex actions on command, on imitation and on using objects, as well as on single but abstract or meaningless movements. Their inability seemed to suggest that they didn't know what to do with their hands or bodies or with objects in their environment. Although complex movements are generally more difficult to perform than simple ones, we have not been impressed by any other substantial group of aphasics or left hemisphere damaged patients in whom only complex movements were impaired with preservation of simple components. This, then, confirms the general impression that true ideational apraxia is rare and usually requires bilateral lesions (similar to visual agnosia).

We also had a case of severe and unusual movement disorder with preserved strength in a patient with cortical degeneration—probably Alzheimer's disease, which may be described as limb-kinetic apraxia. Movements were clumsy, even the elementary ones, as well as those in complex sequences. This was associated with severe bilateral tactile agnosia and constructional apraxia, but no language disturbance.

The special degree of apraxia predicted in conduction aphasics, by

Geschwind (1965), is not substantiated by our results, although our definition of conduction aphasia matches the accepted description in the literature (paraphasic, more or less fluent speech, good comprehension, and poor repetition). In fact, conduction aphasics had higher praxis scores than transcortical sensory aphasics, even though their aphasia was slightly more severe. This is, again, likely related to their better comprehension scores. This study, as well as that made by DeRenzi and Vignolo, points to a factor in apraxia which is beyond auditory–verbal comprehension, but which is, nevertheless, seen in patients with impaired comprehension. It is tempting to extrapolate to a general factor of concept formation or high order cognitive function, which is common to language comprehension and praxis. A similar factor seems to exist in other complex problem solving tasks, such as Raven's Colored Progressive Matrices (Kertesz and McCabe, 1975), which require visuospatial ability rather than movements.

The lack of relationship between the severity of aphasia and gestural performance in the detailed analysis by Goodglass and Kaplan (1963) is probably related to the population studied by them, which was restricted to mild to moderately affected groups. No response to any of the items in the test was excluded as evidence of not comprehending the command. This, again, would exclude patients with low scores, regardless of the cause. Imitation was not retained for more complex movements to the same extent as in the control group. We did not test complex pantomime (e.g., telling a story with gestures), as they have already proven to be an intellectually demanding task. Kimura and Archibald's (1974) lack of correlation between verbal scores and movement imitation may be related treating the small ($N = 15$) left hemisphere group as a whole. The appropriate grouping of a larger population of aphasics may yield more significant correlations with various types of verbal impairment even in their "nonverbal" meaningless hand movements. Some of their hand positions and movements were in fact verbalizable and familiar.

Our study also confirmed the prominence of buccofacial apraxia in transcortical motor and Broca's aphasics. However, this should not lead to equating buccofacial apraxia with the nonfluency and articulatory problems of Broca's aphasia. To consider·apraxia the basic problem in motor aphasia would be to neglect other linguistic, grammatical, and behavioral features of motor aphasia. The relationship of buccofacial apraxia to verbal apraxia, in the sense used by Darley and his associates, may not be causal because of the relatively frequently observed dissociation of the two phenomenon (Goldstein, 1948). Alajouanine and Lhermitte (1960) thought that nonverbal oral apraxia was common in Broca's aphasia, but that it was less complex and could recover quickly, which may account for some of the dissociation. DeRenzi et al. (1966) found a correlation between oral apraxia and the severity of phonemic articulatory problems, but they also had a significant number of exceptions in both directions. They thought it possible that oral nonverbal and speech movement had different mechanisms.

Imitation of oral movements was most impaired in Broca's aphasics, by Poeck and Kerschensteiner (1975). Mateer and Kimura (1977) found nonfluent aphasics impaired on oral movements and repetition of phonemes and syllables. Fluent aphasics were impaired also on the imitation of multiple nonverbal oral movements, which was not accounted for by visual memory span deficits. They hypothesized that simple movements were controlled by the anterior speech zone and multiple movements were programmed or selected by a posterior speech zone. They also admitted however, that the difference may just represent degrees of difficulty.

SUMMARY

Apraxia is defined as a disturbance of purposeful movement without paralysis or comprehension deficit. The complex history of the study of apraxia is reviewed, with an attempt to sort out the ideas generated by the feverish activity at the turn of the century, stimulated by Liepmann and those who argued with him. The controversy continues about ideational apraxia: There are too many divergent definitions of it. Some hold the opinion that it is just a severe variety of ideomotor apraxia. Limb-kinetic apraxia has fallen into disuse, as it is recorded rarely clinically. The left hemisphere is dominant for purposeful movements, not only for speech. The lesions causing apraxia are located in the dominant frontal lobe, in or under the supramarginal gyrus and other speech areas, or in the corpus callosum. The relationship to aphasia is explored in our laboratory and high correlation is found with those aphasic groups with severe comprehension deficit. There is evidence in our and in other studies as well, that this is not simply related to lack of comprehension but to an associated phenomenon.

14

Intelligence and Aphasia

You hear the words inside your head?" he asked. "Well, not exactly "hear", and not exactly "see"–There are–well, sort of shapes–and if you use words you make them clearer, so that they are easier to understand.

The Chrysalids, John Wyndham

THOUGHT AND LANGUAGE

The relationship of thought and speech remains controversial and to a large extent, a philosophical issue. Plato defined thinking as "the conversation which the soul holds with itself". Similarly, monistic philosophers such as Leibnitz, Wordsworth, Ribot, believed that speaking is thinking aloud and thinking is subvocal talking. The dualistic group, Schopenhauer, Berkeley, Binet, and Piaget, believe in the independence of language and thought. Most modern thinkers take a middle of the road approach, like Whitehead: "Let it be admitted that language is not the essence of thought. But this conclusion must be carefully limited. Apart from language, the retention of thought, the easy recall of thought, the interweaving of thought into higher complexity, the communication of thought, are all gravely limited." Most of our thinking is through mental images or verbal symbols although less well-defined processes operate as well, such as daydreaming or automatic decision making. Introspection or "thinking out" any action or plan will shape our thoughts into verbal symbols.

COGNITION AND APHASIA

A unique situation, where language is impaired more or less independently from intelligence, occurs in aphasia. The relationship of the two has been studied a great deal. For direct evidence of the preservation or loss of thought in aphasia, one has anecdotal reports from patients who suffered transient episodes of aphasia or those who recovered from more lasting but milder episodes. These patients and their relatives will usually claim that they had no trouble thinking or formulating what they wanted to say, only their expression suffered. A famous example in the literature is that of Lordat (1843), who was a physician and described his own aphasia as without "any difficulty thinking." There are a few cases of transient aphasia associated with migraine or rapid recovery, who admitted subsequently to "confusion" usually associated with difficulty in understanding what was said to them. We had four such cases, in a series of 20 transient aphasias, in our laboratory. Patients with severe, lasting aphasia usually cannot remember what their thinking process was like at the time of the initial severe impairment. The anecdotal evidence of severe aphasics who were able to return to work or play cards contrasts with the dramatic example of Marie's aphasic cook, who could not fry an egg (Zangwill, 1969). Those who believe that intelligence is profoundly altered in aphasia cite as evidence that aphasics have trouble calculating, putting puzzles together, etc. Trousseau (1864) doubted Lordat's statement and presented aphasics with impaired reading, writing, and calculation as manifestations of impaired intelligence. Broca (1865), on the other hand, said, "When the lesion is quite circumscribed, it is possible that only the language is injured, and intelligence remains intact, as far as we can judge it." His last qualifying clause is most important, because any statement one makes about impaired or retained intelligence depends on how one tests for it. Marie's (1906) sweeping statement of a general intellectual impairment in aphasia has not been accepted by many subsequently. Weisenburg and McBride (1935), who in fact tested aphasics with a wide range of verbal and nonverbal intelligence tests, concluded that intelligence suffers in particular ways. The severity of language disorder was not a regular indicator of the severity of the disturbance in intelligence. Expressive disorders showed a minimum change in intelligence.

MEASURING INTELLIGENCE IN APHASIA

The difficulty of defining intelligence and the lack of agreement even on an operational definition hampers research design and clouds the interpretation of results. Intelligence includes attention, retention, memory, discrimination, abstraction, recall, knowledge, motor skills, integration, problem solving, logic, and planning. A pragmatic, albeit circular, definition of intelligence is what is measured by intelligence tests. This view recognizes that we have been measuring intelligence long before we decided what intelligence really is (Pintner and Paterson, 1923). The question of an overall, general "g" factor of intelligence has not been settled yet. Rather than trying to measure it, most modern investigators are concentrating on specific nonverbal functions in aphasics. Piercy (1969) concluded that the evidence was more consistent with theories which postulate a number of primary abilities than with those with a unitary function. A source of difficulty in assessing intelligence in aphasics is partly that mental processes require the manipulation and expression of verbal, numerical, and spatial material. Each of these are, more or less, sensitive to the aphasic disorder itself. Verbal tests of intelligence are clearly inappropriate in aphasia but the amount of verbalization used to perform the nonverbal tasks remains undetermined. The subjects may have to understand the task and also, verbal feedback may be needed for its performance.

An intellectual defect not directly related to language was postulated in aphasics by Teuber and Weinstein (1956), who found that aphasics performed poorly on "hidden figures." One can argue, however, that the Gottschaldt figures contain objects with verbal labels. Similarly, complex tactile discriminatory tasks were impaired in aphasics (Semmes et al., 1954). When the Wechsler Performance Scale was given to various brain-damaged groups by Orgass et al. (1972), there was no difference between right-and left-damaged groups; but when aphasics were separated, they were worse than right-damaged patients, who were, in turn, worse than left-damaged but nonaphasic patients. An exception was the block design subtest where the right-damaged patients were slightly worse. While the different Wechsler subtests appear to be a measure of global intelligence, they are not homogenous when applied to brain-damaged individuals.

Sex differences in the performance of visuospatial tasks were found by McGlone and Kertesz (1973), who showed that males with right hemisphere lesions had lower scores on Koh's blocks than females. Aphasic females, on the other hand, were the only group with high correlation between severity and the block design test, indicating an asymmetry in the cerebral organization of visuospatial function.

Drawing was correlated with Raven's matrices in aphasics by van Dongen (1974). This is a similar finding to that of Bay (1964) and Zangwill (1969), who said that, in practice, estimates of intelligence in aphasic patients should be based on performance tests only if constructional apraxia has been satisfactorily excluded.

RAVEN'S MATRICES IN APHASIA

One of the most extensively studied, nonverbal tests in aphasia is Raven's Progressive Matrices. No verbal or manual skills are required for its performance, and it is a test of logical reasoning, as well as visuospatial ability.

Conflicting results were obtained by Piercy and Smyth (1962), who found Raven's Matrices to be more affected by the right-sided lesions, and Arrigoni and DeRenzi (1964), who found the performance impaired more by left-sided damage, although there was no difference between aphasics and nonaphasic, left hemisphere injured patients in the latter work. Zangwill (1964) found that for motor aphasics, two of three "jargon," and three of five "amnesic" aphasics performed normally on Raven's Matrices and suggested that failure correlated with constructional apraxia. Studies of DeRenzi and Faglioni (1965), and Colonna and Faglioni (1966), with Raven's Matrices found no difference between aphasics and right hemisphere damaged, nonaphasic patients. DeRenzi and Faglioni (1965) also found that neither aphasia nor the side of the lesion made a difference in the performance. Van Harskamp (1974) used Raven's Matrices and concluded that constructional apraxia interfered with its performance in right brain-damaged patients and aphasia in left brain-damaged patients. Welman and Lanser (1974) administered Raven's Matrices to 39 aphasics—43 percent had poor, 20 percent normal, and 30 percent high scores.

Archibald et al. (1967) classified 29 aphasics as "syntactic, semantic, pragmatic and global" and found that globals scored low on Raven's Colored Progressive Matrices (RCPM). They found a difference between "talking and non-talking" patients. The talking patients were not different statistically from normals and left-brain-damaged nonaphasics.

OUR STUDY WITH THE RCPM

RCPM (Raven, 1965) correlates well with verbal tests of intelligence. It requires no language output or assembly capacity. We chose the colored version, designed for children, because of its simplicity. As a nonverbal measure of intelligence, it appeared appropriate for our aphasic population.

The purpose of our study was to explore intellectual impairment in aphasia, to determine the role of language in the performance of RCPM, and to correlate it with the clinical subgroups of aphasics. Our clinical experience and the publications dealing with intelligence in aphasia suggested that some severely affected aphasics may have relatively well-preserved nonverbal intellectual functions. The lack of agreement in the literature prompted us to choose a sizable, relatively unselected aphasic population, divided into clinical groups on the hypothesis that the performance of some types of aphasics is different from that of others.

The test was administered to 111 aphasics and 52 controls, all of whom also had the Western Aphasia Battery (WAB) (Kertesz and McCabe, 1975). According to the WAB scores, the patients were classified as having global, Broca's, isolation, transcortical motor, transcortical sensory, conduction, Wernicke's, or anomic aphasia. Table 4-2 shows the criteria of taxonomic classification into groups. Some selection took place by not including some of the more severely damaged aphasics, mostly in the global group because they were bedridden or could not attempt the tasks. The majority of patients came from one general hospital, where all aphasics were consecutively examined. Two other hospitals, including a Veteran's hospital, contributed patients, skewing the sex ratio towards males—77:34 = Male:Female. Control Group 1 ($N=19$) consisted of non-brain-damaged, age-matched, hospital population; Control II ($N=18$) non-dominant, hemispheric lesions; Control III ($N=15$) diffusely brain-damaged but nonaphasic patients, whose lesions were not localizable to the hemispheres. Obtunded, psychotic patients, or those with a "language barrier" were excluded. Handedness was determined by questionnaire from the patient or relatives. One hundred and four dextral, six sinistral, and one ambidextrous aphasics, and 49 dextral, two sinistral, and one ambidextrous controls were included. Among the seven left-handed and ambidextrous aphasics, five had right hemisphere, two left hemisphere lesions, and one of the two nonaphasic left-handed controls had a left hemisphere lesion. In five right-handed and one left-handed aphasic, the lesion site could not be determined with the usual neurological methods.

A drawing task was also used to measure "constructional ability" in 149 of the patients. The subject was asked to draw a circle, square, cube, clock, tree, house, and a person, and to bisect a 5-inch line. If he was unable to draw on auditory stimulus, a facsimile was presented for 10 seconds and if the patient failed again, he was asked to copy. The drawings were scored for perspective, completeness, symmetry, and form. Maximum score was 30. If the patient was only able to copy, maximum score was 18.

VISUOSPATIAL PERFORMANCE IN APHASIC GROUPS

The results are summarized in Table 14-1. The subgroups with the low RCPM are on the top, the high RCPM scoring groups are below them, and the control groups are lowermost. Maximum score is 36. These results indicate that global aphasics who are nonfluent, noninformative, have poor comprehension, and cannot repeat or name (see criteria), perform poorly on RCPM (mean score: 3.6). Similarly, a poorer performance on the RCPM was obtained in cortical sensory (Wernicke's) aphasia (mean: 12.1). In contrast to the global group, these patients have fluent speech, at times a great deal of jargon, but they have poor comprehension, repetition, and naming. Transcortical sensory aphasics achieved a low mean, 7.8. These fluent patients retained excellent repetition in face of poor comprehension and naming. We also had one "isolation" aphasic, not included in Table 14.1, whose Raven's score was 6. Common to all these groups is poor comprehension (mean comprehension score below 5.3). Fluency and ability to repeat, which are important factors in separating the language disconnection syndromes, do not seem to be relevant in this "performance" test,

Table 14–1

Means and Standard Deviations of 111 Aphasics and 52 Controls

No.	Aphasic Types	Age*		Raven's**		Comprehension		Drawing**		AQ	
		$\overline{X}$	SD	$\overline{X}$	SD	$\overline{X}$	SD	$\overline{X}$	SD	$\overline{X}$	SD
10	Global	64.5	5.7	3.6	6.2	2.6	1.0	3.4	4.3	9.8	9.1
18	Wernicke's	59.2	9.9	12.1	7.7	4.3	1.8	8.5	7.8	41.2	13.4
5	Transcortical										
	sensory	58.4	12.7	7.8	4.5	5.3	2.2	7.1	4.6	61.3	7.8
27	Broca's	55.1	14.7	16.6	8.5	6.0	2.1	10.9	6.4	28.2	15.8
11	Conduction	66.4	3.5	18.0	7.1	8.4	6.4	15.8	6.8	61.6	4.4
40	Anomic	60.3	9.2	21.8	8.0	9.0	0.6	16.3	5.7	81.4	21.4
19	Control I	60.6	5.3	24.8	6.6	9.8	1.0	22.3	1.5	97.7	19.3
18	Control II	58.2	8.9	17.2	5.5	7.9	6.6	16.5	5.7	96.5	13.3
15	Control III	57.7	12.7	18.3	7.0	9.5	5.5	19.2	5.2	94.1	17.9

*F ratio 0.896 at 8 and 153 df. Not significant at 0.05 level.
**F ratio 9.681 at 8 and 153 df. Significant at 0.01 level.
***F ratio 13.578 at 8 and 149 df. Significant at 0.01 level.

Reprinted with permission of Brain and Language. New York, Academic Press, Vol. 2, 1975, pp. 387–395.

since cortical and transcortical sensory aphasics are quite fluent, and transcortical and isolation patients repeat well.

On the other hand, the RCPM scores of cortical motor (Broca's), transcortical motor, conduction, and anomic aphasics were at par with the scores of the patients with diffuse brain damage but without language impairment (Control Group III); or nondominant hemisphere lesions (Control Group II), and only slightly below those of normal controls (Group I—nonbrain-damaged, age-matched patients) and of the normative data of other investigators [Levinson's (1959) normal mean 24.84]. The mean scores were, respectively, Broca's—16.6, conduction—18.0, and anomic—21.8. Only three transcortical motor aphasics had the RCPM, and their scores—21, 19, 11—were not included in Table 14-1. These uncommon patients say practically nothing spontaneously, but repeat and understand well.

Since comprehension appeared to be the most important single language factor separating the performance of the subgroups on the RCPM and drawing, the results of this subtest on the WAB were included in Table 14-1 for review, although this variable was not independent, of course, from the classification of patients into these groups. The AQ, which is a summary of performance on the language tasks, on the other hand, is independent from the classification criteria for subgrouping aphasics and it is included here as a measure of the "severity" of aphasia. RCPM results do not appear directly related to the severity of aphasia, since Broca's aphasics, who have low total scores, perform as well on the test as conduction or anomic aphasics, who are less severely impaired in their total language performance.

CORRELATION OF RCPM WITH DRAWING, COMPREHENSION, AND AQ

The drawing scores followed closely the pattern of results of the RCPM and were similarly tabulated. Correlation coefficients (Table 14.2), calculated for the whole aphasic population, showed the best correlation between Raven's and drawing scores, followed by Raven's and comprehension, and the least between Raven's and AQ (severity rating).

When the RCPM and drawing scores are subjected to a one-way analysis of variance, the differences are significant at levels better than 0.01 with F ratio of 9.68 at 8 and 153 df for the RCPM, and F ratio of 13.57 at 8149 df for drawing. On the other hand, analysis of variance showed no significant difference between the ages of various groups, an important factor in the performance of RCPM. Once the variance of the Raven's and drawing scores for the population was established, the subgroups could be compared, utilizing the t test (Table 14-3), All aphasic groups appear to perform worse than normal, non-brain-damaged controls, but only global, Wernicke's, and transcortical sensory aphasics, the groups with low comprehension, are significantly below the performance of the nonaphasic, nondominant hemisphere-damaged controls.

The portion of aphasics performing normally on RCPM was calculated for each group by defining normal performance as the same or better than the mean minus one standard deviation from the mean of the normal controls (Group I). The mean was found to be identical to that found by Levinson (1959) for normal-aged population—24.8 (SD-5.3). Forty-two percent of aphasics performed above this level (19.5) on the RCPM. Among globals only 1 percent, transcortical sensory aphasics 0 percent, Wernicke's 5.7 percent, but among Broca's 44.4 percent, conduction 54.5 percent, and anomic aphasics 62.5 percent show normal performance.

Table 14–2
Correlation Coefficient (Pearson r) for Total Aphasic Population:
Mean Scores*

Raven's and drawing	0.680
Raven's and comprehension	0.556
Raven's and AQ (severity)	0.465

*All the correlations are significant at $p \leq 0.01$.

Reprinted with permission of Brain and Language. New York, Academic Press, Vol. 2, 1975, pp. 387–395.

Table 14–3
Levels of Significance on the *t* Test Comparing the Means of
Raven's Scores of Aphasic Groups with Controls*

	Control I	Control II
Global	0.005	0.005
Wernicke's	0.005	0.05
Transcortical sensory	0.005	0.01
Broca's	0.005	NS
Conduction	0.01	NS
Anomic	0.005	NS
Control III	0.01	NS

*The differences between visuospatial function of aphasics and controls depend on the type of aphasia (see text).

Reprinted with permission of Brain and Language. New York, Academic Press, Vol. 2, 1975, pp. 387–395.

DISCUSSION

The performance of RCPM by many aphasics is comparable to a brain-damaged group of controls without language impairment. The only important "language" factor limiting performance seems to be impaired comprehension or another factor which is impaired concurrently with it. This may differ from aphasic comprehension difficulty qualitatively, as illustrated by a few patients who had impaired language comprehension but understood the test and performed normally, and the control patients whose dementia prevented them from performing on the tasks although their language comprehension was still intact. It was also observed repeatedly that normals are able to do the tasks without any verbal instruction whatever, and this suggests that auditory verbal comprehension may not be necessary for its performance. Impaired attention to the task or "set" is often a feature of the same patients who score low on the comprehension tasks as well as on the RCPM. This factor is difficult to quantitate or even define, except in terms of actual performance. A similar deficit in aphasics has been termed "defective organization or selection of material" by Teuber and Weinstein (1956). Raven called the Matrices a "test of observation and clear thinking," requiring "the intellectual capacity to reason by analogy." The above discussed defective factor in some of our aphasics is likely to disrupt this process of "logical reasoning," and also, the selection of the correct response, even though visual perceptual processes may be intact. The extent of "internal verbalization" utilized for the performance of RCPM was thought to be high by Arrigoni and DeRenzi (1964). This may account for the failure of aphasics, but that the relationship is not likely linear is suggested by our data, indicating that some of our more severely affected aphasics (Broca's) perform better than some of those with less overall impairment (Wernicke's, transcortical sensory). Zangwill (1964) also observed the striking phenomenon of the practically speechless patients performing well on the matrices.

There are suggestions in the literature that constructional apraxia seems to be correlated with failure on the RCPM (Zangwill, 1964; Piercy and Smyth, 1962; Arrigoni and DeRenzi, 1964). RCPM scores were correlated with block design scores by Stacey and Gill (1955). We chose drawing as a measure of "constructional apraxia." This task appeared to correlate well with Raven's scores (Table 14-3) and constructional apraxia indeed, may account for some of the difficulties aphasics or nonaphasic controls with right hemisphere damage were having. On the other hand, if the deficit is related entirely to "constructional apraxia", as the correlation with the drawing scores may suggest, then this would be in favor of the bilaterality of constructional praxis, since 105 of 111 of our aphasics had a unilateral left hemisphere lesion, and constructional apraxia and visuospatial abilities have been associated with "nondominant" hemisphere lesions (Zangwill, 1964; Piercy and Smyth, 1962). There is evidence by Arrigoni and DeRenzi (1964), and Poeck et al. (1973) indicating that the "dominant" side also plays a role in constructional praxis.

That many aphasics have the same problem with RCPM and drawing as patients with nonspeaking hemisphere lesions may indicate that both a comprehension related, as well as a "visuospatial" factor is required, or that this visuospatial–nonverbal intelligence factor is distributed in both hemispheres, and unilateral, probably posterior lesions may impair it from either side. The latter suggestion is supported by Teuber and Weinstein (1956), Russo and Vignolo (1967), and Poeck et al. (1973), who showed impaired visuocognitive performances on tasks other than the RCPM by aphasics. It is likely that integration of function of both hemispheres takes place in solving the problems of the RCPM. The results suggest that the hemisphere dominant for language plays an important role in the performance of the so-called "nonverbal" intellectual functions.

Other previously published results of equating aphasic and nonaphasic performance on the test stem from the failure to separate aphasic subgroups. Exclusion of more severely affected aphasics from many of these studies may be also a reason for finding aphasic performance unimpaired. When our anomic, conduction, and Broca's groups are compared with the right hemispheric, brain-damaged group, no significant differences are found, but the difference is substantial for global, Wernicke's, and transcortical sensory aphasia. All aphasic groups differ, to some extent, from non-brain-damaged, age-matched controls; but the numerical differences are much greater in the groups with impaired comprehension than in the others, even though their overall aphasic performance (AQ) is not as severely impaired. Nonverbal "intelligence" is spared in some aphasics more than others, as measured by the RCPM.

One of the most interesting findings in our study was that the impairment on RCPM appears in the same aphasic groups (global, Wernicke's, transcortical sensory) as the impairment in praxis. This confirms the suggestion by Alajouanine and Lhermitte (1964) that only in cases of aphasia with coincident apraxia is performance in nonverbal intelligence appreciably at fault.

Goodglass (1974) felt that language and nonverbal intelligence are independently vulnerable to lesions in the perisylvian zone of the left hemisphere, and aphasia is neither a cause nor an effect of the intellectual deficit. He also thought that it was more common to find severe aphasia in an intellectually well-preserved aphasic than severe intellectual deficit without aphasia, following a focal lesion of the left hemisphere language area.

Basso et al. (1973) went further in their interpretation of intellectual deficit found in aphasics. Their results, with the RCPM given to 55 aphasics and other controls, failed to show correlation with comprehension and naming scores. This result is different from ours and from that of Voinescu and Gheorghita (1974), who also thought that diminished performance on tests of thinking were related to disturbances of reception. The reason for the difference is obscure, but it may relate to population sampling. Leischner and Haberkamp (1974) also found lower scores for "mixed" and "total" aphasics on the Wechsler Performance Scale, administered to 139 aphasics, attributable to receptive disturbances. The Italian group also felt that aphasia was a symptom coincidental with but not influencing the decrement found on the RCPM. They also concluded that the brain is not equipotential for intelligence and that there were two critical areas: One is located in the retrorolandic region of the right hemisphere and is specialized for the intellectual processing of visual data; the other overlaps the language area and is involved in the performance of several different intellectual tasks, verbal as well as nonverbal. The view may be advanced that this region subserves a superordinate, intellectual ability, sharing many of the characteristics attributed to the "g" factor by psychologists.

SUMMARY

Intelligence is closely related to language; some aspects of intelligence are affected in some aphasics. Much of the contradictory evidence about aphasic performance on nonverbal tasks can be clarified when clinically different aphasics are examined separately. Those with poor comprehension seemed to have poor performance on the RCPM, but the severity of aphasia did not seem to be a significant determinant.

The left hemisphere language area plays an important role in the performance of nonverbal tasks which also need intact posterior right hemisphere mediated visuospatial function. There seems to be a general factor of nonverbal intelligence which is not the same as comprehension, but their deficits often overlap.

15

Recovery and Treatment of Aphasia

The temporary nature is one of the most important characteristics in aphasia. . .

Von Monakow (1914)

INTRODUCTION

Neurological and behavioral aspects of recovery from central nervous system (CNS) lesions are of great interest to clinicians following patients, as well as experimenters studying deficits. Few will doubt that recovery from the anoxia, edema, cellular infiltration, and pressure of the acute insult, be it hemorrhage, ischemia, trauma, or any combination of these, often produces significant early improvement in the first 1−3 weeks.

There is another, and indeed so far, unexplained phase of recovery beyond this initial change, lasting for months up to about a year after the insult. It has been described variably depending on etiology and the frequency of repeated observations. The initial phase is maximum in the first 2−3 months, then the rate decreases, and plateauing occurs. Beyond one year, recovery is less likely to occur.

One of the difficulties of observation is that clinicians taking care of the patients in the acute state may not have the opportunity to follow their cases long term, and those in a rehabilitation setting rarely see them at the onset and in the earlier stages of recovery. Therapists interested in rehabilitation may overlook the extent of spontaneous recovery and attribute the gains to treatment. Others interested primarily in diagnosis, pathology, and their classification and measurement may not recognize the changing pattern, and view the neuropsychological deficit as a static one. Nevertheless, considerable literature is accumulating about this important aspect of the nervous system documented in reviews by Stein, Rosen, and Butters (1974), Lebrun and Hoops (1976), Sullivan and Kommers (1977), and Finger (1978). Therapists are realizing that accurate knowledge of the recovery process contributes to the design of the methods and duration of therapy and the allocation of limited resources (Darley, 1972).

RECOVERY FROM APHASIA

Most long-term studies of aphasics were on treated patients, until recently. Vignolo (1964) was the first to include the objective assessment of untreated patients ($N = 27$) at various intervals. Culton (1969) examined spontaneous recovery in 11 aphasics for 2 months post onset, and in a chronic group of ten beyond 11 months. Sarno, Silverman, and Sands (1970) had eight chronic controls (beyond one year onset) followed for "several months" in their study of treatment in global aphasics. Sarno and Levita (1971) studied 14 severe aphasics at onset and 3 and 6 months after. Hagen (1973) had ten matched controls, Basso, Faglioni, and Vignolo (1975) studied 94, and Kertesz and McCabe (1977) 83 patients for spontaneous recovery. Unfortunately, the methods of evaluation were widely differing from the Functional Communication Profile (FCP) to various structured language tasks. The patient populations were not comparable, for some restricted their study to severe aphasics (Sarno et al. 1970 and Sarno and Levita, 1971); others used different classification of their patients such as Hagen (1973), who chose sensorimotor type III impairment (Schuell's system), and Basso et al. (1975), who lumped their patients under Broca's and Wernicke's categories only. We attempted to standardize evaluation and control for the etiology, initial severity, and the type of aphasia as well (Kertesz and McCabe, 1977).

Several important factors in recovery of treated and untreated patients emerge from the literature.

Etiology of Aphasia

Recovery and prognosis significantly differ in various etiologies such as cerebral infarcts, subarachnoid hemorrhage, and trauma. The studies of Butfield and Zangwill (1946), Wepman (1951), and Luria (1970) indicated that post-traumatic patients recovered better than stroke populations (Marks, Taylor, and Rusk 1957; Godfrey and Douglass, 1959). Complete recovery was seen in more than half of our post-traumatic cases (Kertesz and McCabe, 1977). Dramatic spontaneous recovery, such as a global aphasia after a closed head injury improving to a mild anomic state, is not seen in vascular lesions with this extent of initial impairment (Fig. 15-1). Many of these patients were younger, although the scatter of the age factor was considerable. The extent and severity of lesions is variable in our motor vehicle accident population, most of whom had closed head injuries, a few with contusion or subdural hemorrhage.

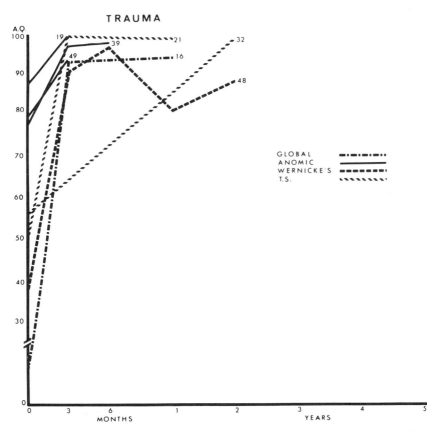

Fig. 15-1.   Individual recovery graphs of posttraumatic patients. The ages are at the end of the lines. AQ is the aphasia quotient (overall score). (Reprinted with permission from Brain 100:1–18, 1977.)

Aphasics after a subarachnoid hemorrhage showed wide variations in their recovery rates, presumably related to the variable extent of their hemorrhage and presence of infarcts or tissue destruction (Fig. 15-2). The prognosis was predictable from the initial scores to some extent. Some of the worst jargon and global patients were seen following ruptured middle cerebral aneurysms.

Types of Aphasia

Differences between types of aphasia occur in recovery also. Head (1926) recognized that some types of aphasia improve more rapidly than others. Weisenburg and McBride (1935), Butfield and Zangwill (1946), Messerli et al.

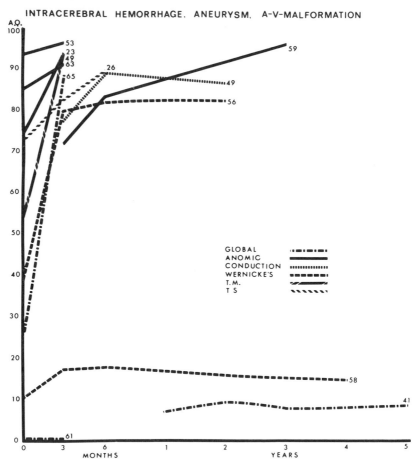

Fig. 15-2. Recovery graphs after intracerebral and subarachnoid hemorrhage. AQ is the overall score (aphasia quotient). (Reprinted with permission from Brain 100:1–18, 1977.)

(1976), and Kertesz and McCabe (1977) considered Broca's or "expressive" aphasics to improve most, while Vignolo (1964) considered expressive disorders to have poor prognosis. Basso et al. (1975) did not find any difference between fluent and nonfluent aphasics. The variability of conclusions reflects problems of classification, e.g., "expressive" disorder includes many different kinds of aphasics. There is universal agreement, however, that global aphasics have poor prognosis.

Initial Severity

Initial severity is closely tied in with the type of aphasia and it is considered to be highly predictive of outcome. (Godfrey, 1959; Schuell et al., 1964; Sands et al., 1969; Sarno et al., 1970; Gloning et al., 1976; Kertesz and McCabe, 1977.) Unfortunately, it is not always taken into consideration in studies of recovery. The most severely affected, although they have a long way to go, show little gain treated or untreated (Sarno et al., 1970). The extent of improvement in mildly affected patients may be small even though they recover completely considering that they were relatively good to begin with (Kertesz and McCabe, 1977).

Time Course

There is a surprising amount of agreement about the time course of the recovery process. A large number of stroke patients recover a great deal in the first two weeks (Kohlmeyer, 1976). The greatest amount of improvement occurs in the first 2 or 3 months after onset (Vignolo, 1964; Cultron, 1969) Sarno and Levita, 1971; Basso et al., 1975; Kertesz and McCabe, 1977) and beyond 6 months the rate of recovery significantly drops (Butfield and Zangwill, 1946; Sands et al., 1969; Vignolo, 1964; Kertesz and McCabe, 1977). Recovery after a year does not seem to occur spontaneously in the majority of cases (Culton, 1969; Kertesz and McCabe, 1977), but some reports note improvement in cases under therapy for many years after the stroke (Schuell et al., 1964; Marks et al., 1957; Smith, 1972; Broida, 1977).

Age, Sex, Intelligence, Education

The influence of age is controversial to some extent. The clinical impression of the younger patient recovering better (Wepman, 1951; Eisenson, 1949; Vignolo, 1964) was confirmed by a reverse correlation between age and initial recovery rates (0–3 months) even if we excluded the post-traumatic group with mean age well below that of the infarct group (Kertesz and McCabe, 1977). This trend just missed being significant statistically and others had the similar lack of correlation between age and recovery in statistical analysis (Sarno and Levita,

1971; Culton, 1971; Smith, 1972). Clinicians will observe remarkably good recovery in elderly patients while some of the young will remain severely disabled. No significant sex differences were found in recovery even though recent studies suggest some asymmetry of brain function, probably involving language organization as well as visuospatial function between men and women (McGlone and Kertesz, 1973). The more bilateral or diffuse representation of language would lead to the expectation of better recovery rates from aphasia in women, but this is not substantiated by our data. Premorbid intelligence, health, and social milieu are considered significant clinically (Darley, 1972). Intellectual and educational level influences the limits of what the patient and relatives consider recovery. Keenan and Brassel's study (1974), on the other hand, indicated that health, employment, and age had little if any prognostic value when compared to factors such as "listening" and "talking" (comprehension and fluency). Similar lack of effect of age, sex, education, occupational status, preillness language proficiency, and current living environment in severe aphasics was found by Sarno et al. (1970b).

Handedness

The data from Subirana (1969) and Gloning et al. (1969) indicate that left-handers recover better from aphasias than right-handers. Gloning (1969) also suggested that left-handers are likely to become aphasic regardless of which hemisphere is damaged. Interestingly, right-handers with a history of left-handedness among parents, siblings, or children, recover, on the average, better than right-handers without such a family history, according to Luria (1970).

Language Components

There is evidence that not only various types of aphasics but also various components of language recover differently. Of course, types of aphasia and various language components are interdependent and sometimes this is ignored in the analysis. Kreindler and Fradis (1968) found that naming, oral imitation, and comprehension of nouns showed the most improvement. Gains in comprehension were greater than in expressive language in the study of Broca's aphasics by Kenin and Swisher (1972), but no such difference was found by Sarno and Levita (1971). Hagen (1973) showed improvement in language formulation, auditory retention, visual comprehension, and visual motor abilities in a 3−6 month postonset period. Ludlow (1977) found the greatest change in digit repetition reverse, identification by sentence, and word fluency in fluent aphasics; digit repetition forward, sentence comprehension, and tactile naming in Broca's aphasics. We studied various language components in four groups of 31 untreated aphasics separated by criteria based on factors independent from those examined. (Lomas and Kertesz, 1978). Comprehension as examined by yes−no questions; sequential commands and repetition were the most improved compo-nents, word fluency was the least. In fact, word fluency remained impaired while all other language factors improved, indicating that it measures something dif-ferent in addition to language, which is corroborated by the observation that it is often impaired in nonaphasic brain-damaged subjects. The highest overall recov-ery scores were attained by the low fluency, high comprehension group. The groups with low initial comprehension showed recovery in yes—no comprehen-sion and repetition tasks, the others with high comprehension recovered in all tasks except word fluency.

Linguistic features of aphasic speech show various patterns of recovery. Ludlow (1977) followed mean sentence length, grammaticability index, and sentence production index as a measure of recovery in Broca's and fluent aphasics. Both groups showed the greatest gains in the second month postonset. Alajouanine (1956) distinguished four stages of recovery in severe expressive aphasia.

1. Differentiation by intonation
2. Decreased automatic utterances
3. Less rigid stereotypic utterances
4. Only volitional slow, agrammatical speech

Kertesz and Benson (1970) pointed out the predictable pattern of linguistic recovery in jargon aphasia. Copious neologistic or phonemic jargon is replaced by verbal paraphasias or semantic jargon and eventually, anomia or more rarely a "pure" word deafness develops. The extraordinary phenomenon of overproduc-tion of jargon is replaced by anomic gaps or circumlocutions, indicating the recovery of regulatory or inhibitory systems.

RECOVERY STUDY WITH THE WAB

Prognosis

We assessed the prognosis of stroke patients with aphasia using 67 patients who had an initial examination, as well as a follow-up test at least one year after (Kertesz and McCabe, 1977). The Aphasia Quotient (AQ), a summary of the subtests of the Western Aphasia Battery (Kertesz and Poole, 1974) measured at the end of this long term follow-up (average 28.6 month), was used to categorize the outcome (Table 15-1). Almost all of the global aphasics remained poor. Broca's and Wernicke's aphasics showed a wider range of outcome. Some pa-tients with Wernicke's aphasia retain fluent jargon under pressure for many months. After a while, they lose their phonemic paraphasias; their language deficit consists of verbal substitutions and anomia. Broca's aphasics have an intermediate outlook just about evenly divided between fair and good recovery.

Table 15–1
Final Outcome of Aphasia

Group	N	0–25 (Poor)	25–50 (Fair)	50–75 (Good)	75–100 (Very good)
Global	16	13	2	0	1
Broca's	12	0	6	6	1
Conduction	6	0	1	1	4
Wernicke's	13	4	6	3	0
Isolation	1	0	1	0	0
Transcortical motor	2	0	0	2	0
Transcortical sensory	3	0	0	1	2
Anomic	13	0	0	3	10
Total	67	17 (25.4%)	16 (23.9%)	16 (23.9%)	18 (26.9%)

(Adapted with permission from Brain 100:1–18, 1977.)

Anomic, conduction, and transcortical aphasics have a uniformly good prognosis, the majority of cases showing excellent spontaneous recovery. Some of the completely recovered patients were not even included in this analysis because they were not tested again after their three months' repeat scores were normal (almost half of anomics). Of the total of 67, 25 percent had poor, 24 percent fair, 24 percent good, and 27 percent excellent prognosis.

Evolution of Syndromes

The evolution of aphasic syndromes and the patterns of transformation from one clinically distinct group into another, as defined by the subscores on subsequent examinations, were also studied (Table 15-2). It appeared that anomic aphasia is a common end stage of evolution in addition to being a common aphasic syndrome *de novo*. Four of 13 Wernicke's, four of eight transcortical and isolation, four of 17 Broca's, two of eight conduction, and one of 22 global aphasias evolved into anomic aphasia. Complete recovery from aphasia depends on the difficult definition of normal language function. We used an arbitrary cutoff AQ of 93.8 (see Chapter 4). This was the actual mean of the standardization group with brain-damaged but clinically judged nonaphasic patients (Kertesz and Poole, 1974). Final AQs indicated that 12 anomic, five conduction, two transcortical sensory, and one transcortical motor aphasic reached this criterion of recovery. Although this represents only 21 percent of the 93 total, it is 62.5 percent of the conduction, 50 percent of the transcortical, and 48 percent of the anomic patients (Table 15-2). Reversal of the direction on evolution from the patterns described (Table 15-2) may occur with an extension of a stroke or tumor. For instance, if an anomic aphasic becomes nonfluent or the jargon becomes

Table 15–2
Evolution of Aphasia

Initial Classification	Endstage	Percent recovered completely
Globals (22) ⟶	2 Broca	
	1 Transcortical motor	
	1 Conduction	
	1 Anomic	
Broca's (17) ⟶	1 Transcortical motor	
	3 Anomic	
Conduction (8) ⟶	2 Anomic	
	5 Nonaphasic	(62.5%)
Wernicke's (13) ⟶	1 Global	
	1 Transcortical sensory	
	4 Anomic	
Isolation (2) ⟶	1 Anomic	
Transcortical motor 3 ⟶	2 Anomic	
	1 Nonaphasic	
(6)	2 Nonaphasic	(50%)
Transcortical sensory 3 ⟶	1 Anomic	
Anomic (25) ⟶	12 Nonaphasic	(48%)
Total 93		21%

(Adapted with permission from Brain 100:1–18, 1977.)

more neologistic, one of the above should be considered. Leishner (1976) also studied the transformation of aphasic syndromes 3 months post stroke, specifying the degree of improvement at the same time.

Recovery Rates

Recovery rates appeared to relate clearly to the time of examination after onset. Therefore, we took the differences between the AQs of the first test, and the one 3 months later as the rate for the first interval, the 3–6 months' test as the second, and between 6 months and the last test which may be anywhere up to five years, as the third interval recovery rate. In Table 15-3, the recovery rates for each subgroup are displayed. Only those patients (36) were included who had been examined within 45 days of onset, and subsequently within the specified time, and had stable infarcts or hemorrhages (CVA). The degree of improvement was by far the greatest in the first interval, that is, between the first test within a month and a half from onset and 3 months later, but some recovery was noted in

Table 15–3

Mean Rates of Recovery

Type of Aphasia	Mean AQ	Initial Age	N	0–3 Months	N	3–6 Months	N	6–12 or more
Global (spontaneous)	24.1	53.8	5	5.16	4	−1.35	2	−0.2
(treated)	21.4	66.4	5	16.82*	5	−2.88*	4	10.65**
Broca's (spontaneous)	35.6	54	4	36.8	2	1.0	3	4.63
(treated)	—	54.4	0	—	1	0.8*	2	7.6*
Conduction	60.5	55.6	4	34.9	3	9.4	2	5.0
Wernicke's	34.0	60.9	4	14.9	1	1.6	1	21.2
Anomic	76.9	64.0	14	7.9	4	2.1	3	2.5
Total			36	16.64	20	1.52	17	7.34

*No significant difference at $p = 0.05$ between spontaneous and treated.
**Significant
(Adapted with permission from Brain 100:1–18, 1977.)

all subsequent intervals. That the improvement was greater in the third interval than in the second is probably the result of including some long-term patients in this group.

The differences in recovery rates between various types of aphasia are evident from Table 15-3. The Kruskal–Wallis nonparametric one-way analysis of variance was performed on the improvement scores for the first 3 months. The analysis proved to be significant $(H^1 - 27.28, df = 5, P < 0.01)$ indicating that there are some significant differences between groups of aphasics—untreated globals, treated globals, Broca's conduction, Wernicke's and anomics. Following this overall test of significance the Mann–Whitney U tests were employed in conjunction with the procedure recommended by Ryan (1962) to discover which groups differed significantly in their recovery rates. Both the untreated globals and anomics improved significantly less than the Broca's ($P < 0.02$ for untreated globals and $P < 0.04$ for anomics) and the conduction aphasics ($P < 0.04$ for both untreated globals and anomics). There were no significant differences in the other comparisons including that between treated and untreated globals ($P < 0.05$). The highest rates of recovery were shown by Broca's ($X = 36.8$) and conduction aphasics ($X = 34.9$); the lowest recovery rate by untreated global ($X = 5.16$) and anomic aphasics ($X = 7.9$). Recovery rates should not be confused with the level of recovery which is much higher among anomic aphasics.

In the global "long term period," the treated group showed higher recovery rate, but one aphasic was probably not truly global to begin with (the line ending in 72, in Fig. 15-3), but his initial scores were depressed because of nonlanguage factors. It is notable that only nonfluent aphasics (Global and Broca's) received treatment in this population. The reasons for this are multiple, such as the associated hemiplegia which will keep this type of aphasic in a hospital longer, and the more rapid recovery of others.

Recovery Patterns

The patterns of recovery in CVA, according to the type of aphasia, are illustrated in Figs. 15-3−15-7. The ages of patients are at the end of the lines. Each aphasic in the study is represented in one of the graphs. The interrupted lines indicate the duration of speech therapy.

1. *Global* aphasics (*N* = 22) who understand little or nothing and speak only in stereotyped utterances, show limited recovery as a rule, with a few exceptions mentioned above. Individual recovery graphs of the patients followed from the onset, who were included in Table 15-3, are displayed in Fig. 15-3.

2. *Broca's* aphasics (motor aphasia) (*N* = 17); patients with poor output but good comprehension who showed the highest recovery rates (Fig. 15-4). The initial scores were somewhat better than global aphasics. Those showing the best improvement were also the youngest. These patients are easily recognizable by experienced clinicians. They are attentive, well aware of their speech difficulty, and often clearly frustrated by it; most of them make an effort to correct their speech. In the few treated patients, therapy only began at 6 months. The course of their recovery did not seem to be different from the untreated group.

3. *Conduction* aphasics (central aphasia) (*N* = 8) show a favorable spontaneous recovery pattern (Fig. 15-5); their speech is characterized by many phonemic paraphasias, fair fluency, good comprehension, but poor repetition. They often show the phenomenon of phonemic anticipation or repeated related paraphasias to approach a target word, such as "spark . . . bark . . . spork . . . fork" (the "conduites d'approche").

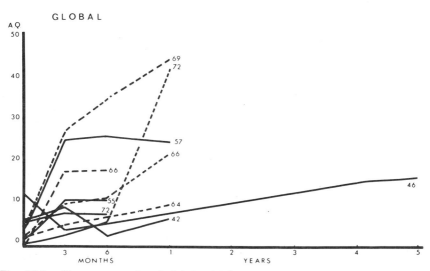

Fig. 15-3. Recovery graphs of global aphasics. Interrupted lines indicate duration of speech therapy. AQ is the aphasia quotient. (Reprinted with permission from Brain 100:1−18, 1977.)

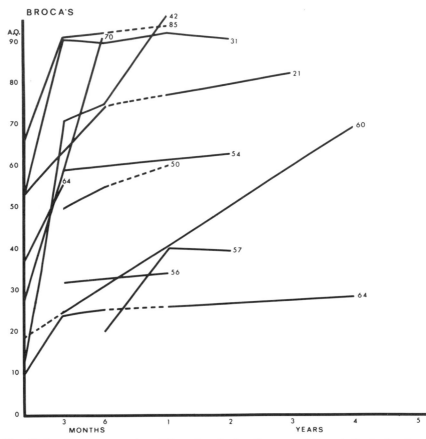

Fig. 15-4.   Recovery graphs of Broca's aphasics. Interrupted lines indicate duration of speech therapy. AQ is the aphasia quotient.

4. *Wernicke's* aphasics (Sensory aphasia) ($N = 13$) seemed to have a bimodal pattern of recovery (Fig. 15-6). Some Jargon aphasics improve little and retain fluent jargon under pressure for many months, one as long as 2 years. After a while, they lose their phonemic paraphasias and their language deficit consists of semantic substitutions and anomia. Those of the Wernicke's group with higher initial scores and less jargon obviously do better. Age in this group seems to be an important prognostic factor as well, as older patients remained more disabled.

5. *Transcortical* Aphasics ($N = 6$) have not been widely appreciated. These patients often show quick recovery rather early in their course (Fig. 15-5). Transcortical Motor aphasics who may be quite mute and cannot even say their name or address, but will surprisingly repeat a complicated sentence, can be confidently assured of recovery within weeks. Transcortical Sensory

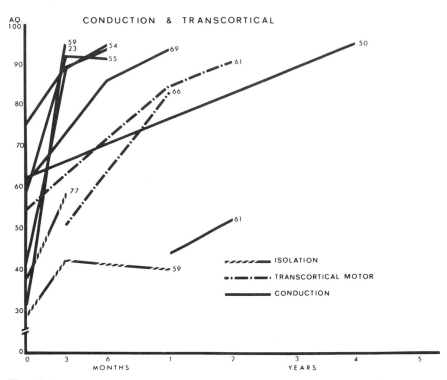

Fig. 15-5.   Recovery graphs of Conduction and Transcortical aphasics. AQ is the aphasia quotient.

aphasics have fluent, irrelevant, paraphasic speech with poor comprehension, but excellent repetition, and they are often seen in trauma. Their prognosis is good. Isolation syndrome ($N = 2$) (Geschwind, Quadfasel, and Segarra, 1968) has not been seen often enough to draw reliable conclusions, but they recover to some extent, although not as well as the other transcortical syndromes.

6. *Anomic* aphasia ($N = 25$) is the mildest language impairment. The patients have high scores to begin with and they often recover completely (Fig. 15-7). Some naming difficulty and circumlocutory speech may persist a long time and may prevent employment, especially if associated with alexia and agraphia.

At a first glance, the recovery curves appear variable, but certain overall patterns clearly emerge. Initial severity is undoubtedly the most important simple factor, followed by the configuration of clinical and linguistic features which constitute the type of aphasia. The time course of recovery is quite characteristic, much of it occurring in the first three months after brain damage and plateauing, and in some cases, showing slow changes beyond 6 months. The etiology is an

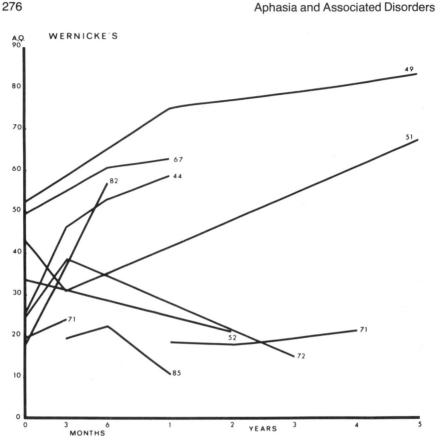

Fig. 15-6.   Recovery graphs of Wernicke's aphasics. AQ is the aphasia quotient.

important consideration, and posttraumatic patients must be studied separately. Age, sex and handedness seem less crucial variables, although we did not have enough left-handers to contribute to this issue. The predictability of the evolution in various forms of aphasia is an important clinical feature. It is more useful to consider these changes in the syndromes as a reflection of the underlying process rather than as evidence against the differences between aphasic groups. The extent of spontaneous recovery is such in aphasia that any serious study of classification localization or treatment has to consider it and control for it in the presentation of results.

LANGUAGE THERAPY

Treatment of aphasics is an established practice, even though only a few studies considered spontaneous recovery in assessing the efficacy of therapy. The first systematic study of treatment, by Butfield and Zangwill (1964), did not have

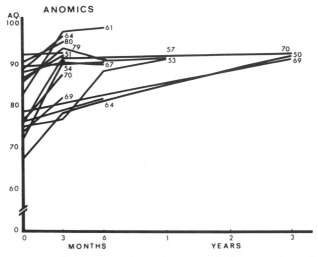

Fig. 15-7. Recovery graphs of Anomic aphasics. Note that only the top of AQ scale is used in the coordinate. (Reprinted with permission from Brain 100:1−18, 1977.)

untreated controls but an attempt was made to describe the method of therapy; mainly the use of oral drills, and transmodal cues. Gains after 6 months were attributed to therapy, assuming that further spontaneous recovery was not significant at that time. Vignolo (1946), who studied treated and untreated patients did not find a significant difference between these groups but suggested that therapy between second and sixth months may have optimal effect. Sarno et al. (1970) compared only global aphasics, who underwent stimulation therapy and programmed instruction, with untreated controls. They found no significant difference.

There are two controlled studies in the literature presenting evidence that therapy is effective: the first by Hagen (1973), who studied ten treated aphasics matched in severity and type (sensorimotor type III of Schuell) to ten untreated ones, and found significantly better recovery in language formulation, speech production, reading comprehension, spelling, and arithmetic in the treated group, mostly in the first 6 months of treatment. Auditory comprehension, auditory retention, visual comprehension, and visual motor abilities improved equally in the treatment and control group. All patients were included in the study at 3 months; treatment began at 6 months after the stroke. The second, by Basso, Faglioni, and Vignolo (1975), had 91 treated aphasics and 94 controls, who could not come for therapy, for family or logistical reasons. A significant effect of therapy was shown on the oral expression of aphasics in a minimum of 6 months of therapy and a negative effect of the duration of aphasia before therapy began. Unfortunately, the design lumped all aphasics into two categories, possibly allowing more global or severe jargon aphasics to be included into the untreated sample. This is bound to occur in everyday therapy situations, as the therapists are much less likely to persist with global or severe jargon patients who do not progress. Another important problem of this retrospective study is that instead of controlling the time of inclusion after the onset, it examined the "effect of this variable" on improvement. This, in fact, resulted in allowing the early group, when spontaneous recovery is greatest, to be weighted in favor of the treated and the late group, when recovery is less likely to occur, to be loaded with untreated patients. To design a study of treatment of aphasia, it is essential to match patients for initial severity, type, etiology, and time from onset. Hagen's study is the only one complying with this so far, but his method of selection of "sensorimotor type III" patients is not defined anywhere.

Pizzamiglio et al. (1976) examined the recovery of comprehension in 64 aphasics, classified as Broca's (30), Wernicke's (12), global (10), transcortical sensory (four), amnestic (six), and conduction (two) aphasia, 3 months apart, with tests for phonetic, semantic, and syntactic discriminations (4, 4, and 2 picture choices). Severity of aphasia was not controlled and only Broca's group was divided into those under or over 12 months since onset. Broca's aphasics showed significant changes on the phonetic and syntactic tests and Wernicke's improved on the semantic test. Gloning et al. (1976) determined the outcome of aphasia in 107 patients: 46 recovered "fully." Initial improvement (spontaneous recovery) and, to a lesser extent, speech therapy were positive factors in recovery. Trauma and vascular etiology were mixed, and speech therapy was not randomly allocated. Messerli et al. (1976) selected 53 patients who benefited from speech therapy for a retrospective analysis of factors: They found that severity and type of aphasia were the most important variables and that Broca's and Wernicke's aphasics improved the most. The presence of apraxia and deficits of operational intelligence were poor prognostic factors. The recovery of two Japanese—American polyglots was reported to be parallel except for Japanese writing, which seemed to improve later, when Japanese instruction was started (Watamori and Sasanuma, 1978).

A cooperative study of aphasia therapy, by Wertz et al. (1978), followed stroke patients undergoing stimulus—response speech therapy and compared them to the results of "social interaction" group therapy. Each group, containing 29 patients, received 8 hours/week, for 11—44 weeks, according to their preliminary report (a paper presented to the Annual Meeting of the American Association for the Advancement of Science, Washington, D C, February, 1978). The results showed significant gains, as measured by the PICA, in both groups, but individually treated patients did better. Other measures, such as RCPM, showed less overall improvement. Maximum improvement occurred in the first 3 months. Significant improvement occurred in the language performance between 26 and 48 weeks in both groups; it was assumed that spontaneous recovery was not operational at that time. This allowed the authors only to speculate about the efficacy of therapy, since no true control group was studied. One could interpret the data, however, that the social interaction group was, in effect, a control group, and that more structured speech therapy did not contribute much more to recovery.

Therapy itself is most complex and difficult to standardize. It is said that there are as many varieties of aphasia treatment as there are aphasics. Therapists are reluctant to follow rigidly prescribed treatment programs, pointing out the need to tailor therapy to the needs of the individual. Not only the methods, but the content differs considerably, creating overlapping categories. Lately, psycholinguistic principles have been contributing increasingly to the content of therapy. The following main methods of therapy are presently in use. The first two are considered to be used by most therapists (Darley, 1975).

Stimulation Approach

Wepman (1951) recognized that aphasics are, in fact, stimulated rather than educated during treatment. Familiar materials, relevant to the patient, are used without pressure and with reinforcing acceptance of every response. Schuell's (1964) approach is similar:

1. Use intensive *auditory stimulation* with meaningful patterns and high frequency words, adjusting the rate, loudness, and length of presentation to the needs of each patient
2, Use highly repetitive stimulation
3. Elicit rather than force some response to every stimulus
4. Stimulate more responses than correct errors
5. Use different language modalities for facilitation: spelling aloud to help writing, writing to help auditory retention, etc.

Various forms of the specific stimulation approachs were defined by Taylor (1964):

1. *Association approach:* Attempting to elicit associated words by structuring sessions around families of words and semantic units such as body parts, furniture, etc., using the maximum possible word environments for each target word.
2. *Situational approach:* Everyday situations are acted out, facilitating functionally useful learning vocabulary or statements.
3. *Minimal differences approach:* Similar sounding words and similar looking written material are used as stimuli for teaching.

Other varieties of stimulation appear to be less structured. These are variously called:

1. *"Environmental stimulation":* Everybody around the patient talks to him as much as possible.
2. *"Rapport approach":* There is a warm relationship between the clinician and the patient without regard to the content and method of contact.

3. *"Socialization approach"*: Individual or group sessions include informal "fun" activities.
4. *"Interest approach"*: Subjects are discussed which relate to the patients' previous group or individual work activities and interests.
5. *"Psychotherapeutic approach"*: Problems of anxiety and loss of self-esteem are focused on and corrected.

Programmed Instruction Approach

The desired language behavior is defined and programs to reach it are constructed. Martha Taylor Sarno and associates defined and developed this approach (Taylor, 1964). Many individual steps from preverbal programs to practicing syntax are used to achieve the desired language behavior (Sarno et al., 1970). Although such a program is repeatable and quantifiable, it is very difficult to design and to persist with. This is also called the psycholinguistic approach when careful attention is directed to the rules of language and the language deficit itself. Goda (1962) advocated using the patients own spontaneous speech to design programs and drill material. Language Oriented Therapy, as described by Shewan (1978), also uses an operant paradigm while the content is based on the knowledge about language impairment in aphasics. It considers the language modalities and the level at which the patient should be trained. The criteria for moving from one level to another are predetermined. The purpose is to teach strategies rather than responses.

Various other, more or less distinct, therapeutic approaches can be identified from the literature. This is far from a complete catalogue.

Deblocking Method

Weigl (1968) described a special kind of stimulation which uses an intact channel to eliminate a block in understanding or expression via other channels. A response is evoked in an intact channel (e.g., recognition of a printed word) just before presenting the same stimulus to a blocked channel (auditory comprehension).

Preventive Method

This is a specific application of linguistic theory by Beyn and Shokhor-Trotskaya (1966). Instead of object naming, they worked on expressions as a whole, preventing the occurrence of telegraphic speech.

Compensatory Approach

This encourages the patient to use his own compensatory strategies, e.g., the patient who needs repetition to understand is encouraged to ask for it. Patients with word-finding difficulty are encouraged to circumlocute (Holland, 1977).

Operant Conditioning with Automatic Teaching Machines

These have been described by Keith and Darley (1967). Patients universally and understandably prefer human contact!

Melodic Intonation Therapy (MIT)

This therapy has been tried for global aphasics (Sparks et al., 1974) based on evidence that many severely affected aphasics can sing words better than speak, and that musical, tonal abilities are subserved by the right hemisphere. The patient intones a melody for simple statements (like opera).

Visual Communication (VIC)

Nonverbal symbols were used to train global aphasics to express themselves, based on the demonstration that the chimpanzee can be taught a nonverbal communication system (Glass et al., 1973). Gardner et al. (1976) taught patients to recognize and maniupulate symbols to respond to commands, answer questions, describe his actions, and express desires and feelings. A similar approach is the use of hand signals to teach global aphasics basic communication (Eagleson et al., 1970).

Visual Action Therapy

Helm and Benson (1978) presented a study of severely affected global aphasics who were not able to benefit from traditional treatment until they responded to visual matching of objects to pictures and actions.

Drug Treatment

Drug treatment of aphasia included dexamethasone, sodium amytal, priscol, meprobamate, hyperbaric oxygen, with unimpressive results.

Direct Psychotherapy and Hypnosis

This has been used also, and at times, considered useful to reduce the emotional problems of aphasics and to facilitate recovery.

Special Therapies for Various Modalities

These have appeared, for example, for "verbal apraxia" (Rosenbeck et al., 1973) or for retraining of writing (Hatfield and Weddell, 1976).

Brookshire (1977) attempted to analyze the relationship between clinician and patient behavior. He is developing a system for recording and coding the events during therapy. He has aptly stated that "a definite study of the effects of treatment on recovery from aphasia will be impossible without some means of describing objectively and unambiguously the exact nature of the treatment program or programs employed in the study."

SUMMARY

Recovery from aphasia depends on etiology, initial severity, and type of aphasia and follows a predictable time course in strokes. Age, handedness, intelligence, and education are less definite factors. Recovery is greater in trauma, more variable in subarachnoid hemorrhage. Initial severity is highly predictive of outcome. The evolution from one aphasic type to another occurs in a characteristic pattern. Anomic aphasia is a common end stage of Wernicke's, conduction, transcortical, and at times, Broca's aphasias. Complete recovery occurred in many conduction, transcortical, and anomic aphasics. Global and some Wernicke's aphasics have poor, Broca's aphasics intermediate prognosis. The recovery rates are highest in the first 3 months, still significant in the second, but slow after 6 months, and plateau after a year from onset. The highest recovery rates were shown by Broca's and Conduction aphasics.

There are many forms of speech therapy; stimulation and programmed instruction are the most often used. The impact of therapy is difficult to separate from spontaneous recovery but at least two controlled studies suggest a positive effect in contrast to another on global aphasics with negative results.

16

Recovery of Associated Disorders

It does not suffice to destroy an organ to understand what functions it serves

Claude Bernard (1865)

THEORETICAL AND EXPERIMENTAL CORRELATES OF RECOVERY

Rigid localization of function in the nervous system is hardly compatible with repeated observations of recovery of function, after destroying those parts of the nervous system held responsible. One of the earliest opponents of phrenological localization was Flourens (1824), who demonstrated recovery after ablative experiments in pigeons. Lashley's (1938) well-known theory of *equipotentiality* of cortical function is based on similar extensive ablations, consistent with recovered function. He also found 18 cases in the literature in which he could estimate the magnitude of the lesions in the left frontal lobe and the degree of recovery from motor aphasia, obtaining a negative correlation of 0.9 (the smaller the lesion the greater the recovery). He considered this analogous to the correlation between remaining intact cortical tissue and the amount of learning in animals.

The *substitutionist* theory of recovery has never been precisely formulated. Fritsch and Hitzig (1870) thought that the other hemisphere was taking over the motor functions of cortical lesions in dogs. However, this was not confirmed by destroying the analogous opposite side in adult animals. In man, there is evidence that the right hemisphere is capable of assuming some speech function, such as comprehension (nouns better than verbs) and automatic nonpropositional speech, from hemispherectomies (Smith, 1966) and callosal sections (Gazzaniga, 1970). Kinsbourne (1971) argued that the right hemisphere may be the source of some aphasic speech. In the adult, however, the extent to which this recovery occurs is finite, both in cases of hemispherectomies and many aphasics. In fact, the behavior of hemispherectomized patients with no cortical tissue left is very similar to global aphasics with extensive infarction of the sylvian area. This indicates that the remaining language function of global aphasics is probably entirely subserved by the right hemisphere. That restitution of speech is often due to the activity of the opposite hemisphere is known as Henschen's axiom. Henschen (1922) gave credit to Jackson, Wernicke and other contemporaries for this principle. Nielsen (1946) further advocated the idea that recovery occurs to a large extent by the variable capacity of the right hemisphere to develop speech. Geschwind (1969) also believes in the considerable amount of individual variation in hemispheric substitution. Some people can make use of certain commissural connections more than others, and some cortical mechanisms on the right hemisphere can be more easily activated. Munk (1881) thought that regions of the brain previously ''not occupied'' could assume certain functions (''vicarious functioning''). Lashley (1938) considered that preservation of part of a system concerned with the same function is necessary. However, ''reverse ablations'' indicate that certain areas which are needed for recovery do not contribute to the normal function (Bucy, 1934). Clinically, it is evident that right hemisphere lesions will not cause aphasia, even though the right hemisphere subserves some language functions.

Transfer of function occurs more easily in the immature nervous system. This *plasticity of function* has been demonstrated in experiments by Kennard (1943), who found that unilateral lesions in precentral areas in infant animals have minimal effects compared to adults. In children under the age of 5, up to 10–12, at times, the rate of recovery from aphasia is excellent (Basser, 1962; Hecaen, 1976). Maturation of the left hemisphere seems to inhibit the right hemisphere, and lesions in the left speech area, when they occur early in life, preempt this inhibition on the right and sparing of language or recovery occurs. There is, however, a reduction in overall intellectual capacity due to ''crowding'' in the right hemisphere (Milner, 1974).

The functional plasticity of the young may depend on the microneurons of type II cells of Golgi (Hirsch and Jacobson, 1974). These cells remain adaptive while the long axon cells responsible for the major transmission of information in and out of the CNS are under early and exacting genetic control and specification. The state of flexibility for these microneurons may be terminated in the teens in man by hormonal changes, explaining the age limit of relocalization of language. Acquisition of a foreign language without an accent also appears to be limited by puberty interestingly enough. Pertaining to this is the experimental evidence showing that bird song acquisition depends on hormone levels (Nottebohm, 1970).

Hierarchical representation of function at different levels of the nervous system was proposed by Jackson (1873). Damage at a higher level releases the lower ones from inhibition and leads to "compensation". More recently, Geschwind (1974) cited examples of neuronal systems that could be released in turn to take over where the ones above are destroyed. The slowing of the system is the price exacted for plasticity.

Diaschisis is a term coined by Van Monakow (1914), who postulated that damage to parts of the nervous system deprives the other areas from the usual stimulation and creates a state of shock. Eventually, the undamaged portions of the brain could resume normal functioning as the effect of diaschisis subsided. Bilateral reduction of cerebral blood following cerebral infarct could be one of the phenomena underlying diaschisis (Meyer, 1970). This is known to persist up to 2 months. Release of catecolamines during this period has also been demonstrated; whether it is a cause or an associated phenomenon is largely unknown (Meyer, 1974). Diaschisis is more marked after sudden lesions, such as infarcts, or trauma. Tumors often grow slowly, minimizing the effect of diaschisis. Large tumors within speech areas may not produce deficits due to the *"serial lesion" phenomena* reported by Ades and Raab (1946). Two-stage removal was much less damaging than the same area destroyed at once. Dax (1865), in describing the 40-odd observations of left hemisphere lesions (published posthumously by his son, after Broca's discovery) also suggested that left hemisphere disease may not alter speech if the lesion developed slowly. Von Monakow (1914) also noted that aphasia may be absent in Broca's area with slowly growing tumors. The neural shock or diaschisis is avoided in slowly growing or multistage lesions.

Regeneration in the mammalian CNS is not comparable to that in the peripheral nervous system. Axonal regrowth was found, however, in ascending catecholaminergic fibers. Growing axons tend to invade vacant terminal space (Schneider, 1973). The recently discovered phenomenon of *collateral sprouting* could be the underlying mechanism of recovery and even diaschisis in certain instances (Liu and Chambers, 1958). Both regenerative and collateral sprouting has been demonstrated by Moore (1974). Collateral sprouting, whether from intact axons or collaterals of the damaged axons, seems to be more important. *Central denervation hypersensitivity* (Cannon and Rosenbluth 1949) could explain why some central structures would become more responsive to remaining stimulations after damage, therefore promoting recovery. Remaining fibers from the damaged area could produce a greater effect on the denervated region, achieving the same result. The opposite effect of denervation hypersensitivity has also been argued. The initial hypersensitivity would induce inhibition of function (diaschisis), and the appearance of collateral sprouting would put an end to the denervation and the accompanying inhibition.

Pharmacological aspects or recovery are most complex. Cholinergic agents (Ward and Kennard, 1942), anticholinesterases (Luria et al., 1969), amphetamines (Braun et al., 1966) accelerate recovery; barbiturates (Watson and Kennard, 1945) slow recovery. Catecholamines may act as inhibitors (Meyer, 1974), and bicuculline as a disinhibitor of recovery (Duffy et al., 1976).

Anatomical variations of the speech areas and the role of less lateralization in left-handers could contribute to the variable extent of recovery from lesions which appear to be identical (Luria, 1970). The nature of the injury may provide another anatomical variable. Rubens (1977) explained the dramatic recovery from thalamic hemorrhage on the basis of the nervous structures being pushed aside rather than destroyed, as in an ischemic infarct, and which therefore allow for more recovery. Kohlmeyer (1976) considered that recanalization of the occluded artery contributes to the frequent recovery in the first two weeks after stroke.

Functional compensation employs a behavioral rather than a neural model. Substituted maneuvers or tricks have been described and documented by Sperry (1947). Instead of rerouting connections, the brain-damaged organism develops new solutions to problem using residual structures. Luria (1969) formulated the theory of *"retraining"* which claims that the dynamic reorganization after injury is promoted by specific therapy. Recovery by using alternate pathways may occur in man, such as the use of ipsilateral corticospinal system by the speaking hemisphere to carry out commands in patients with callosal lesions (Geschwind, 1974).

Motivational factors were found to be powerful in changing postlesion behavior in animals, and this has shown to be important in the recovery of human deficits as well. Karl Lashley illustrates this in a poignant anecdote: He bet a patient of Dr. Franz, who could not learn the alphabet after 900 repetitions, 100 cigarettes that he could not learn it in a week. "After 10 trials he was letter perfect, and remembered it until the debt was paid." Many patients, after hospitalization, develop functional disorders superimposed upon the organic, and they are likely to have a passive attitude and depression. This lack of motivation may be changed, producing recovery. The experiments of Franz and Odin (1917) to force the use of paralyzed limbs is evidence that intense motivation is really effective in compensating for organic defects. Stoicheff (1960) provided interesting evidence for the effect of positive and negative verbal comments on the performance of aphasics.

The psychological processes of motivation, relearning, and environmental enrichment may be superimposed on physiological ones. In the serial lesion paradigm, interoperative exposure to light stimulation was necessary to achieve visual recovery in occipital lesions (Meyer et al., 1958). Greater environmental stimulation attenuates postlesion maze learning deficit in rats, according to Finger (1978).

RECOVERY OF NONVERBAL FUNCTION

Very little information is available concerning the recovery of nonverbal intelligence in patients, in contrast to the increasing literature on recovery and treatment of aphasia. Previous studies found performance on Raven's Colored Progressive Matrices (RCPM) impaired in a general aphasic population (see Chapter 14). Culton (1969) used Raven's Standard Progressive Matrices in 11 aphasics and found considerable recovery of nonverbal performance in the group, 2 months postonset, and no recovery in the group beyond 11 months. Campbell and Oxbury (1976) examined right hemisphere damaged patients 3–4 weeks and 6 months after a stroke, with verbal and nonverbal tasks, including block design and matrices. Those with neglect on drawing, on the initial test, remained impaired on visuospatial tests 6 months later, in spite of the resolution of neglect. Other reports describe inattention up to 12 years after onset (Zarit and Kahn, 1974). Nonverbal intellectual function, or performance skills on the Wechsler Adult Intelligence Scale, took longer to recover than verbal intelligence in trauma, as measured by Bond (1975). The most rapid period of recovery occurred during the first 6 months and more slowly reached a maximum at 24 months. Psychosocial outcome, affected by personality and intellectual changes, correlated negatively with the duration of posttraumatic amnesia. Mandleberg and Brooks (1975) found that recovery of performance IQ continued over 3 years in severe trauma.

Our own previously published analysis of RCPM performance and language function suggested that impaired comprehension is the most prominent subtest correlating with RCPM, and that aphasics with initially poor comprehension (global, Wernicke's, transcortical sensory aphasias) show poorer performance on the RCPM (Kertesz and McCabe, 1975). The hypothesis occurred to us that recovery of language function, especially comprehension, should be paralleled by recovery of nonverbal performance, as measured by the RCPM, if these neuropsychological functions or their disturbances are related.

RECOVERY OF NONVERBAL FUNCTION IN APHASIA

We undertook studying recovery of visuospatial nonverbal function with the RCPM and correlated it with various language functions in the aphasic stroke patients. They were right-handed and had a single vascular episode in the left hemisphere, as proven by hemiplegia or isotope scan. The initial portion of this study included 49 aphasics who had both the RCPM and the Western Aphasia Battery, our standardized aphasia test, within 1 month of onset of their stroke and also 3 months later. Thirty-three aphasics had 3−6 month, and 29 had 6−12 month, recovery studies. Twenty aphasics were examined at all intervals. We divided the aphasics into taxonomic groups according to their performance on the subtests of our aphasia battery (see Table 4-2). Recovery curves of language total (AQ), comprehension total (COMT.), RCPM, block design, and drawing, for each aphasic type were constructed. The raw scores were converted to percentages of the possible total. Each patient had an initial examination, within 30 days of onset for classification. However, not all patients were examined in each interval. The interrupted sections in the graphs indicate that the patients participating in each time interval were to some extent different. This also explains why the starting points of some parameters are different from the end values of the previous interval. The continuous graphs indicate the same individuals throughout all the intervals of recovery.

We were unable to control the effect of speech therapy on the language recovery in this study, as the duration and frequency of the therapy were extremely variable. Only about 35 percent of patients received therapy in this group and most of them only in the first few weeks of hospitalization.

Global aphasics (Fig. 16-1) show recovery from deficient performance on the RCPM, which is parallel to that of language in the first 3 months, but surpasses it in the 3−6 month poststroke interval. In the 6−12 month interval, the RCPM and language reach a plateau. Drawing and block design recover more in the later intervals, but not quite to the same extent as the RCPM.

Broca's aphasics (Fig. 16-2) show dramatic language recovery, but have only modest improvement in the RCPM in all three intervals, although drawing and block design recovery rates are higher in the first 3 months. It should be considered that they start off with higher RCPM scores than others.

Wernicke's aphasics (Fig. 16-3) have poor recovery of RCPM and block design, as compared to language function. The variation among individual patients is considerable. The drawing scores show some decline in 3−6 months, but only three patients were studied in this interval.

Conduction aphasics (Fig. 16-4) also show more recovery in language than in the RCPM, but the number of patients is too small to draw conclusions. It appears that block design and drawing do not change significantly, but they are rather high to begin with in this group.

Transcortical Sensory aphasics (Fig. 16-5) show parallel recovery from language and performance in the first three months. The numbers are too small for any conclusions subsequently.

Anomic aphasics (Fig. 16-6) show lower scores and rates of recovery in performance than in language, but their starting scores are relatively high with correspondingly less recovery.

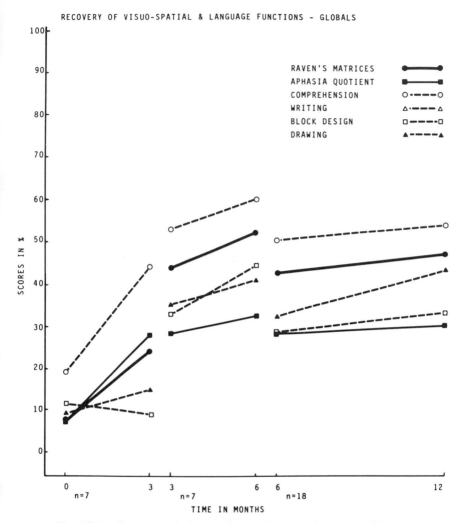

Fig. 16-1. Recovery of visuospatial and language functions—Global.

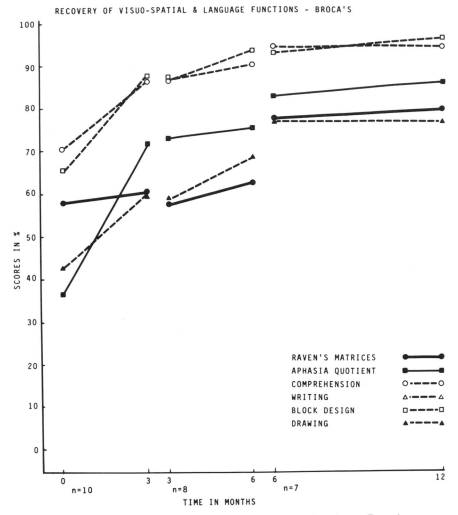

RECOVERY OF VISUO-SPATIAL & LANGUAGE FUNCTIONS - BROCA'S

Legend:
- RAVEN'S MATRICES ●————●
- APHASIA QUOTIENT ■————■
- COMPREHENSION ○·————○
- WRITING △·————△
- BLOCK DESIGN □————□
- DRAWING ▲————▲

SCORES IN %

TIME IN MONTHS

n=10   n=8   n=7

Fig. 16-2.   Recovery of visuospatial and language functions—Broca's.

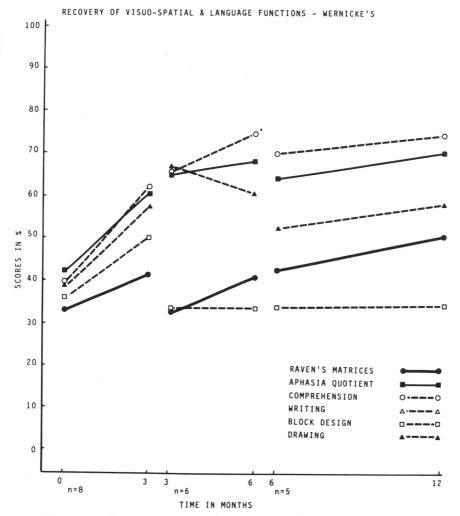

Fig. 16-3.   Recovery of visuospatial and language functions—Wernicke's.

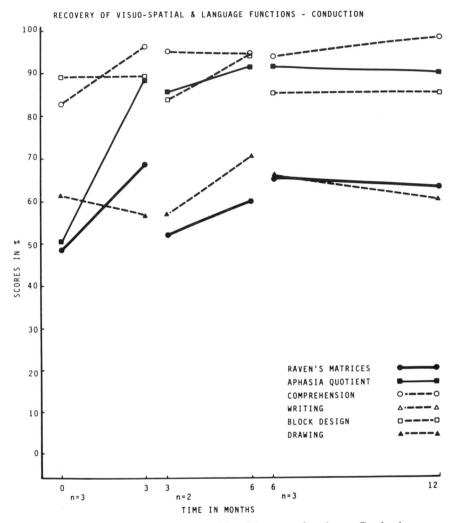

RECOVERY OF VISUO-SPATIAL & LANGUAGE FUNCTIONS - CONDUCTION

Fig. 16-4.   Recovery of visuospatial and language functions—Conduction.

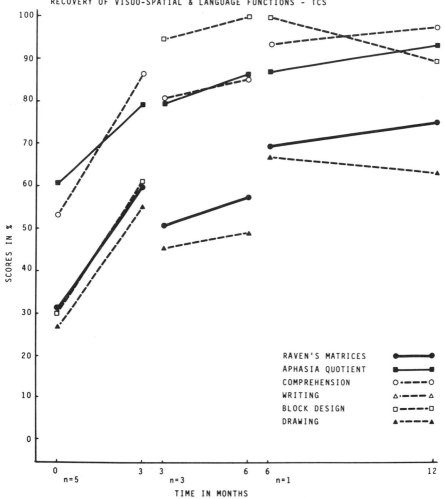

Fig. 16-5. Recovery of visuospatial and language functions—TCS.

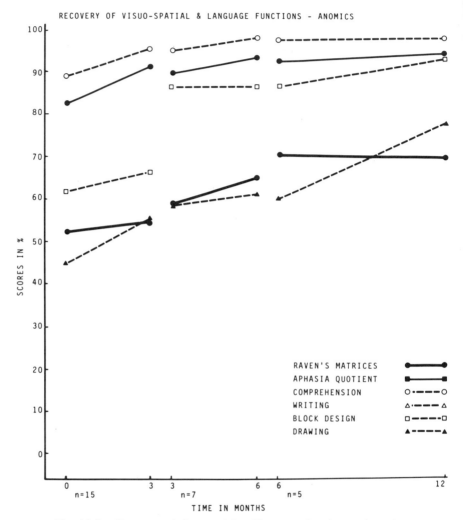

RECOVERY OF VISUO-SPATIAL & LANGUAGE FUNCTIONS - ANOMICS

TIME IN MONTHS

Fig. 16-6.   Recovery of visuospatial and language functions—Anomics.

All aphasics who were followed through all three intervals, 0−3, 3−6, and 6−12 months postonset, were considered together ($N = 20$). This was a fairly representative sample of the aphasic population: three global, six Broca's, four Wernicke's, five anomic, and two conduction aphasics. The recovery rates were lower for the RCPM for the first 3 months, but it continued to rise at nearly the same rate in the second interval, in contrast to language, which plateaued after 3 months (Fig. 16-7). The recovery from visuospatial intelligence in

RECOVERY OF VISUOSPATIAL FUNCTION AND LANGUAGE
IN APHASICS

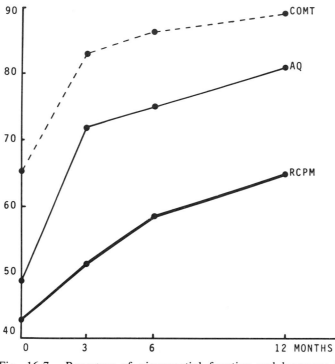

Fig. 16-7. Recovery of visuospatial function and language in aphasics. N = 20.

aphasics seemed to continue, even in the 6−12 month interval. Recovery rates for language and RCPM were significant at $P \leq 0.05$ in all intervals, as calculated by the repeated measures t test (see Table 16-1). The recovery rates are the differences of mean scores calculated as percentages of the maximum of each parameter measured.

The correlation of RCPM recovery rates in aphasics with the recovery of various language parameters measured by the WAB reveals that the correlations are the most significant in the 0−3 month period; this is the time for the highest recovery rates (Table 16-2). Reading, responsive speech, sentence comprehension, word recognition, and object naming are correlated most significantly ($p \leq 0.01$), and sentence completion, repetition, AQ, drawing, and praxis correlate at $p \leq 0.05$. In the 3−6 month period only reading, and in the 6−12 month period only responsive speech, correlated at $p \leq 0.05$ level.

Table 16–1

Recovery Rates of Language and RCPM in Aphasics

Interval in months	N	Comprehension	AQ	RCPM
0–3	20	17.6**	23.5**	8.6*
3–6	20	3.3**	3.6**	7.1**
6–12	20	2.5*	4.4**	6.3**

*$p \leq 0.05$.   **$p \leq 0.01$.

The recovery rates are differences of mean scores (percentages of the maximum) with the significance of difference measured by the t test for each interval.

Table 16–2

Correlation of RCPM and WAB Subtests Recovery

Subtests	Intervals		
	0–3 Months N=49	3–6 Months N=33	6–12 Months N=29
Information content	0.18	0.19	0.29
Fluency	0.01	0.09	−0.06
Yes–no comprehension	−0.00	−0.05	−0.00
Word recognition	0.40**	0.19	0.09
Sentence comprehension	0.40**	−0.11	0.21
Repetition	0.33*	0.18	−0.12
Object naming	0.39**	−0.01	0.34
Word fluency	0.14	−0.10	0.08
Sentence completion	0.28*	0.13	−0.07
Responsive speech	0.41**	0.25	0.37*
Aphasia quotient	0.33*	0.26	0.27
Reading	0.45**	0.35*	0.09
Writing	0.29	0.08	0.04
Praxis	0.32*	0.37	0.14
Drawing	0.37*	0.04	−0.01
Block design	0.18	−0.47*	0.45
Calculation	0.10	−0.13	−0.05

*$p \leq 0.05$.   **$p \leq 0.01$.

The Pearson r correlation coefficients are calculated for each interval and subtest.

RECOVERY OF VISUOSPATIAL AND CONSTRUCTIONAL FUNCTIONS IN RIGHT HEMISPHERE LESIONS

We followed the visuospatial, constructional, and language functions of 18 right hemisphere damaged patients who were right-handed and clinically not aphasic. Not all patients could be seen in all intervals; therefore, the recovery curve is discontinuous. Although these results are considered preliminary, they represent a contrast to the aphasic recovery group that is worth examining.

RCPM, drawing, and block design show significant and comparable recovery in the $0-3$ month interval (Fig. 16-8). RCPM recovery is less in a $3-6$ months' interval and subsequently at $6-12$ months. Drawing scores are variable, with deterioration in the $3-6$ month interval and recovery in the $6-12$ month period. The control language tests remain unimpaired, but initially impaired writing scores show a rise paralleling block design. The means of recovery rates were compared with a multiple measures t test (Table 16-3). Only the RCPM and drawing recovery rates were significant at $0-3$ months' interval.

The recovery rates of RCPM were correlated with the recovery of reading, writing, praxis, drawing, block design, and calculation in the $0-3$, $3-6$, and $6-12$ month intervals. The only significant correlation occurred in the $3-6$ month interval, with the recovery of writing (Table 16-4).

RECOVERY OF PRAXIS IN APHASICS

Recovery from apraxia has not been documented systematically, so far. We had the opportunity to follow 50 aphasics with the complete apraxia battery in $0-3$ months, 25 in $3-6$ months, 15 in $6-12$ months, and 13 of these patients are included in all the intervals. The details and rationale of assessing praxis are discussed in Chapter 12. In our test, 20 commands are given for upper limb, buccofacial, instrumental (transitive), and complex performances. The patient is scored 3 for acceptable, 2 for approximate performance, 2 for imitation only, and 1 for approximate performance on imitation or if performed with the actual object. Recovery from praxis closely parallelled language function in all aphasic groups.

Global aphasics ($N = 8$) have somewhat better recovery in praxis in the $3-6$ and $6-12$ month intervals than in total language scores. The praxis recovery curve parallels comprehension more than the other language subtests (Fig. 16-9). Recovery continues in the third interval.

Broca's aphasics ($N = 9$) have steeper initial language recovery but subsequent rates are similar for praxis and language (Fig. 16-10). Praxis and com-

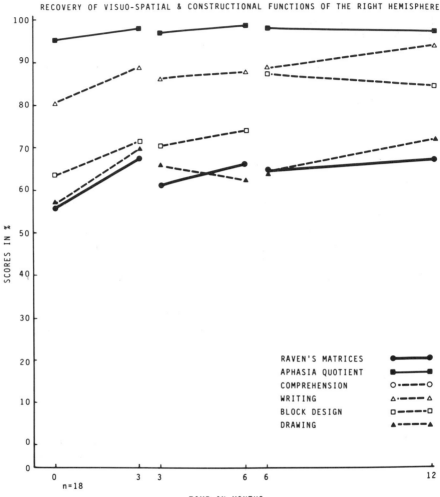

Fig. 16-8.   Recovery of visuospatial and construction functions of the right hemisphere.

prehension have higher initial levels and have less to rise to recovery in this group.

Wernicke's aphasics (N = 5) have similar recovery rates of praxis as Broca's aphasics, even though the patterns of language recovery are substantially different (Fig. 16-11).

Conduction aphasics (N = 4) show a modest amount of recovery from both praxis and language function except for repetition which improves to a greater extent initially (Fig. 16-12).

Table 16–3

Recovery Rates of RCPM, Drawing, Block Design, Writing, and
AQ in Nondominant Lesions

Interval in months	N	RCPM	Drawing	Blocks	Writing	AQ
0–3	18	11.2**	12.2**	8.0	1.83	1.73
3–6	12	5.1	–5.0	3.7	1.28	1.1
6–12	7	2.8	6.6	–3.2	13.5	–1.0

*$p \leqslant 0.05$.   **$p \leqslant 0.01$.

The recovery rates are differences of mean scores (percentages of the maximum) with the significance of difference measured by the t test for each interval.

Transcortical Sensory aphasics ($N = 6$) were only followed in the first interval in sufficient numbers to make it worthwhile to present their recovery curves. They have relatively good praxis to begin with which does not recover as much as comprehension or the aphasia quotient in this group (Fig. 16-13).

Anomic aphasics ($N = 18$) show no recovery in praxis in contrast to the improvement in other parameters, but they have practically normal praxis scores to start with (Fig. 16-14). This is a ceiling effect observed in other groups as well, related to good initial scores and, therefore, a smaller room for improvement. This has to be taken into consideration when one interprets the relatively low rates of recovery seen in the less severely impaired patients.

The recovery rates of the 13 patients who were followed in all three intervals are summarized in Table 16-5 and in Fig. 16-15. The distribution of these patients were: four globals, four Broca's, one Wernicke's, and four anomics. These are quite parallel to the recovery rates of language (AQ) and comprehension and, to a great extent, similar to reading and writing recovery, discussed in the subsequent section. The initial recovery of praxis may not be as rapid as language, but it continued to rise slightly.

Table 16–4

Correlation of Performance Subtests and RCPM Recovery in
Nondominant Lesions

Intervals	N	Reading	Writing	Praxis	Drawing	Block design	Calculation
0–3 months	18	–0.03	–0.05	0.11	0.15	0.18	0.01
3–6 months	12	0.08	0.73*	–0.17	0.44	–0.16	–0.06
6–12 months	6	0.16	0.10	0.07	–0.26	0.27	0.54

*$p < 0.01$.

The Pearson r correlation coefficient is significant only for writing.

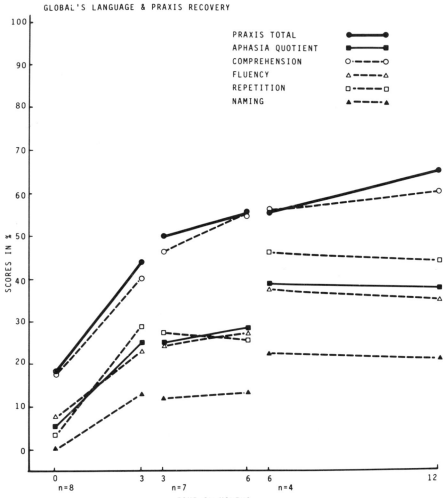

Fig. 16-9.   Global's language and praxis recovery.

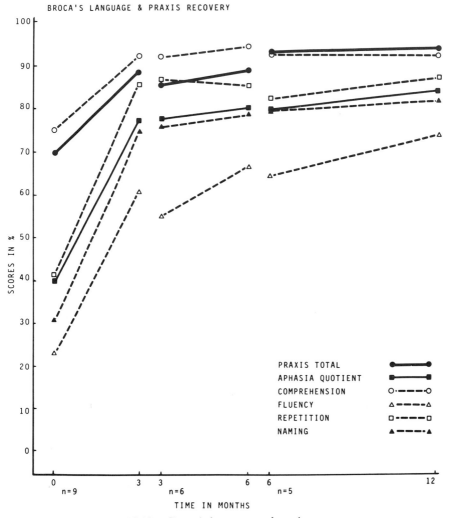

Fig. 16-10.   Broca's language and praxis recovery.

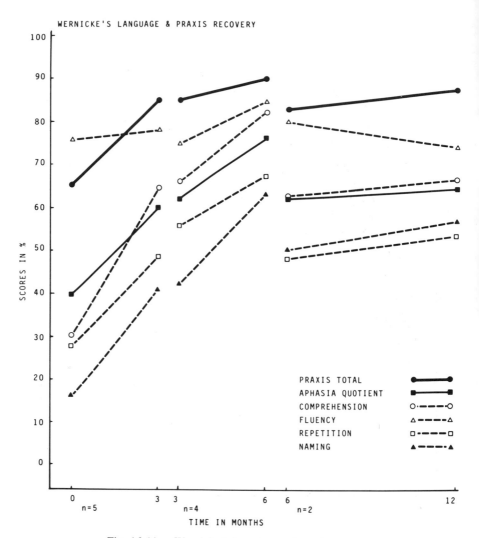

Fig. 16-11. Wernicke's language and praxis recovery.

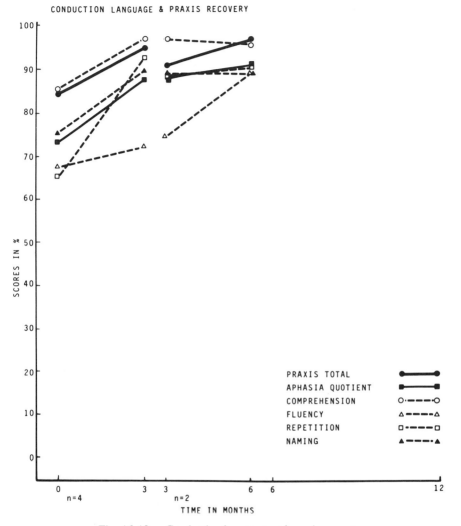

Fig. 16-12. Conduction language and praxis recovery.

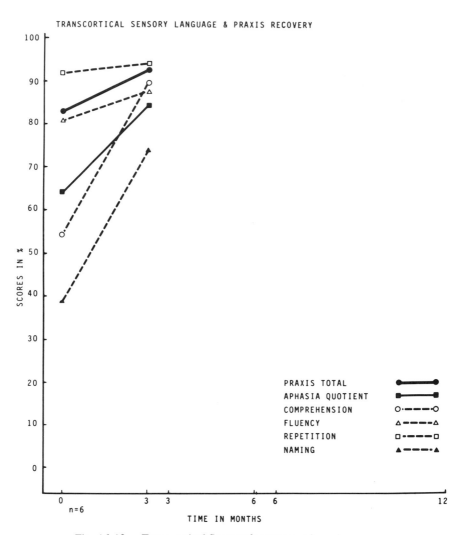

Fig. 16-13.   Transcortical Sensory language and praxis recovery.

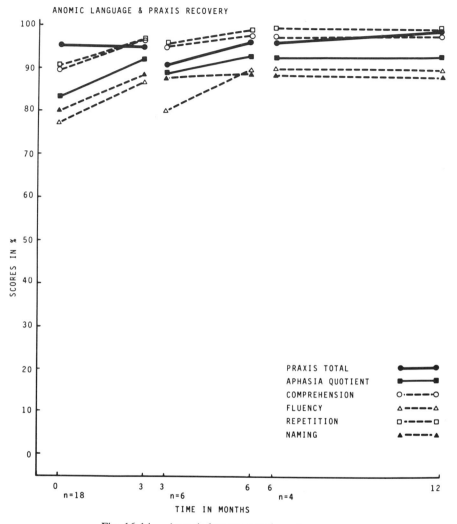

Fig. 16-14.　Anomic language and praxis recovery.

Table 16–5
Recovery Rates of Praxis

	0–3	3–6	6–12
Upper limb	17.4*	4.1	3.1
Buccofacial	23.1*	−3.1	4.6
Instrumental	25.7*	4.1	4.7
Complex	15.9	8.7	5.6
Praxis total	20.5*	3.5	4.5*
AQ	28.0**	3.5*	1.7
Comprehension	21.8**	4.5*	2.4

$*p \leq 0.05$. $**p \leq 0.01$.   df = 12.

The recovery rates are differences of mean scores (percentages of the maximum) with the significance of difference measured by the t test for each interval.

RECOVERY OF READING, WRITING, AND CALCULATION

Recovery from alexia, agraphia, and acalculia has not been studied systematically. Newcombe et al. (1976) drew recovery curves for the performance of two patients who were followed for 6 months and 4 years, respectively, after removal of occipital lesions (abscess and meningioma). Without language therapy, the rate of recovery of the ability to read word lists was maximal initially, and decelerated until 8 to 10 weeks after surgery, at which time a slower rate was achieved. Object naming curves of the patient with an abscess showed slower recovery and more residual errors, in contrast to a post traumatic case, which showed better recovery of naming.

We had 69 aphasics in whom reading, writing, and calculation were examined at successive intervals. Not all of them could be followed for a whole year; therefore, the numbers and starting points varied in each interval. When recovery rates of reading, writing, and calculation are examined in different groups of aphasics, these were found to parallel language recovery with some important variations.

1. *Global aphasia* ($N = 9$) shows very little change in writing and calculation in contrast to the significant recovery in comprehension and reading (Fig. 16-16).
2. *Broca's aphasia* ($N = 13$) recovers substantially in all parameters, although somewhat less in writing and calculation. The rate of recovery in reading and writing is as high in the 0−3 month interval as in spoken language. Practically all recovery seems to occur in this first 3 months, and the curve flattens in the second 3−6 month interval (Fig. 16-17).

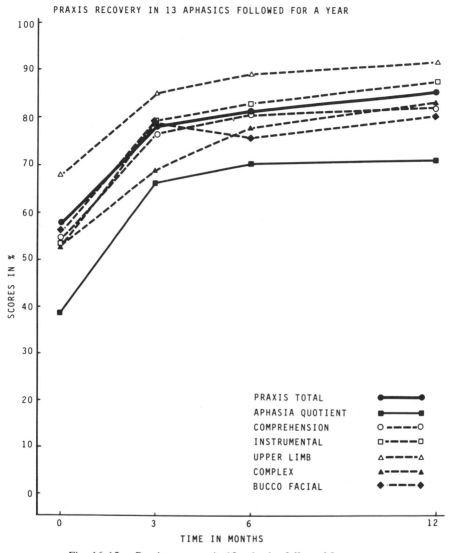

Fig. 16-15.   Praxis recovery in 13 aphasics followed for a year.

3. *Wernicke's aphasia* (N = 7) having reading and writing recovery rates parallel to other language parameters. Writing is low as in the other groups (Fig. 16-18).

4. *Conduction aphasia* (N = 6) shows that reading and calculation are close to language, while writing scores are substantially lower, although the rate of recovery is about the same (Fig. 16-19).

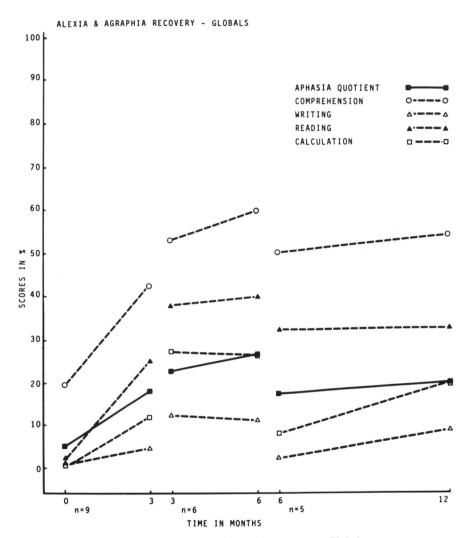

Fig. 16-16.   Alexia and agraphia recovery—Globals.

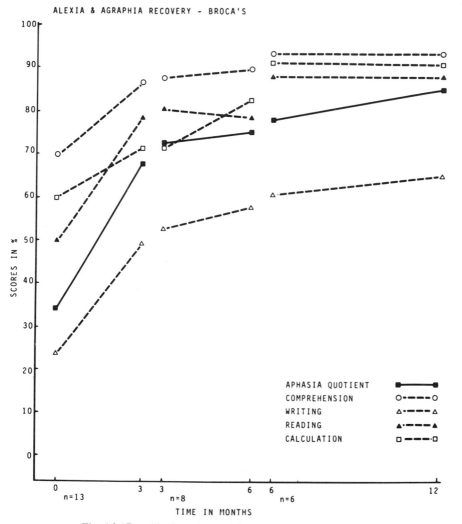

ALEXIA & AGRAPHIA RECOVERY - BROCA'S

APHASIA QUOTIENT	■———■
COMPREHENSION	O·—━·O
WRITING	△·—━·△
READING	▲·—━·▲
CALCULATION	□·—━·□

SCORES IN %

TIME IN MONTHS

n=13   n=8   n=6

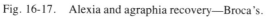

Fig. 16-17.   Alexia and agraphia recovery—Broca's.

309

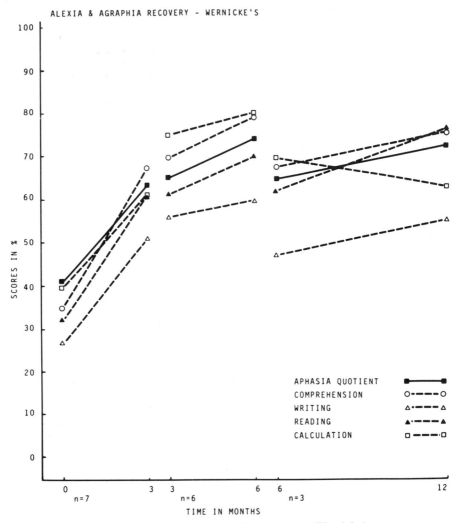

Fig. 16-18.   Alexia and agraphia recovery—Wernicke's.

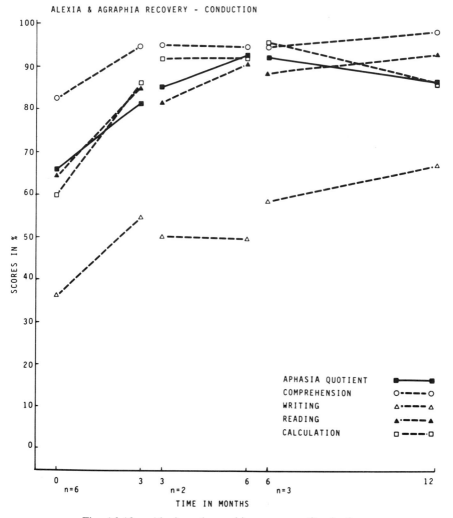

ALEXIA & AGRAPHIA RECOVERY - CONDUCTION

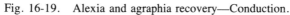

Fig. 16-19. Alexia and agraphia recovery—Conduction.

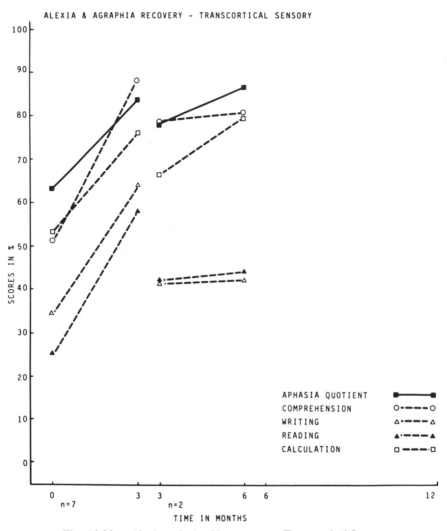

Fig. 16-20.   Alexia and agraphia recovery—Transcortical Sensory.

5. *Transcortical Sensory aphasia* ($N = 7$) shows good recovery in reading, writing and in language scores in the first 3 months. There were not enough patients in the subsequent intervals to justify comments (Fig. 16-20).

6. *Anomic aphasia* ($N = 20$) has similar recovery in reading and calculation to language, but writing rises steeply in the first interval from its relatively low starting level. (Fig. 16-21).

We followed 20 aphasics with the reading and writing tasks, as well as the other subtests of the WAB, for each of the 0−3, 3−6, and 6−12 month inter-

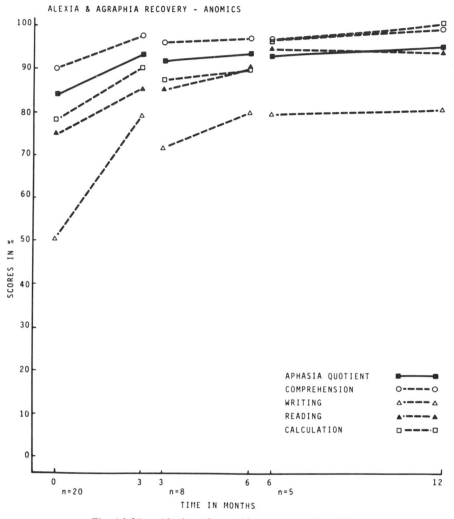

ALEXIA & AGRAPHIA RECOVERY - ANOMICS

APHASIA QUOTIENT	■——■
COMPREHENSION	O----O
WRITING	△·---△
READING	▲·---▲
CALCULATION	□---·□

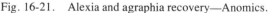

Fig. 16-21.   Alexia and agraphia recovery—Anomics.

vals. This group consisted of: three globals, six Broca's, three Wernicke's, two
conductions, one transcortical sensory, one transcortical motor, and four
anomic aphasics. The recovery curves are displayed in Fig. 16-22. The recovery
curves are parallel in all subtests, except calculation, where the initial curve is
not as steep and more recovery is seen in 3—6 months than in the other parameters. Recovery is significantly greater in the first 0—3 months. Levels of significance in a repeated measures t test were calculated for all subtests (Table 16-6),
indicating highly significant recovery in the first 3 months, followed by moderate
recovery in language, reading, and writing, but not significant in calculation. In

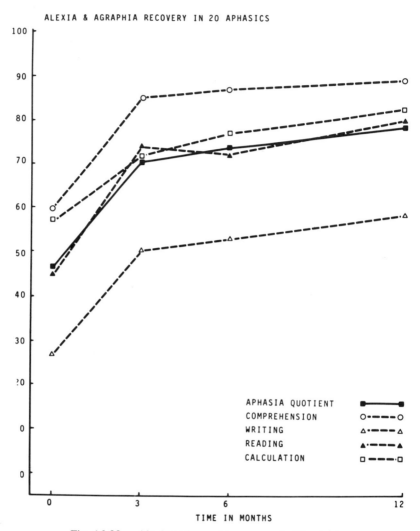

Fig. 16-22.   Alexia and agraphia recovery in 20 aphasics.

Table 16–6
Recovery Rates of Alexia and Agraphia in Aphasics

	Intervals in months ($N=20$)		
	0–3	*3–6*	*6–12*
Reading	28.9**	6.5*	2.45
Writing	15.95**	4.2*	5.3**
Calculation	17.16*	6.15	3.43
Comprehension	25.08**	1.85	2.13
AQ	24.0**	2.98*	4.05*

$*p \leq 0.05.$ $**p \leq 0.01.$ df = 19.

The recovery rates are differences of mean scores (percentages of the maximum) with the significance of difference measured by the *t* test for each interval.

the third interval, the recovery rates are similarly low. The writing subtest scores are consistently lower in all intervals even though their recovery rates are parallel with the rest of the parameters, reflecting the usually severe involvement of writing in aphasia discussed in Chapter 12.

DISCUSSION

The recovery of nonverbal visuospatial function appears to be more or less parallel with language in the total aphasic groups. Differences appear in the first 3 months where RCPM scores improve less than language. This seems to be related to large gains in comprehension by global, Broca's and Wernicke's aphasics in this period. The recovery of constructional ability (block design and drawing) seems less uniform among aphasic groups. Global aphasics recover very little initially, and one wonders if the task is more difficult for global aphasics because of the necessity to manipulate the blocks and the pen besides the visuospatial perceptual elements. However, the difference is not explained entirely by praxis since that was shown to recover quite parallel with language.

The inter-relationship of language functions with visuospatial and constructional tasks is well documented and discussed in detail in Chapter 14. It is possible that a common cognitive factor underlies these processes, accounting for the similarity in their impairment and recovery. Equally plausible is the explanation of anatomical contiguity. The lesions affecting language and the associated performance functions overlap to a great extent as far as we can determine with our present, rather crude methods. Are the same neuronal systems subserving both kinds of cognitive function or are the anatomical systems so close geographically or physiologically that the lesions affect them all? We simply do not know. There is one important overriding distinction, however, indicating a fundamental difference between performance and language function: Right (nondominant) hemisphere lesions substantially impair the former but not the latter. This is not to say, of course, that the right hemisphere has no role in language or in the recovery of language, as there is ample evidence to the contrary. Notwithstanding minor changes in written language after right hemisphere lesions and instances of mixed dominance, the fact remains that the left hemisphere specializes in language and praxis to a much greater extent than other associated functions. One may regard it, therefore, as contrary to expectation to observe similar recovery curves in visuospatial and constructional function, and in language. If nonverbal visuospatial function is bilaterally represented, why does it not recover much more rapidly than language function? A reasonable explanation for the similarity of recovery seems that the element of cognitive impairment with left hemisphere lesions is common with language functions. This commonality suggests that clinicians and researchers may use these nonverbal functions as a control measure of spontaneous recovery and contrast it with the treated language functions.

SUMMARY

The extent of recovery in the higher order nervous system is considerable even though much of it remains a mystery. It seems that one part of the system can substitute for the other and that the homologous portions of the opposite hemisphere are often implied. The evidence for this is substantial, but certain aspects of hemispheric specialization especially the limitation of recovery in the mature individual remains the subject of intense interest.

The recovery of nonverbal, visuospatial functions, praxis, reading, writing, and calculation are reviewed and our data are presented. Recovery of nonverbal function in aphasia varies significantly in each group; in global aphasics it surpasses language recovery, but in other groups it tends to lag behind. RCPM recovery correlates most with reading, comprehension, and naming subtests in the first interval. Visuospatial and constructional functions recover significantly in right hemisphere lesions in the first 3 months but subsequently the change is less significant. Recovery from apraxia closely paralleled language function recovery in all groups. A study of recovery of reading, writing, and calculation indicated a similar parallel with some variations discussed. These recovery studies can be helpful to the clinician in formulating prognosis and planning therapy.

REFERENCES

Ades, HW, Raab, DH: Recovery of motor function after two-stage extirpation of area 4 in monkeys. J Neurophysiol 9: 55−60, 1946

Ajuriaguerra, J de, Hécaen H: Le cortex cérébral. Masson et Cie, Paris, 1964

Ajuriaguerra, J de, Hécaen, H, Angelergues R: Les apraxies, variétés cliniques et latéralisation lésionnelle. Rev Neurol 102: 494−566, 1960

Alajouanine, T: Verbal realization in aphasia. Brain 79: 1−28, 1956

Alajouanine, T, Castaigne, P, Lhermitte, F, Escourolle, R, Ribaucourt, B de: Étude de 43 cas d'aphasie post-traumatique. Confrontation anatomo-clinique et aspects evolutifs. L'encéphale 46:1−45, 1957

Alajouanine, T, Lhermitte, F: Nonverbal communication in aphasia, in DeReuck A & O'Connor M (eds): Disorders of Language. London, Churchill, 1964

Alajouanine, T, Lhermitte, F. Ribaucourt-Ducarne, B de: Les alexies agnosiques et aphasiques, in Les grandes activités du lobe occipital. Paris, Masson & Cie, 1960

Alajouanine, T, Ombredane, A, Durand, M: Le syndrome de la desintegration phonetiques dans l'aphasie. Paris, Masson, 1939

Albert, ML, Bear D: Time to Understand. A case study of word deafness with reference to the role of time in auditory comprehension. Brain 97:373−384, 1974

Albert, M L, Soffer, D, Silverberg, R, et al: The anatomical basis of visual agnosia. Abstr Neurol 28:395, 1978

Albert, M L, Yamadori, A, Gardner, H, Howes, D: Comprehension in alexia. Brain 96:317−328, 1973

Ammon, KH, Godehardt, E: Paraphasie und Form der Aphasie: eine Clusteranalyse bei unausgelesenen Patienten, in G. Peuser (ed), Brennpunkte der Patholinguistik. Munchen, Wilhelm Fink Verlag, 1978

Archibald, Y, Wepman, J, Jones, LV: Nonverbal cognitive performance in aphasic and nonaphasic brain-damaged patients. Cortex 3:275−294, 1967

Aristotle: (Analytica Posteriora), in McKeown, R (ed): Introduction to Aristotle, New York, Random House, 1947

Arrigoni, G, DeRenzi, E: Constructional apraxia and hemispheric locus of lesion. Cortex 1:170−197, 1964

Basser, LS: Hemiplegia of early onset and the faculty of speech with special reference to the effects of hemispherectomy. Brain 85:427−460, 1962

Basso, A, DeRenzi, E, Faglioni, P, et al: Neuropsychological evidence for the existence of cerebral areas critical to the performance of intelligence tasks. Brain 96:715−728, 1973

Basso, A, Faglioni, P, Vignolo, LA: Etude coutrôlée de la reéducation du langage dans l'aphasie: Comparaison entre aphasiques traités et non-traitée. Rev Neurol 131:607−614, 1975

Basso, A, Taborelli, A, Vignolo, L A: Dissociated disorders of speaking and writing in aphasia. J Neurol Neurosurg Psychiatry 41:556−563, 1978

Bastian, H: Aphasia and Other Speech Defects. H.K. Lewis, London, 1898

Bay, E: Aphasia and intelligence. Int J Neurol 4:252−264, 1964

Bay, E: Principles of classification and their influence on our concepts of aphasia, in DeReuck, AVS, O'Connor, M (eds): Disorders of Language. London, Churchill, 1964, p 122−139

317

Breckner, M: The biological way of thought. New York, Columbia University Press, 1959, pp 200

Bell, D S: Speech functions of the thalamus inferred from the effects of thalomotomy. Brain 91:619−638, 1968

Benedikt, M: Über Aphasie, Agraphie und verwandte pathologische Zustande. Wien Med Pr 6:1865

Benson, D F: Fluency in aphasia: Correlation with radioactive scan localization. Cortex 3:373−394, 1967

Benson, D F: The third alexia. Arch Neurol 34:327−331, 1977

Benson, D F, Denckla, M B: Verbal paraphasia as a source of calculation disturbance. Arch Neurol 21:96−102, 1969

Benson, D F, Geschwind, N: The alexias, in Vinken, P and Bruyn, G (eds): Handbook of Clinical Neurology, vol. 4. Amsterdam, North-Holland. 1969, p 112

Benson, D F, Geschwind, N: Developmental Gerstmann syndrome. Neurology 20:293−298, 1970

Benson, DF and Geschwind, N: The aphasias and related disturbances in Baker, AB, Baker, LH (eds): Clinical Neurology, Vol. 1. Harper and Row, 1977

Benson, D F, Patten, D H: The use of radioactive isotopes in the localization of aphasia-producing lesions. Cortex 3:258−271, 1967

Benson, D F, Sheremata, W A, Bouchard, R, et al: Conduction aphasia—A clinicopathological study. Arch Neurol 28:339−346, 1973

Benson, D F, Weir, W F: Acalculia: Acquired anarithmetia. Cortex 8:465−472, 1972

Bentler, P M: A lower-bound method for the dimension-free measurement of internal consistency. Soc Sci Res 1:343−357, 1972

Benton, A L: The fiction of the "Gerstmann syndrome." J Neurol Neurosurg Psychiatry 24:176−181, 1961

Benton, A L: Contributions to aphasia before Broca. Cortex 1:314−327, 1964

Benton, A L: Problems of test construction in the field of aphasia. Cortex 3:32, 1967

Benton, A L: Development of a multilingual aphasia battery progress and problems. J Neurol Sci 9:39−48, 1969

Benton, A L: Reflections on the Gerstmann syndrome. Brain Lang 4:45−62, 1977

Bernard, C: Introduction à l'étude de la médecine expérimentale, 1865, Paris. Reissued Paris: Garnier-Flammarion, 1966

Beyn, E S. Shokhor-Trotskaya, M K: The preventive method of speech rehabilitation in aphasia. Cortex 2:96−108, 1966

Boller, F, and Green E: Comprehension in severe aphasia. Cortex, 8, 382−394, 1972

Boller, F, Kim, Y, Mack, JL: Auditory comprehension in aphasia, in Whitaker, H, Whitaker, H (eds): Studies in Neurolinguistics, Vol. 3. New York. Academic Press, 1978

Boller, F, Vignolo, L A: Latent sensory aphasia in hemisphere damaged patients. An experimental study with the token test. Brain 89/4:815−830, 1966

Bond, M R: Assessment of psychosocial outcome after severe head injury, in Outcome of Severe Damage to the Central Nervous System. Amsterdam, Elsevier, 1975

Botez, M I, Barbeau, A: Role of subcortical structures, and particularly of the thalamus, in the mechanisms of speech and language. Int J Neurol 8:300−320, 1971

Blumstein S: A Phonological Investigation of Aphasic Speech. Janua Linguarum Series Minor 153. The Hague: Mouton, 1973

Blumstein, S E, Baker, E, Goodglass, H: Phonological factors in auditory comprehension in aphasia. Neuropsychologia 15:19−30, 1977

Brain, W R: Visual disorientation with special reference to lesions of the right cerebral hemisphere. Brain 64:244−272, 1941

Brain, W R: Speech Disorders. London, Butterworths, 1961

Bramwell, B: A remarkable case of aphasia: Acute and complete embolic softening of the left motor vocal speech center (Broca's convolution) in a right handed man! Transient motor aphasia marked inability to name objects and especially persons; considerable agraphia and slight word blindness. Brain 21:343−373, 1898

Braun, J J, Meyer, P M, Meyer, D R: Sparing of a brightness habit in rats following visual decortication. J Comp Physiol Psychol 61:79−82, 1966

Broadbent, W H: Cerebral mechanism of speech and thought. Med Chir Trans 55:145−194, 1872

Broca, P: Remarques sur le siège de la faculté du langage articulé, suivies d'une observation d'aphemie (perte de la parole). Bull Soc Anat (Paris), 36:330−357, 1861

Broca, P: Sur le siège de la faculté du langage articulé. Bull Anthropol 6:377−393, 1865

Broida, H: Language therapy effects in long term aphasia. Arch Phys Med Rehabil 58:248−253, 1977

Brookshire, R H: Aphasia. Minneapolis, BRK 1973

Brookshire, R H: A system for recording events in patient−clinician interactions during aphasia treatment sessions, in Rationale for Adult Aphasia Therapy. Omaha, University of Nebraska Medical Center, 1977

Brown, J W: Aphasia, Apraxia and Agnosia—Clinical and theoretical Aspects. Springfield, Ill, Thomas, 1972

Brown, W S, Marsh, J T, Smith, J C: Contextual meaning effects on speech-evoked potentials. Behav Biol 9:755−761, 1973

Buchsbaum, M, Fedio, P: Hemispheric differences in evoked potentials to verbal and nonverbal stimuli in the left and right visual fields. Physiol Behav 5:207−210, 1970

Bucy, P C: The relation of the premotor cortex to motor activity. J Nerv Ment Dis 79:621−630, 1934

Bugiano, O, Conforto, C, Sacco, G: Aphasia in thalamic hemorrhage. Lancet:1052, 1969

Burckhardt, G: Ueber Rindenexcisionen, als Beitrag zur operativen Therapie der Psychosen. Allg Z Psychiatr 47:463−548, 1891

Butfield, E, Zangwill, O L: Re-education in aphasia: a review of 70 cases. J Neurol Neurosurg Psychiatry 9:75−79, 1946

Callaway, E, Harris, P R: Coupling between cortical potentials from different areas. Science 183:873−875, 1974

Campbell, D C, Oxbury, J M: Recovery from unilateral visuospatial neglect. Cortex 12:303−312, 1976

Cannon, WF and Rosenbluth, A: The Supersensitivity of Denervated Structures. New York: Macmillan, 1949

Carmon, A, Lavy, S, Gordon, H, et al: Hemispheric differences in rCBF during verbal and non-verbal tasks, in Ingvar, D H, Lassen, N A (eds) Brain work. Alfred Benzon Symposium VIII, Copenhagen, Munksgaard, 1975

Cattell, R B, Coulter, M A: Principles of behavioural taxonomy and the mathematical basis of the taxonomic computer program. Br J Math Statist Psychol 19:237−269, 1966

Chaika, E: A linguist looks at "schizophrenic" language. Brain & Lang 1:257−276, 1974

Chedru, F, Geschwind, N: Writing disturbances in acute confusional states. Neuropsychologia 10:343−353, 1972

Ciemins, V A: Localized thalamic hemorrhage. A case of aphasia. Neurology 20:776−782, 1970

Cohen, R, Engel, D, Kelter, S, et al: Validity of the Sklar aphasia scale. J Speech Hear Res 20/1:146−154, 1977

Colonna, A, Faglioni, P: The performance of hemisphere-damaged patients on spatial intelligence tests. Cortex 2:293−307, 1966

Conrad, K: New problems of aphasia. Brain 77/4:491−509, 1954

Cooley, W W, Lohnes, P R: Multivariate procedure for the behavioral sciences. New York, Wiley, 1962

Critchley, M: The Parietal Lobes. London, Arnold, 1953

Critchley, M: The neurology of psychotic speech. Brit J Psychiat 110:353−364, 1964

Critchley, M: The enigma of Gerstmann's syndrome. Brain 89:183−198, 1966

Critchley, M: Aphasiology and Other Aspects of Language. London, Arnold, 1970

Critchley, M: Articulatory defects in Aphasia: The problem of Broca's aphemia, in Aphasiology, London, Arnold, 1970.

Crockett, D J: A comparison of empirically derived groups of aphasic patients on the N.C.C.E.A. J Clin Psychol 33:194−198, 1977

Crockett, H G, Estridge, N M: Cerebral hemispherectomy. Bull Los Angeles Neurol Soc 16:71−87, 1951

Culton, G L: Spontaneous recovery from aphasia. J Speech Hear Res 12:825−832, 1969

Culton, G L: Reaction to age as a factor in chronic aphasia in stroke patients. J Speech Hear Dis 36:563−564, 1971

Dandy, W E: The effect of total removal of the left temporal lobe in a right handed individual: localization of areas of the brain concerned with speech. J Nerv Ment Dis 74:739−742, 1931

Darley, F L: Diagnosis and Appraisal of Communication Disorders. Englewood Cliffs, N J, Prentice Hall, 1964

Darley, F L: The efficacy of language rehabilitation in aphasia. J Speech Hear Dis 37:3−22, 1972

Darley, F L: Treatment of acquired aphasia, in W.S. Friedlander (ed): Advances in Neurology, vol. 7. Current reviews of higher nervous system dysfunction. New York, Ravens, 1975

David, M, Hecaen, H, Angelergues, R, et al: Les tumeurs occipitales. Neuro-Chir 1:85−108, 1955

Davis, K R, Juan, M T, New, P F J, Schnur, J A, and Roberson, G H: Cerebral infarction diagnosis by computerized tomography—analysis and evaluation of findings. Am J Roentgenol 124/4:643−660, 1975

Davison, C, Goodhart, S P, Needles, W: Cerebral localization in cerebrovascular disease. Assoc Res Nerv Ment Dis 13:Chapter 14, 435−465, 1934

Dax, M: Lésions de la moitié gauche de l'encéphale coincidant avec l'oubli des signes de la pensée (lu à Montpellier en 1836). Gaz Hebd 2ème série (1865)2

Dejerine, J: Des différentes variétés de cécité verbale. Mem Soc Biol:1−30, 1892

Dejerine, J: L'aphasie motrice et sa localisation corticale. L'encéphale 2:471−520, 1907

Dejerine, J: Semeiologie des affections du système nerveux. Paris, Masson, 1914

Dennis, M: Dissociated naming and locating of body parts after left anterior temporal lobe resection: An experimental case study. Brain Lang 3:147−163, 1976

Denny-Brown, D: The nature of apraxia. J Nerv Ment Dis 126:9−32, 1958

DeRenzi, E, Faglioni, P: The comparative efficiency of intelligence and vigilance tests in detecting hemispheric cerebral damage. Cortex 1:410−433, 1965

DeRenzi, E, Faglioni, P: Normative data and screening power of a shortened version of the Token Test. Cortex 14:41−49, 1978

DeRenzi, E, Pieczuro, A, Vignolo, L A: Oral apraxia and aphasia. Cortex 2:50−73, 1966

DeRenzi, E, Pieczuro, A, Vignolo, L A: Ideational apraxia: A quantitative study. Neuropsychologia 6:41−52, 1968

DeRenzi, E, Vignolo, L: The token test: A sensitive test to detect receptive disturbances in aphasics. Brain 85:665−678, 1962

Dubois, J, Hécaen, H, Angelergues, R, Chatelier, M, Marcie, P: Etude neurolinguistique de l'aphasie de conduction. Neuropsychologia 2:9−44, 1964

Dubois, J, Hécaen, H, Marie, P: L'agraphie "pure." Neuropsychologia 7:271−286, 1969

Dubois-Charlier, F: Etude neurolinguistique du problème de l'alexie pure. These de doctorat de IIIème cycle, Faculté des Lettres et Sciences Humaines, Paris X, 1970

Duffy, F H, Snodgrass, S R, Burchfiel, J L, et al: Pharmacological reversal of deprivation amblyopia in the cat. Paper presented to Twenty eight Annual Meeting, American Academy of Neurology, Toronto, 1976

Durbin, M, Martin, RL: Speech in mania: syntactic aspects. Brain Lang 4:208−218, 1977

Eagleson, H M, Vaughn, G R. Knudson, A B C: Hand signals for dysphasia. Arch Phys Med 51:111−113, 1970

Eisenson, J: Prognostic factors related to language rehabilitation in aphasic patients. J Speech Hear Dis 14:262−264, 1949

Eisenson, J: Examining for Aphasia; A Manual for the Examination of aphasia and related disturbances. New York, Psychological Corporation, 1954

Emerick, L L: Appraisal of Language Disturbances. Test Protocol. Marquette, Mich, Northern Michigan U, 1971

Erkulvrawatr, S: Alexia and left homonymous hemianopia in a non-right-hander. Ann Neurol 3:549−552, 1978

Exner, S: Untersuchungen ueber die Localisation der Functionen in der Grosshirnrinde des Menschen. Wien, Braunmueller, 1881

Ferguson, J H, Boller, F: A different form of agraphia: Syntactic writing errors in patients with motor speech and movement disorders. Brain Lang 4:382−389, 1977

Finger, S: Environmental attenuation of brain lesion symptoms, in Finger, S (ed): Recovery from Brain Damage. New York, Plenum, 1978

Finkelnburg, F: Ueber Aphasie und Asymbolie nebst Versuch einer Theorie der Sprachbildung. Arch Psychiat 6:1876

Fisher, C M: The pathologic and clinical aspects of thalamic hemorrhage. Trans Am Neurol Assoc 84:56−59, 1959

Flourens, P: Recherches expérimentales sur les propriétés et les fonctions du système nerveux dans les animaux vertébrés. Paris. Crevot, 1824

Foerster, O: Motorische Felder und Bahnen, in Bumke, O, Foerster, O (eds): Handbuch der Neurologie, vol. 6. Berlin, Springer, 1936, pp. 1–357

Foix, C: Nouveau Traité de Médecine, vol. 18. Paris, Masson et Cie, 1928, p. 135

Franz, S I, Oden, R: On cerebral motor control: The recovery from experimentally produced hemiplegia. Psychobiol 1:3–18, 1917

French, L A, Johnson, D R, Brown, I A, et al: Cerebral hemispherectomy for control of intractable convulsive seizures. J Neurosurg 12:154–164, 1955

Fritsch, G T, Hitzig, E: Uber die elektrische Erregbarkeit des Grosshiars. Arch Anat Physiol:300–332, 1870

Gado, M H, Coleman, R E, Merlis, A L, Alderson, P O, Lee, K S: Comparison of computerized tomography and radionucleide imaging in "Stroke." Stroke 7:109–113, 1976

Galin, D, Ornstein, R: Lateral specialization of cognitive mode: an EEG study. Psychophysiology 9:412–418, 1972

Gardner, H, Albert, M L, and Weintraub, S: Comprehending a word: The influence of speed and redundancy on auditory comprehension in aphasia. Cortex, 11, 155–162, 1975

Gardner, H, Denes, G, Zurif, E: Critical reading at the sentence level in aphasia. Cortex 11:60–72, 1975

Gardner, H, Zurif, E: Critical reading of words and phrases in aphasia. Brain Lang 3:173–190, 1976

Gardner, H, Zurif, E B, Berry, T, et al: Visual communication in aphasia. Neuropsychologia 14:275–292, 1976

Gazzaniga, M S: The Bisected Brain. New York, Appleton, Century & Crofts, 1970

Gazzaniga, M, Velletri Glass, A, Sarno, M T, Posner, J B: Pure word deafness and hemispheric dynamics: a case history. Cortex 9:136–143, 1973

Gerstmann, J: Fingeragnosie. Wien Klin Wochenschr 40:1010–1012, 1924

Gerstmann, J: Fingeragnosie und isolierte Agraphie ein neues Syndrom. Z ges Neurol Psychiat 108:152–177, 1927

Gerstmann, J: Zur Symptomatologie der Hirnläsionen im Übergangsgebiet der unteren Parietal-und mittleren Occipitalwendung. (Das Syndrom: Fingeragnosie, Rechts–Links–Storung, Agraphie, Akalkulie.) Nervenarzt 3:691–695, 1930

Gerstmann, J: Syndrome of finger agnosia, disorientation for right and left, agraphia and acalculia (local diagnostic value). Arch Neurol Psychiat (Chicago) 44:398–408, 1940

Gerstmann, J, Schilder, P: Über eine besondere Gangstörung bei Stirnhirnerkrankung. Wien Med Wochenschr 76:97–102, 1926

Geschwind, N: The anatomy of acquired disorders of reading, in Money J (ed): Reading Disability. Baltimore, Johns Hopkins, 1962

Geschwind, N: Sympathetic dyspraxia. Trans Am Neurol Assoc 88:219–220, 1963

Geschwind, N: Disconnexion syndromes in animals and man. Brain 88:237–294, 585–644, 1965

Geschwind, N: Problems in the anatomical understanding of the aphasias, in Benton, A (ed); Contributions to Clinical neuropsychology. Chicago, Aldine, 1969

Geschwind, N: Late Changes in the Nervous System: An Overview, in Plasticity and Recovery of Function in the Central Nervous System. New York, Academic, 1974

Geschwind, H: The apraxias: Neurological mechanisms of disorders of learned movement. Am Sci 63:188−195, 1975

Geschwind, N: personal communication, 1979

Geschwind, N, Fusillo, M: Color naming defects in association with alexia. Arch Neurol (Chicago) 15:137−146, 1966

Geschwind, N, Kaplan, E: A human cerebral deconnection syndrome. Neurology (Minneapolis) 12/10:675−685, 1962

Geschwind, N, Quadfasel, F, Segarra, J: Isolation of the speech area. Neuropsychologia 6:327−340, 1968

Gilmour, J S L: A taxonomic problem. Nature 139:1040−1042, 1937

Gloning, I, Gloning, K, Hoff, H: Neuropsychological Symptoms and Syndromes in Lesions of the Occipital Lobe and Adjacent Areas. Paris, Gauthier Villars, 1968

Gloning, I, Gloning, K, Haub, G, et al: Comparison of verbal behaviour in right-handed and non-right-handed patients with anatomically verified lesions of one hemisphere. Cortex 5:43−52, 1969

Gloning, I, Gloning, K, Weingarten, K, Berner, P: Über einen Fall mit Alexie der Brailleschrift. Wien 7. Nervenheilk 10:260−273, 1955

Gloning, K: As quoted by Benson, D F, Geschwind, N from: The alexias, in P. Vinken, G. Bruyn (eds): Handbook of Clinical Neurology. Amsterdam, North-Holland, 1969

Gloning, K, Trappl, R, Heiss, W D, et al: Prognosis and speech therapy in aphasia, in Lebrun, Y, Hoops, R (eds): Neurolinguistics (vol. 4), Recovery in Aphasics. Amsterdam, Swets & Zeitlinger, B V, 1976

Glass, A V, Gazzaniga, M S, Premack, D: Artificial language training in global aphasics. Neuropsychologia 11:95−103, 1973

Goda, S: Spontaneous speech, a primary source of therapy material. J Speech Hear Dis 27:190−192, 1962

Godfrey, C M, Douglass, E: The recovery process in aphasia. Can Med Assoc J 80:618−624, 1959

Goldstein, K: Die Transkortikalen Aphasien. Fischer, Jena, 1915

Goldstein, K: Das Wesen der amnestischen Aphasie. Schweiz Arch Neurol Psychiatr 15:163−175, 1924

Goldstein, K: Language and Language Disturbances. New York, Grune & Stratton, 1948

Goldstein, M N: Auditory agnosia for speech ("Pure Word Deafness"). Brain Lang 1:195−204, 1974

Gonzalez, C F, Grossman, C B, Palacios, E: Computed Brain and Orbital Tomography—Technique and Interpretation. New York. Wiley, 1976

Goodglass, H: Are aphasia and intelligence causally related? in Lebrun, Y, Hoops, R (eds): Neurolinguistics (ed 2) Intelligence and Aphasia. Amsterdam, Swets & Zeitlinger B V, 1974

Goodglass, H, Barton, M, Kaplan, E: Sensory modality and object naming in aphasia. J Speech Hear Res 11:488−496, 1968

Goodglass, H, Gleason, J, Hyde, M: Some dimensions of auditory language comprehension in aphasia. J Speech Hear Res 13:595−606, 1970

Goodglass, H, Hyde, M, Blumstein, S: Frequency, picture-ability and availability of nouns in aphasia. Cortex 5:104−119, 1969

Goodglass, H, Kaplan, E: Assessment of Aphasia and Related Disorders. Philadelphia, Lea & Febiger, 1972

Goodglass, H, Kaplan, E: Disturbance of gesture and pantomime in aphasia. Brain 86/

4:703−720, 1963

Goodglass, H, Klein, B, Carey, P, et al: Specific semantic word categories in aphasia. Cortex 2:74−89, 1966

Goodglass, H, Quadfasel, F A, Timberlake, W H: Phrase length and the type of severity of aphasia. Cortex 1:133−153, 1964

Greenblatt, S: Alexia without agraphia or hemianopsia. Brain 96:307−316, 1973

Greenblatt, S: Subangular alexia without agraphia or hemianopsia. Brain Lang 3:229−245, 1976

Grewel, F: The acalculias, in Vinken, P J, Bruyn, G W (eds): Handbook of Clinical Neurology. Vol 4. Amsterdam, North-Holland, 1969

Hagen, C: Communication abilities in hemiplegia: Effect of speech therapy. Arch Phys Med Rehabil 54:454−463, 1973

Hatfield, F, Weddell, R: Re-training in writing in severe aphasia, in Neurolinguistics Lebrun, Y, Hoops, R (eds. 4), Recovery in Aphasics. Amsterdam, Swets & Zeitlinger, B V, 1976

Hawkins, D: The Language of Nature. San Francisco, Freeman, 1964, pp 372

Head, H: Aphasia and Kindred Disorders of Speech. Cambridge, Cambridge University Press, 1926

Hécaen, H: Clinical symptomatology in right and left hemisphere lesions, in Mountcastle, V (ed): Interhemispheric Relations and Cerebral Dominance. Baltimore, Johns Hopkins, 1962

Hécaen, H: Aspects des troubles de la lecture (alexies) au cours des lésions cérébrales en foyer. Word 23:265−287, 1967

Hécaen, H: Introduction a la neuropsychologie. Paris, Larousse, 1972

Hécaen, H: Acquired aphasia in children and the ontogenesis of hemispheric functional specialization. Brain Lang 3:114−134, 1976

Hécaen, H, Angelergues, R: Localization of symptoms in aphasia, in de Reuck, A V S, O'Connor, M (eds): CIBA Foundation Symposium: Disorders of Language. London, Churchill, 1964

Hécaen, H, Angelergues, R, Douzens, J A: Les agraphies. Neuropsychologia (Oxford) 1:179−208, 1963

Hécaen, H, Angelergues, R, Houllier, S: Les variétés cliniques des acalculies au cours des lésions retro-rolandiques: approche statistique du problème. Rev Neurol 105:85−103, 1961

Hécaen, H, Consoli, S: Analyse des troubles du langage au cours des lésions de l'aire de Broca. Neuropsychologia 11:371−388, 1973

Hécaen, H, Gimeno, A: L'apraxie idéomotrice unilatérale gauche. Rev Neurol 102:648−653, 1960

Hécaen, H, Gruner, J: Alexie "pure" avec intégrité du corps calleux, in Michel, F, Schott, B (eds): Les syndromes de disconnexion calleuse chez l'homme. Lyon, Hôpital Neurologique, 1975

Hécaen, H, Kremin, H: Neurolinguistic Research on Reading Disorders Resulting from Left Hemisphere Lesions: Aphasic and "Pure" Alexia, in Whitaker, H, Whitaker, H (eds): Studies in Neurolinguistics, vol. 2. New York, Academic, 1976

Heilbroner, K: 1907, as quoted by Kleist, K, in Kortikale (innervatorische) Apraxie. Jahrb Psychiat Neurol 28:46−112, 1907

Heilman, K M: Ideational apraxia—a re-definition. Brain 96/4:861−864, 1973

Heilman, K M: A tapping test in apraxia. Cortex 11:259−263, 1975

Heilman, K M, Coyle, J M, Gonyea, E F, et al: Apraxia and agraphia in a left-hander. Brain 96:21−28, 1973

Heilman, K M, Gonyea, E F, Geschwind, N: Apraxia and agraphia in a right-hander. Cortex 10:284−288, 1974

Heilman, K M, Rothi, L, Campanella, D, Wolfson, S: Wernicke and global aphasia without alexia. Arch Neurol 36:129−133, 1979

Heilman, K M, Safran, A, Geschwind, N: Closed head trauma and aphasia. J Neurol Neurosurg Psychiat 34:265−269, 1971

Heilman, K M, Valenstein, E: Auditory neglect in man. Arch Neurol 26:32−35, 1972

Heimburger, R F, Demeyer, W, Reitan, R M: Implications of Gerstmann's syndrome. J Neurol Neurosurg Psychiatr 27:52−57, 1964

Helm, N, Benson, F: Visual Action Therapy for Global aphasia. Presentation in the Academy of Aphasia, Chicago, October 16th, 1978

Henschen, S E: Klinische und Anatomische Beiträge zur Pathologie des Gehirns, vols. 5−7. Stockholm, Nordiska Bokhandel n, 1920−1922

Hier, D B, Mohr, J P: Incongruous oral and written naming. Evidence for a subdivision of the syndrome of Wernicke's aphasia. Brain Lang 4:115−126, 1977

Hill, A B: Principles of Medical Statistics. New York, Oxford University Press, 1971

Hinshelwood, J: Letter, Word and Mind-Blindness. London, Lewis, 1900

Hinshelwood, J: Congenital Word-Blindness. London, Lewis, 1917

Hirsch, H V B, Jacobson, M: The perfect brain, in Gazzaniga M S, Blakemore, C B (eds): Fundamentals of Psychobiology. New York, Academic, 1974

Hoff, H, Gloning, I, Gloning, K: Das Pötzlsche Syndrome. Wien Klin Wochenschr 74:684−687, 1962

Holland, A: Communicative Ability in Daily Living: Its measurement and observation. Paper presented Academy of Aphasia, Montreal, 1977

Holland, A L: Some practical considerations in aphasia rehabilitation, in Sullivan, M, Kommers, M S (eds): Rationale for Adult Aphasia Therapy. University of Nebraska Medical Center, 1977

Howes, D: An approach to the quantitative analysis of word blindness, in Money, J (ed): Reading Disability. Baltimore, Johns Hopkins, 1962

Howes, D, Geschwind, N: Quantitative studies of aphasic language. Assoc Res Nerv Ment Dis 42:229−244, 1964

Howes, D, Green, E: Expressive aphasia from posterior cerebral lesions: A reevaluation of conduction or central aphasia. Paper presented at Academy of Aphasia, Rochester, New York, 1972

Hubel, D, Wiesel, T: Receptive fields and functional architecture in two nonstriate visual areas (18 and 19) of the cat. J Neurophysiol 28:229−289, 1965

Huber, W, Stachowiak, F J, Poeck, K, et al: Die Wernicke's Aphasie. J Neurol 210:77−97, 1975

Ingvar, D H, Schwartz, M S: Blood flow patterns induced in the dominant hemisphere by speech and reading. Brain 97:273−288, 1974

Isserlin, M: Aphasie, in Bumke, O, Foerster, O (eds): Handbuch der Neurologie, vol. 6. Berlin, Springer, 1936, p 627−806

Jackson, H: Remarks on those cases of disease of the nervous system in which detect of expression is the most striking symptom. Med Times Gaz, 1866

Jackson, H J: Case of large cerebral tumour without optic neuritis and with left hemiplegia and imperception. London Ophthal Hosp Rep 8:434−442, 1876

Jackson, H J: On affections of speech from disease of the brain. Brain 1:304−330, 1878

Jackson, J H: Clinical remarks on cases of defects of expression (by words, writing, sings, etc.) in diseases of the nervous system. Lancet: 604−605, 1864

Jackson, J H: On the anatomical and physiological localization of movements in the brain. Lancet 1:84−85, 162−164, 232−234, 1873

Jakobson, R: Towards a linguistic typology of aphasic impairments, in De Reuck, A V S, O'Connor, M (eds): Disorders of Language. London, Churchill, 1964, pp 21−42

Jefferson, G: Jacksonian epilepsy. A background and a postscript. Postgrad Med J, London 11:150−162, 1935

Jefferson, G: Localization of function in the cerebral cortex. Br Med Bull 6:333−340, 1950

Johns, DF, Lapointe, LL: Neurogenic disorders of speech, in Whitaker, H, Whitaker, HA (eds): Studies in Neurolinguistics, vol. 1.New York, Academic, 1976, pp 161−199

Kanzer, M: Early symptoms of aphasia with brain tumours. J Nerv Ment Dis 95:702−720, 1942

Karis, R, Horenstein, S: Localization of speech parameters by brain scan. Neurology 26:226−230, 1976

Keenan, J, Brassell, E: Aphasia Language Performance Scales (ALPS). Murfreesboro, Tennessee, Pinnacle, 1975

Keenan, S S, Brassel, E G: A study of factors related to prognosis for individual aphasic patients. J Speech Hear Dis 39:257−269, 1974

Keith, R L, Darley, F L: The use of a specific electric board in rehabilitation of the aphasic patient. J Speech Hear Dis 32:148−153, 1967

Kenin, M, Swisher, L: A study of pattern of recovery in aphasia. Cortex 8:56−68, 1972

Kennard, M A, McCulloch, W S: Motor response to stimulation of cerebral cortex in absence of areas 4 and 6 (Macaca mulatta). J Neurophysiol 6:181−190, 1943

Kerschensteiner, M, Poeck, K, Brunner, E: The fluency−nonfluency dimension in the classification of aphasic speech. Cortex 8:233−247, 1972

Kertesz, A: Visual agnosia: The dual deficit of perception and recognition. Cortex (in press, 1979)

Kertesz, A, Benson, D F: Neologistic jargon: A clinicopathological study. Cortex 6:362−386, 1970

Kertesz, A, Ghent, C, Poole, E: Localization of lesions in aphasia. Neurol India Proc III:463−465, 1973

Kertesz, A, Lesk, D, McCabe, P: Isotope localization of infarcts in aphasia. Arch Neurol 34:590−601, 1977

Kertesz, A, McCabe, P: Intelligence and aphasia: Performance of aphasics on Raven's Coloured Progressive Matrices (RCPM). Brain Lang 2:387−395, 1975

Kertesz, A, McCabe, P: Recovery patterns and prognosis in aphasia. Brain 100:1−18, 1977

Kertesz, A, Phipps, J B: Numerical taxonomy of aphasia. Brain Lang 4:1−10, 1977

Kertesz, A, Poole, E: The aphasia quotient: The taxonomic approach to measurement of aphasic disability. Can J Neurol Sci 1:7−16, 1974

Kimura, D: Dual functional asymmetry of the brain in visual perception. Neuropsychologia 4:275−285, 1966

Kimura, D: The Neural Basis of Language Qua Gesture, in Whitaker, HA, Whitaker, H (eds): Studies in Neurolinguistics, vol. 2. New York, Academic, 1976, p 146

Kimura, D, Archibald, Y: Motor function of the left hemisphere. Brain 97:337–350, 1974

Kinkel, W R, Jacobs, L: Computerized axial transverse tomography in cerebrovascular disease. Neurology 26:924–930, 1976

Kinsbourne, M: The minor cerebral hemisphere as a source of aphasic speech. Arch Neurol 25:302–306, 1971

Kinsbourne, M, Rosenfield, D B: Agraphia selective for written spelling. Brain Lang 1:215–225, 1974

Kinsbourne, M, Rosenfield, D B: Agraphia selective for written spelling. Brain Lang 1:215–225, 1974

Kinsbourne, M, Warrington, E K: A disorder of simultaneous form perception. Brain 85:461–486, 1962

Kinsbourne, M, Warrington, E: A study of finger agnosia. Brain 85:47–66, 1962

Kleist, K: Korticale (innervatorische) Apraxie. Jahrb Psychiatr Neurol 28:46–112, 1907

Kleist, K: Über Leitungsaphasie und grammatische Störungen. Monatsschr Psych Neurol 40:118–199, 1916

Kleist, K: Gehirnpathologie. Leipzig, Barth, 1934

Kleist, K: Sensory aphasia and amusia. Translated by Fish, F J and Stanton, J B: The Myeloarchitectonic Basis. Oxford, Pergamon, 1962

Klein, R, Harper, J: The problem of agnosia in the light of a case of pure word deafness. J Ment Sci 102:112–120, 1956

Klor, B M, Friedman, P, Shewan, C M: A standardization of a task for auditory comprehension of sentences for adult aphasics. Paper presented, American Speech and Hearing Association, 1976

Kohlmeyer, K: Lokaldiagnose ischämischer Insulte anhand aphasischer und anderer neuropsychologischer Syndrome. Med Klin 64/45:2079–2086, 1969

Kohlmeyer, K: Dynamic speech studies by measurement of regional cerebral blood flow in aphasic and nonaphasic cases, in Harper et al. (eds): Blood Flow and Metabolism in the Brain. Edinburgh, Churchill–Livingstone, 1975

Kohlmeyer, K: Aphasia due to focal disorders of cerebral circulation: Some aspects of localization and of spontaneous recovery, in Lebrun, Y, Hoops, R (eds): Neurolinguistics, vol. 4, Recovery in Aphasics. Amsterdam, Swets & Zeitlinger B V, 1976

Konorski, J: In Brain Mechanisms and Learning. Oxford, Council for International Organization of Medical Sciences, 1961

Kotani, S: A case of alexia with agraphia. J J Exp Psychol 2:333–348, 1935 (in Japanese)

Kreindler, A, Fradis, A: Performances in Aphasia. A Neurodynamical, Diagnostic and Psychological Study. Paris, Gauthier–Villars, 1968

Kreindler, A, Gheorghita, N, and Voinescu, I: Analysis of verbal reception of a complex order with three elements in aphasics. Brain 94:375–386, 1971

Kussmaul, A: Die Störungen der Sprache. Versuch einer Pathologie der Sprache. Leipzig, Vogel, 1877

Larsen, B, Skinhoj, E, Endo, H: Localization of basic speech functions as revealed by rCBF measurements in normals and in patients with aphasia, in Meyer, A S, Lechner, M, Revich M (eds): Cerebral Vascular Disease. Eighth International Salzburg Conference, Amsterdam–Oxford, 1977

Larsen, B, Skinhoj, E, Lassen, N A: Variation in regional cortical blood flow in the right and left hemisphere during automatic speech. Brain 101:193−211, 1978

Lashley, K S: Factors limiting recovery after central nervous lesions. J Nerv Ment Dis 88:733−755, 1938

Lebrun, Y, Hoops, R: Neurolinguistics (ed 4), Recovery in Aphasics. Amsterdam, Swets & Zeitlinger, B V, 1976

Lecours, A R, Vanier-Clement, M: Schizophasia and jargon aphasia. Brain Lang 3:516−565, 1976

Leischner, A: Die Störungen der Schriftsprache (Agraphie und Alexie). Stuttgart, Verlag Georg Thieme, 1957

Leischner, A: The agraphias in Vinken, P J, Bruyn, G W (eds): Handbook of Clinical Neurology, vol. 4. Amsterdam, North-Holland, 1969

Leischner, A: Uber den Verlauf und die Einteilung der aphasischen Syndrome. Arch Psychiat Nervenkr 216:219−231, 1972

Leischner, A: Aptitude of aphasics for language treatment, in Lebrun, Y, Hoops, R (eds): Recovery in Aphasics. Amsterdam, Swets & Zeitlinger BV, 1976, pp 112−124

Leischner, A, Haberkamp, H: The influence of nonverbal factors on the performance of IQ of aphasics, in Lebrun, Y, Hoops, R (eds): Neurolinguistics (ed 2), Intelligence and Aphasia. Amsterdam, Swets & Zeitlinger B V, 1974

Leonhard, K: Reine Agraphie und konstruktive Apraxie als Ausdruck einer Leitungsstörung. Arch Psychiatr Nervenkr: 471−503, 1952

Lesser, R: Linguistic Investigations of Aphasia. Arnold, London, 1978

Levinson, B M: A comparison of the Coloured Progressive Matrices (CPM) with the Wechsler Adult Intelligence Scale (WAIS) in a normal aged white male population. J Clin Psychol 15:288−291, 1959

Lewandowsky, M, Stadelmann, E: Über einen bemerkenswerten Fall von Hirnblutung und uber Rechenstorungen bei Herderkrankung des Gehirns. J Psychol Neurol (Leipiz) 11:249−265, 1908

Lhermitte, F, Lecours, A R, Ducarne, B, et al: Unexpected anatomical findings in a case of fluent jargon aphasia. Cortex 9:436−449, 1973

Lichtheim, L: On Aphasia. Brain 7:443, 1885

Liepmann, H: Das Krankheitsbild der Apraxie (''motorischen asymbolie''). Monatsschr Psychiatr Neurol, Bd VIII, 1900. Monographie, Berlin, 1900

Liepmann, H: Die linke Hemisphäre und das Handeln. Münch Med Woensch 2:2375 −2378, 1905

Liepmann, H: Drei Aufsatze aus dem Apraxiegebiet. Berlin, Karger, 1908

Liepmann, H: Diseases of the brain, in Barr, C W (ed): Curschmann's textbook on Nervous Diseases, vol. 1. Philadelphia, Blakiston, 1915, pp 467−551

Liepmann, H: Apraxie. Ergeb Gesamten Med 1:516−543, 1920

Liepmann, H, Maas, O: Ein Fall von linksseitiger Agraphie und Apraxie bei rechtsseitiger Lähmung f. J Psychol Neurol 10:214−227, 1907

Liepmann, H, Storch, E: Der mikroskopische gehirnbefund bei dem Falle Gorstelle. Monatsschr Psychiatr Neurol 11:115−120, 1902

Lissauer, H: Ein Fall von Seelenblindheit nebst einem Beitrag zur Theorie derselben. Arch Psychiatr Nervenkr 21:2−50, 1889

Liu, C N, Chambers, W W: Intraspinal sprouting of dorsal root axons. Arch Neurol (Chicago) 79:46−61, 1958

Lomas, J, Kertesz, A: Patterns of spontaneous recovery in aphasic groups: A study of adult stroke patients. Brain Lang 5:388−401, 1978

Lordat, J: Analyse de la parole pour servir à la théorie de divers cas d'alalie et de paralalie (de mutisme et d'imperfection de parler) que les nosologistes ont mal connus. J Med. Pratique Montpellier 7:333−353, 417−433, 1843

Low, W, Wada, J A, Fox, M: Electroencephalographic localization of the conative aspects of language production in the human brain. Trans Am Neurol Assoc 98:129−133, 1973

Ludlow, C: Recovery from Aphasia: A foundation for treatment. In Rationale for Adult Aphasia Therapy, Sullivan, M A, Kommers, M S (eds). University Medical Center, 1977.

Luria, A: Factors and forms of aphasia, in Disorders of Language. London, Churchill, 1964

Luria, A P: Higher Cortical Functions in Man. New York. Basic Books, 1966.

Luria, A R: Traumatic Aphasia. Hague, Mouton, 1970

Luria, A R: Neuropsychological studies on aphasia, in Hoops, R, Lebrun, Y (eds), Neurolinguistics 6, Amsterdam, Swets & Zeitlinger B V, 1977

Luria, A R, Naydin, V L, Tsvetkova, L S et al: Restoration of higher cortical function following local brain damage, in Vinken, P J, Bruyn, G W (eds): Handbook of Clinical Neurology, vol 3. Amsterdam, North-Holland, 1969

Luria, A, Tsevtkova, L: The mechanisms of dynamic aphasia. Foundations of Language 4:296−307, 1968

Mack, J L, Boller, F: Associative visual agnosia and its related deficits: The role of the minor hemisphere in assigning meaning to visual perceptions. Neuropsychologia 15:345−349, 1977

Maly, J, Turnheim, M, Heiss, W D, et al: Brain perfusion and neuropsychological test scores: A correlation study in aphasics. Brain Lang 4:78−94, 1977

Mandleberg, I A, Brooks, D M: Cognitive recovery after severe head injury. J Neurol Neurosurg Psychiatry 38:1121−1126, 1975

Marcuse, H: Apraktische Symptome bei einem Fall von seniler Demenz. Zentralbl Nerv Heilk Psychiatr 27:737−751, 1904

Marie, P: Révision de la question de l'aphasie: La troisiéme circonvolution frontale gauche ne joue aucun rôle spécial dans la fonction du langage. Sem Med 21:241−247, 1906, May 23

Marie, P: Révision de la question de l'aphasie: l'aphasie de 1861 à 1866: essai de critique historique sur la genere de la doctrine de Broca. Sem Med Paris: 26, 565−571, 1906

Marie, P, Foix, C: Les aphasies de guerre. Rev Neurol 24:53−87, 1917

Marinesco, G, Sager, O, Kreindler, A: Etudes electroencéphalographiques; electroencéphalogrammes dans l'aphasie. Bull Acad Med Paris 116:182, 1936

Marks, M M, Taylor, M L, Rusk, L A: Rehabilitation of the aphasic patient: a survey of three years' experience in a rehabilitation setting. Neurology 7:837−843, 1957

Marshall, J, Newcombe, F: Patterns of paralexia: A psycholinguistic approach. J Psycholinguist Res 2:175−200, 1973

Martin, A D: Aphasia testing: A second look at the Porch index of communicative ability. J Speech Hear Dis 42/4:547−562, 1977

Maspes, P E: Le syndrome expérimental chez l'homme de la section du splenium du corps calleux: alexie visuelle pure hémianopsique. Rev Neurol 80:100−113, 1948

Mateer, C, Kimura, D: Impairment of nonverbal oral movements in aphasia. Brain Lang 4:262−276, 1977

Matsumiya, Y, Tagiliasco, V, Lombroso, C T, et al: Auditory evoked response: meaningfulness of stimuli and interhemispheric asymmetry. Science 175:790−792, 1972

Maximilian, V A, Prohovnik, I, Risberg, J et al: Regional blood flow changes in the left cerebral hemisphere during word pair learning and recall. Brain Lang 6:22−31, 1978

Mazzocchi, F, Vignolo, L A: Computer assisted tomography in neuropsychological research: a simple procedure for lesion mapping. Cortex 14:136−144, 1978

Messerli, P, Tissot, A, Rodriguez, J: Recovery from aphasia: Some factors of prognosis, in Lebrun, Y, Hoops, R (eds): Neurolinguistics 4, Recovery in Aphasics. Amsterdam, Swets & Zeitlinger, B V, 1976

McAdam, D W, Whitaker, H A: Language production: electroencephalographic localization in the normal human brain. Science 172:499−502, 1971

McGlone, J, Kertesz, A: Sex difference in cerebral processing of visuospatial tasks. Cortex 9:313−320, 1973

McKissock, W, Paine, K W E: Primary tumours of the thalamus. Brain 81:41−63, 1958

Messina, A V, Chernik, N L: Computed tomography: The "resolving" intracerebral hemorrhage. Radiology 118:609−613, 1975

Mettler, R A: Selective Partial Ablation of the frontal cortex: A correlative study of the effects on human psychotic subjects. New York, Hoeber, 1949

Meyer, A: The frontal lobe syndrome, the aphasias and related conditions. A contribution to the history of cortical localization. Brain 97:565−600, 1974

Meyer, D R, Isaac, W, Maher, B: The role of stimulation in spontaneous reorganization of visual habits. J Comp Physiol Psychol 51:546−548, 1958

Meyer, J S, Shinohara, Y, Kanda, T, et al: Diaschisis resulting from acute unilateral cerebral infarction. Arch Neurol 23:241−247, 1970

Meyer, J S, Welch, K M A, Okamoto, S, et al: Disordered neurotransmitter function. Brain 97:655−664, 1974

Meynert, T: Ein Fall von Sprachstorung anatomisch begrundet. Med Jahrb Zschr Ges Arzte 12:152−187, 1866

Meynert, T: Klinische Vorlesungen uber Psychiatrie. Wien 1890, S, 270

Mills, C K: The anatomy of the cerebral cortex and the localization of its functions, in Dercum, F X (ed): A Textbook on Nervous Diseases by American Authors. Edinburgh & London, Pentland, 1895

Milner, B: Hemispheric specialization: scope and limits, in Schmitt, F O, Worden, F G (eds): The Neurosciences: Third Study Program. Cambridge, M I T Press, 1974

Mishkin, M, Forgays, D G: Word recognition as a function of retinal locus. J Exp Psychol 43:43−48, 1952

Mohr, J P: Broca's area and Broca's aphasia, in Whitaker, H, Whitaker, H A (eds): Studies in Neurolinguistics, vol 1. New York, Academic , 1976, pp 201−235

Mohr, J P, Pessin, M S, Finkelstein, S, et al: Broca aphasia: Pathologic and Clinical Aspects. Neurology 28:311−324, 1978

Mohr, J P, Watters, W C, Duncan, G W: Thalamic hemorrhage and aphasia. Brain Lang 2:3−17, 1975

Monakow, C von: Die Lokalisation im Grosshirn und der Abbau der Funktionen durch corticale Herde. Bergmann, Wiesbaden, 1914

Monrad-Krohn, G H: The prosodic quality of speech and its disorders. Acta Psych et Neurol Scand 22:255—269, 1947

Moore, R Y: Central Regeneration and Recovery of Function: The Problem of Collateral Reinnervation in Plasticity and Recovery of Function in the Central Nervous System. New York, Academic, 1974

Morlass, J: Contribution à l'étude de l'apraxie. Paris, Legrand, 1928

Morrell, L K, Huntington, D A: Electrocortical cortical localization of language production. Science 174:1359—1360, 1971

Morrell, L K, Salamy, J G: Hemispheric asymmetry of electrocortical response to speech stimuli. Science 174:164—166, 1971

Mountcastle, V B, Rose J E: Touch and kinesthesis, in Field, J (ed): Handbook of Physiology, vol. 1. Washington, D C, American Physiological Society, 1960, pp 387—430

Moutier, F: L'aphasie de Broca. Paris, Steinheil, 1908.

Munk, H: Ueber die Funktionen der Grosshirnrinde. Gesammelte Mitteilungen aus den Jahren 1877—1880. Berlin, Hirschwald, 1881

Naeser, M A, Hayward, R W: Lesion localization in aphasia with cranial computed tomography and the Boston Diagnostic Aphasia Exam. Neurology 28:545—551, 1978

Nathan, P W: Facial apraxia and apraxic dysarthria. Brain 70:449—478, 1947

Needham, L, Swisher, L P: A comparison of three tests of auditory comprehension for adult aphasics. J Speech Hear Dis 37:123—131, 1972

New, PFJ, Scott, WR: Computed Tomography of the Brain and Orbit. Baltimore, Williams & Wilkins, 1975

Newcombe, F, Marshall, J: Stages in recovery from dyslexia following a left cerebral abscess. Cortex 9:329—332, 1973

Newcombe, F B, Oldfield, R C, Wingfield, A: Object naming by dysphasic patients. Nature (London) 207:1217—1218, 1965

Nielsen, J M: The unsolved problems in aphasia alexia resulting from a temporal lesion. Bull Los Angeles Neurol Soc 4:168—183, 1939

Nielsen, J M: Agnosia, apraxia, aphasia. New York, Hoeber, 1946

Nothnagel: Uber die Lokalisation der Gehirnkrankheiten. VI Kongress Inn. Med. Wiesbaden, 1887

Nottebohm, F: Ontogeny of bird song. Science 167:950—956, 1970

Nunnally, J C: Psychometric Theory. New York, McGraw-Hill, 1967

Ogle, J W: Aphasia and agraphia in St. George's Hospital. Rep Med Res Coun (London) 2:83—122, 1867

Ojemann, G A: Subcortical language mechanisms, in Whitaker, H, Whitaker, H (eds): Studies in Neurolinguistics, vol. 1. New York, Academic, 1976

Ojemann, G A, Fedio, P, Van Buren, J: Anomia from pulvinar and subcortical parietal stimulation. Brain 91:99—116, 1968

Ojemann, G A, Whitaker, H A: Language localization and variability. Brain Lang 6:239—260, 1978

Oppenheimer, D R, Newcombe, F: Clinical and Anatomic Findings in a Case of Auditory Agnosia. Arch Neurol 35:712—717, 1978

Orgass, B, Hartje, W, Kerschensteiner, M, et al: Aphasie und nichtsprachliche Intelligenz. Nervenarzt 43:623—627, 1972

Orloci, L: An agglomerative method for the classification of plant communities. J Ecol 55:193−205, 1967a

Orloci, L: Data centering: A review and evaluation with reference to component analysis. Syst Zool 16:208−212, 1976b

Osgood, C E, Miron, M S (eds): Approaches to the study of aphasia. Urbana, University Illinois Press, 1963

Oxbury, J, Oxbury, S, Humphrey, N: Varieties of colour anomia. Brain 92:847−860, 1969

Parker, H M: J Australian College of Speech Therapists 20:104−106, 1970

Penfield, W, Rasmussen, T: The Cerebral Cortex of Man. New York, MacMillan, 1950

Penfield, W, Roberts, L: Speech and Brain Mechanisms. Princeton, N J, Princeton Univ Press, 1959

Peritz, G: Zur Pathopsychologie des Rechnens. Dtsch Z Nervenheilkd 61:234−340, 1918

Phipps, J B: Dendrogram topology. Syst Zool 20:306−308, 1971

Pick, A: Studien über motorische Aphasie. Wien, 1905.

Pick, A: Studien über motorische Apraxie und ihre nahestehenden Erscheinungen. Leipzig, Deuticke, 1905

Pick, A: Die agrammatischen Sprachstörungen. Berlin, Springer, 1913

Pick, A: Aphasie, in Bumke, O, Foerster, O (eds): Handbuch der Normalen und Pathologischen Physiologie, vol. XV. Berlin, Springer, 1931

Pieczuro, A, Vignolo, L A: Studio sperimentale sull'aprassia ideomotoria, Sist Nerv 19:131−143, 1967 as quoted in Heiluan 1975

Piercy, M: Neurological aspects of intelligence, in Vinken, P J, Bruyn, G W (eds): Handbook of Clinical Neurology, vol. 3. Amsterdam, North-Holland, 1969

Piercy, M, Smyth, V O G: Right hemisphere dominance for certain nonverbal intellectual skills. Brain 85:775−789, 1962

Pintner, R, Paterson, D: A Scale of Performance Tests. New York, Appleton, 1923

Pizzamiglio, L, Appicciafuoco, A: Semantic comprehension in aphasia. J Commun Disord, 3, 280−288, 1971

Pizzamiglio, L, Appicciafuoco, A, Razzano, C: Recovery of comprehension in aphasic patients, in Lebrun, Y, Hoops, R (eds): Recovery in Aphasics, Neurolinguistics (ed 4). Amsterdam, Swets & Zeitlinger B V, 1976

Poeck, K, Kerschensteiner, M: Analysis of the sequential motor events in oral apraxia, in Zulch, Creutzfeldt, Galbraith (eds): Cerebral localization. Berlin, Springer−Verlag, 1975

Poeck, K, Kerschensteiner, M, Hartje, W, et al: Impairment in visual recognition of geometric figures in patients with circumscribed retrorolandic brain lesions. Neuropsychologia 11:311−317, 1973

Poeck, K, Orgass, B: Gerstmann's syndrome and aphasia. Cortex 2:421−437, 1966

Poeck, K, Orgass, B: Gerstmann syndrome without aphasia: Comments on the paper by Strub and Geschwind. Cortex 11:291−295, 1975

Poppelreuter, W: Die psychischen Schädigungen durch Kopfschuss im Kriege 1914−1916, vol. 1. Die Störungen der niederen und hoheren Sehleistungen durch Verletzungen des Occipitalhirns. Leipzig, Voss, 1917

Porch, B E: The Porch Index of Communicative Ability: Administration, Scoring and Interpretation. Palo Alto, Calif., Consulting Psychologists, 1971

Raven, J C: Guide to Using the Coloured Progressive Matrices. London, Lewis, 1965

Rochford, G, Williams M: Studies in the development and breakdown of the use of names. J Neurol Neurosurg Psychiatry 25:228−233, 1962

Rosenbeck, J C, Lemme, M L, Ahern, M B, et al: A treatment for apraxia of speech in adults. J Speech Hear Dis 38:462−472, 1973

Rosenfield, B B, Goree, J A: Angiographic localization of aphasia. Paper presented to the Academy of Neurology, Bal Harbour, Florida, May 1, 1975

Rothmann, M: Lichtheimsche motorische Aphasie. Z Klin Med 60:87−121, 1906

Rubens, A B: Aphasia with infarction in the territory of the anterior cerebral artery. Cortex 11:239−250, 1975

Rubens, A B: Transcortical motor aphasia, in Whitaker, H, Whitaker, H A (eds): Studies in Neurolinguistics. New York, Academic, vol. 1. 1976, pp 293−303

Rubens, A: The role of changes within the central nervous system during recovery from aphasia, in Sullivan, M, Kommers, M S (eds): Rationale for Adult Aphasia Therapy. University of Nebraska Medical Center, 1977

Russell, W R, Espir, M L E: Traumatic Aphasia. London, Oxford Univ Press, 1961

Russo, M, Vignolo, L A: Visual figure-ground discrimination in patients with unilateral cerebral disease. Cortex 3:113−127, 1967

Sands, E, Sarno, M T, Shankweiler, D: Long-term assessment of language function in aphasia due to stroke. Arch Phys Med Rehabil 50:202−207, 1969

Sarno, M T: The functional communication profile. Manual of directions. Rehabilitation Monograph 42. New York, Institute of Rehabilitation Medicine, 1969

Sarno, M T, Levita, E: Natural course of recovery in severe aphasia. Arch Phys Med Rehabil 52:175−179, 1971

Sarno, M T, Silverman, M, Levita, E: Psychosocial factors and recovery in geriatric patients with severe aphasia. J Am Geriatr Soc 18:405−409, 1970b

Sarno, M T, Silverman, M, Sands, E: Speech therapy and language recovery in severe aphasia. J Speech Hear Res 13:607−623, 1970

Sasanuma, S: Kanji and kana processing in alexia without agraphia. Logoped−Phoniatr Ann Bull., University of Tokyo 7:77−92, 1973

Sasanuma, S, Fujimura, O: Selective impairment of phonetic and nonphonetic transcription of words in Japanese aphasic patients: kana versus kanji in visual recognition and writing. Cortex 7:1−18, 1971

Sasanuma, S, Fujimura, O: An analysis of writing errors in Japanese aphasic patients: kanji versus kana words. Cortex 8:265−282, 1972

Schaltenbrand, G: The effects of stereotaxic electrical stimulation in the depth of the brain, Brain 88:835−840, 1965

Schilder, P: Fingeragnosie, Fingerapraxie, Fingeraphasie. Nervenarzt 4:625−629, 1931

Schiller, F: Aphasia studied in patients with missile wounds. J Neurol Neurosurg Psychiatry 10:183, 1947

Schneider, G E: Early lesions of superior colliculus: Factors affecting the formation of abnormal retinal projections. Brain Behav Evol 8:73−109, 1973

Schuell, H: The Minnesota test for differential diagnosis of aphasia. Minneapolis, Univ Minnesota Press, 1965

Schuell, H: A short examination for aphasia. Neurology (Minneapolis) 7:625−634, 1957

Schuell, H, Jenkins, J J: Reduction of vocabulary in aphasia. Brain 84:243−261, 1961

Schuell, H M, Jenkins, J J, Carroll, J B: A factor analysis of the Minnesota test for differential diagnosis of aphasia. J Speech Hear Res 5:349−369, 1962

Schuell, H, Jenkins, J J, Jimenez-Pabon, E: Aphasia in Adults: Diagnosis, Prognosis and Treatment. New York, Hoeber Medical Division, Harper & Row, 1964

Schuster, P, Taterka, H: Beitrag zur Anatomie und Klinik der reinen Worttaubheit. Z Neurol Psychiatr 105:494−538, 1926

Schwab, O: Uber vorübergehende aphasische Störungen nach Rindenexzision aus dem linken Stirnhirn bei Epileptikern. Dtsch Z Nervenheilkd 94:117−184, 1927

Selby, G: Stereotaxic surgery for the relief of Parkinson's disease. II. An analysis of the results of a series of 303 patients (413 operations). J Neurol Sci 5:343−375, 1967

Semmes, J, Weinstein S, Ghent, L, et al: Performance on complex tactual tasks after brain injury in man: analysis by locus of lesion. Am J Psychol 67:220, 1954

Shallice, T, Warrington, E K: Auditory−verbal short-term memory impairment and conduction aphasia. Brain Lang 4:479−491, 1977

Shelburne, S A: Visual evoked responses to word and nonsense syllable stimuli. Electroencephalogr Clin Neurophysiol 32:17−25, 1972

Shewan, C M: Error patterns in auditory comprehension of adult aphasics. Cortex 12:325−336, 1976

Shewan, C: Personal communication, 1978

Shewan, C M, Canter, G J: Effects of vocabulary, syntax and sentence length on auditory comprehension in aphasic patients. Cortex 7:209−226, 1971

Shipps, F C, Madeira, J T, Huntington, H W: Atlas of Brain Anatomy for EMI Scans. Springfield, Illinois, Thomas, 1975

Simonyi, G, Palotas, G: Zur taktilen Alexie. Nervenarzt 30:341−345, 1969

Sittig, O: Storung des Ziffernschreibens und Rechnens bei einem Hirnverletzten. Monatsschr Psychiatr Neurol 49:299−306, 1921

Sittig, O: Über Apraxie. Berlin, Karger, 1931

Sklar, M: Sklar Aphasia Scale: Protocol Booklet. Beverly Hills, Calif, Western Psychological Services, 1973

Smith, A: Speech and other functions after left (dominant) hemispherectomy. J Neurol Neurosurg Psychiatry 29:467−471, 1966

Smith, A, Chamoux, R, Leri, J, et al: Diagnosis, intelligence and rehabilitation of chronic aphasics. Ann Arbor, University of Michigan Department of Physical Medicine & Rehabilitation, 1972

Smyth, G E, Stern, K: Tumors of the thalamus—A clinico-pathological study. Brain 61:339−374, 1938

Sneath, P H A, Sokal, R R: Numerical Taxonomy, The Principles and Practice of Numerical Classification. San Francisco, Freeman, 1973

Soh, K, Larsen, B, Skinhoj, E, et al: Regional cerebral blood flow in aphasia. Arch Neurol 35:625−632, 1978

Sparks, R, Helm, N, Albert M: Aphasia rehabilitation resulting from melodic intonation therapy. Cortex 10:303−316, 1974

Spellacy, F, Spreen, O: A short form of the Token Test. Cortex 5:390−397, 1969

Sperry, R W: Effect of crossing nerves to antagonistic limb muscles in the monkey. Arch Neurol Psychiatr 58:452−473, 1947

Sperry, R W, Gazzaniga, M C: Language following surgical disconnection of the hemispheres, in Millikan, C, Darley, F (eds): Brain Mechanisms Underlying Speech and Language. New York, Grune & Stratton, 1967

Sperry, R W, Gazzaniga, M S, Bogen, J E: Interhemispheric relationship: the neocortical commissures; syndromes of hemispheric disconnection, in Vinken, P J, Bruyn, G W (eds): Handbook Clinical Neurology, vol. 4. Amsterdam, North-Holland, 1969, pp 273−290

Spreen, O, Benton, A L: Neurosensory Center Comprehensive Examination for Aphasia. Victoria, B C, University of Victoria Press, 1968

Spreen, O, Benton, A, Fincham, R: Auditory agnosia without aphasia. Arch Neurol 13:84−92, 1965

Sroka, H, Solsi, P, Bortstein, B: Alexia without agraphia with complete recovery. Confin Neurol 35:167−176, 1973

Stacey, C L, Gill, M: The relationship between Raven's Coloured Progressive Matrices and two tests of general intelligence for 172 subnormal adult subjects. J Clin Psychol 11:86−87, 1955

Starr, M A: The pathology of sensory aphasia, with an analysis of fifty cases in which Broca's center was not diseased. Brain 12:82−101, 1889

Stein, D G, Rosen, J J, Butters, N (eds): Plasticity and Recovery of Function in the Central Nervous System. New York, Academic, 1974

Stengel, E, Patch, I C L: Central aphasia associated with parietal syndromes. Brain 78:401−416, 1955

Stoicheff, M L: Motivating instructions and language performance of dysphasic subjects. J Speech Hear Res 3:75−85, 1960

Strub, R L, Gardner, H: The repetition defect in conduction aphasia—amnestic or linguistic? Brain Lang 1:241−255, 1974

Strub, R, Geschwind, N: Gerstmann syndrome without aphasia. Cortex 10:378−387, 1974

Subirana, A: Handedness and cerebral dominance, in Vinken, P J, Bruyn, G W (eds): Handbook of Clinical Neurology, vol. 4. New York, Elsevier, 1969

Sullivan, M, Kommers, M S (eds): Rationale for Adult Aphasia Therapy. University of Nebraska Medical Center, 1977

Suter, C: Anomic aphasia—Differential diagnosis and cerebral localization of lesion in twenty cases. J Am Med Assoc 151:462−468, 1953

Szirtes, J, Vaughan, J R: Topographic analysis of speech-related cerebral potentials. Electroencephalogr Clin Neurophysiol 34.754, 1973

Taylor, M L: Language therapy, in Burr, H G (ed): The Aphasic Adult: Evaluation and Rehabilitation. Charlottesville, Wayside, 1964

Taylor, M L: A measurement of functional communication in aphasia. Arch Phys Med Rehabil 46:101−107, 1965

Teuber, H L, Weinstein, S: Ability to discover hidden figures after cerebral lesions. Arch Neurol. Psychiatry 76:369−379, 1956

Teyler, T J, Roemer, R A, Harrison, T F, et al: Human scalp-recorded evoked-potential correlates of linguistic stimuli. Bull Psychon Soc 1:333−334, 1973

Thorndike, E L, Lorge, I: The teacher's word book of 30,000 words. New York, Teachers College Press, Columbia University, 1968

Tikofsy, R S, Kooi, K A, Thomas, M H: Electroencephalographic findings and recovery from aphasia. Neurology (Minneapolis) 10:154−156, 1960

Trescher, J H, Ford, F R: Colloid cyst of the third ventricle. Report of a case. Arch Neurol Psychiatry 37:959−973, 1937

Trousseau, A: Clinique médicale de l'Hôtel-Dieu de Paris. Paris, Baillière, 1861−1864

Tuke, J B, Fraser, J: Case with a lesion involving Broca's convolution without Broca's aphasia. J Ment Sci (London) 18:46−56, 1872

Tzortis, C, Albert, M L: Impairment of memory for sequences in conduction aphasia. Neuropsychologia 12:355−366, 1974

Van Buren, J, Borke, R C: Alterations in speech and the pulvinar. Brain 92:255−284, 1969

Van Dongen, H: Impairment of drawing and intelligence in aphasic patients, in Lebrun, Y, Hoops, R (eds): Neurolinguistics (ed 2), Intelligence and Aphasia. Amsterdam, Swets & Zeitlinger, B V, 1974

Van Harskamp, F: Some considerations concerning the utility of intelligence tests in aphasic patients, in Lebrun, Y, Hoops, R (eds): Neurolinguistics (ed 2), Intelligence and Aphasia. Amsterdam, Swets & Zeitlinger, B V, 1974

Verhas, M, Schoutens, A, Demol, O, et al: Study in cerebrovascular disease: Brain scanning with technetium 99^m pertechnetate: Clinical correlations. Neurology 25:553−558, 1975

Vignolo, LA: Evolution of aphasia and language rehabilitation: a retrospective exploratory study. Cortex 1:344−367, 1964

Vignolo, L: Auditory agnosia: A review and report of recent evidence, in Benton, A (ed): Contributions to Clinical Neuropsychology. Chicago, Aldine, 1969

Vogt, O, Vogt, C: Die myeloarchitektonische Felderung des Strinhirns. J Psychol Neurol Leipzig 15, 221, 1910, as quoted by Kleist

Voinescu, I, Gheorghita, N: Thinking by aphasics, in Lebrun, Y, Hoops, R (eds): Neurolinguistics (ed 2), Intelligence and Aphasia. Amsterdam, Swets & Zeitlinger, B V, 1974

Wagenaar, E, Snow, C, Prins, R: Spontaneous speech of aphasia patients: A psycholinguistic analysis. Brain Lang 2:281−303, 1975

Ward, A A Jr, Kennard, M A: Effect of cholinergic drugs on recovery of function following lesions of the central nervous system. Yale J Biol Med 15:189−229, 1942

Ward, J: Hierarchical grouping to optimize on function. Amer Statistical Assn J 58:236−244, 1963

Warrington, E K, Shallice, T: The selective impairment of auditory-verbal short-term memory. Brain 92:885−896, 1969

Watamori, T S, Sasanuma, S: The recovery processes of two English−Japanese bilingual aphasics. Brain Lang 6:127−140, 1978

Watson, C W, Kennard, M A: The effect of anticonvulsant drugs on recovery of function following cerebral cortical lesions. J Neurophysiol 8:221−231, 1945

Weigl, E: On the problem of cortical syndromes, in Simmel, M L (ed): The Reach of Mind. New York, Springer, 1968

Weigl, E., Bierwisch, M: Neuropsychology and linguistics: Topics of common research. Found Lang 6:1−18, 1970

Weigl, E, Fradis, A: The transcoding processes in patients with agraphia to dictation. Brain Lang 4:11−22, 1977

Wiesenburg, T, McBride, K: Aphasia. New York, Commonwealth Fund, 1935

Welman, A, Lanser, J: Intelligence or intellectual tests in aphasic patients, in Lebrun, Y, Hoops, R (eds): Neurolinguistics (ed 2) Intelligence and Aphasia. Amsterdam, Swets & Zeitlinger, B V, 1974

Wepman, J M: Recovery from Aphasia. New York, Ronald, 1951

Wepman, J M, Jones, L V: The Language Modalities Test for Aphasia (LMTA). Chicago, Education—Industry Service, 1961

Wernicke, C: Der aphasische symptomenkomplex. Cohn & Weigart, Breslau, in Boston Studies on the Philosophy of Science, vol. IV. Dordrecht, Reidel, 1874, p 196

Wernicke, C: Die neueren Arbeiten uber Aphasie. Fortschr Med 4:371—377, 1886

Wernicke, C: The Symptom—Complex of Aphasia in Diseases of the Nervous System, ed. by A Church. Appleton, New York, 265—324, 1908

Wernicke, C: Grundris der Psychiatrie 1900, as quoted by Kleist (1911): Der Gang und der gegenwartige Stand der Apraxieforschung. Ergeb Neurol. Psychiatr 1:342—452

Wertz, R T, Collins, M J, Brookshire, R H, et al: The Veterans Administration Cooperative Study on Aphasia: A comparison of Individual and Group Treatment. Presentation to the Academy of Aphasia

Whitaker, H: A case of the isolation of the language function, in Whitaker, H, Whitaker, H (eds): Studies in Neurolinguistics, vol. 2. New York, Academic, 1976

Whitaker, H, Ojemann, G A: Graded localisation of naming from electrical stimulation mapping of left cerebral cortex. Nature 270:50—51, 1977

Wing, S D, Norman, D, Pollock, J A, Newton, T H: Contrast enhancement of cerebral infarcts in computed tomography. Radiology 121:89—92, 1976

Wood, C C, Goff, W R, Day, R S: Auditory evoked potentials during speech perception. Science 173:1248—1251, 1971

Woods, B T, Poppel, E: Effect of print size on reading time in a patient with verbal alexia. Neuropsychologia 12:31—41, 1974

Yarnell, P, Monroe, P, Sobel, L: Aphasia outcome in stroke: A clinical neuroradiological correlation. Stroke 7:516—522, 1976

Zaidel, D, Sperry, R W: Some long-term motor effects of cerebral commissurotomy in man, Neuropsychologia 15:42—48, 1977

Zaidel, E: Auditory vocabulary of the right hemisphere following brain bisection or hemidecortication. Cortex 12:187—211, 1976

Zangwill, O L: Le problème de l'apraxie ideatoire. Rev Neurol 102:595—603, 1960

Zangwill, O L: Intelligence in aphasia, in DeRueck, A V S, O'Connor, M (eds): Disorders of Language. CIBA Foundation Symposium, Boston, Little Brown, 1964

Zangwill, O: Intellectual status in aphasia, in Vinken, P, Bruyn, G (eds): Handbook of Clinical Neurology, vol 4. Amsterdam, North-Holland, 1969

Zangwill, O L: Excision of Broca's area without persistent aphasia, in Zulch, K J, Creutzfeldt, O, Galbraith, G C (eds). Cerebral Localization. New York, Springer Verlag, 1975

Zarit, S H, Kahn, R L: Impairment and adaptation in chronic disabilities: spatial inattention. J Nerv Dis 159:63—72, 1974

Zollinger, R: Removal of left cerebral hemisphere. Arch Neurol Psychiatry 34:1055—1064, 1935

Zurif, E B, Caramazza, A: Psycholinguistic Structures in Aphasia: Studies in Syntax and Semantics, in Whitaker, H, Whitaker, H (eds): Studies in Neurolinguistics, vol. 1. New York, Academic, 1976

Glossary of Some
Less Familiar Terms

Acanthomeatal Line. A line that connects the outer corner of the eye with the external auditory meatus. A surface equivalent (although not quite the same) of the orbitomeatal line.

Adynamic Aphasia. Same as transcortical motor aphasia. Adynamic refers to the main feature. The difficulty of initiating speech.

Agrammatism. Telegraphic speech due to brain injury or disease, in which the grammatical modifiers are missing with relative preservation of nouns and verbs or substantive words.

Anagram Letters. A selection of individual movable letters for testing graphic competence without actual writing.

Anarthria. Marie's term for a pure motor disorder of speech. Also used for a severe, complete dysarthria.

Angular Gyrus. A convolution of the inferior parietal lobule surrounding the posterior end of the first temporal fissure. *See also* Fig. 9-1 in text.

Anosognosia. Impaired or absent recognition of one's own disease.

Aphasia Quotient (AQ). The total score of the language subtests of the Western Aphasia Battery. A measure of language impairment expressed as a percentage of normal.

Aphemia. Broca's term for severe nonfluent aphasia. Also used to describe "pure word dumbness" or "pure motor aphasia."

Auditory Sequencing. Comprehension of sequentially heard items. It is similar to auditory retention span and is often tested with sequential commands.

Categorical Defect. Henry Head's concept of the two-way defect of word ing and of comprehending certain categories of words.

Centrum Semiovale. The large white matter region between the lateral cortex and the basal ganglia, containing many long tracts and long association fibers.

Conduit d'approche. The French term for phonemic approximations. A patient approaches a target word by approximately similar sounding phonemes.

Constructional Apraxia. The inability to draw or to put blocks or sticks together. This is often more of a visuospatial deficit than a true apraxia, and it is often produced by lesions from either side of the brain.

Contiguity or Combination Disorder. The difficulty to combine substantive words in a contiguous fashion, as seen in nonfluent Broca's aphasia. This disorder is similar to that of agrammatism.

Coronal. A cut of the brain that is parallel to the face and perpendicular to the lateral view and the horizontal cut.

Cortical Quotient (CQ). The total score on the Western Aphasia Battery, including the nonverbal tests expressed as a percentage of normal.

Crossed Aphasia. A right-handed person who becomes aphasic from a right hemisphere lesion. (The opposite situation—that of a left-handed aphasic with a left-sided lesion—is much more common.)

Cytoarchitectonics. The mapping of regions of the brain according to the neuronal architecture.

Echolalia. The pathological repetition of words.

Fluency. The rate, amount, and quality of language output.

Fluency in Controlled Association. *See* Word Fluency.

Functional Communication. Functional Speech. The communicative value of speech and gestures usually in relation to spontaneous communication and preferably in the natural environment of the patient.

Grammatical Modifiers. Auxiliary or connecting words, pronouns, articles, and prepositions.

Grapheme. Independent units of writing corresponding to phonemes in spoken language.

Homunculus. "A little man" representing a functional map drawn on the cortex, usually from stimulation studies.

Information Content. A measure of the communicative value of a spontaneous speech sample on the WAB.

Ingravescent Aphasia. Mild or latent aphasia, seen at early stages of tumor or with recovery from stroke or trauma.

Isolation Syndrome. Isolation of the speech area from other association areas of the brain. Also called mixed transcortical aphasia.

Literal Paraphasia. Errors representing changes in phonemes (letters). This contrasts with verbal paraphasia, which is the substitution of words.

Major Hemisphere. One of the two cerebral hemispheres that is the more dominant for language; usually the left one.

Mosaicism. Detailed mapping of brain function, sharply delineated on the surface of the brain.

Morpheme. The smallest contrastive unit of grammar that is capable of altering meaning. An example of a "free" morpheme is *boat*. It can stand alone. An example of a "bound" morpheme is *s*. An example of both types of morphemes can be found in *boats*.

Myeloarchitectonics. The mapping of various regions of the brain which myelinize (deposit insulating material on the nerve fibers) at different times.

Neologism. Meaningless words, which are common in jargon aphasia.

Nosology. The study of disease entities.

Operculum. The inside surfaces of the sylvian fissure surrounding the insula (the island of Reil).

Orbitomeatal Line. A line that connects the floor of the orbit with the external auditory meatus on the skull x-ray.

Pallilalia. Pathological repetition of syllables or phonemes.

Paralexia. A reading error. Also a variety of misreading, which is related to spatial neglect or visual field defect.

Paragraphia. Writing errors.

Paraphasia. Speech errors.

Parasagittal. The plane parallel to the front to back axis; usually refers to structures adjacent to the interhemispheric fissure.

Perisylvian. The structures around the sylvian fissure.

Phonematic Aphasia. A disorder similar to "phonetic" disintegration of language. A term used in French literature to designate agrammatism and literal paraphasias in conduction and Broca's aphasia.

Phoneme. The smallest independently pronounced sound of speech that is capable of signaling a difference in meaning. (For example, the word *shoot* has five letters, three phonemes and only one syllable. A letter may represent more than one phoneme, as in *a*).

Phonetic Association. The selecting of a spoken word from an array of similarly sounding words.

Planum Temporale. The triangular portion of the inside of the temporal lip (operculum) of the sylvian fissure behind the primary auditory cortex (Heschl's gyrus).

Procrustean Beds. Henry Head's sarcastic reference to the mythological figure who stretched or shortened his guests to fit his beds. The term refers to categories of aphasia and the efforts to fit patients into them.

Propositional speech. Jackson's term for sentences conveying new ideas in contrast to automatic or emotional speech. The same sentence can represent both propositional and automatic speech, depending on the context.

Prosody. Inflection and melody of speech.

Pseudobulbar Paralysis. Difficulty in speaking or swallowing due to impaired (upper motor neurone) innervation of the bulbar (medullary) centers.

Rolandic Fissure. The central fissure of Rolando, which connects the sylvian fissure with the interhemispheric fissure on the lateral surface of the brain separating the frontal and parietal lobes. It runs obliquely and is difficult to identify at times.

Schizophasia. The jargon produced by psychotics which is similar to, yet distinct from, neologistic jargon aphasia.

Selection or Similarity Disorder. Fluent Aphasia in which the selection of substantive words is impaired and the wrong (paraphasic) choice is often made.

Semantic Disintegration of Language. Wernicke's aphasia and jargon in the French literature.

Simultanagnosia. The failure of recognition of a whole picture at once with some recognition of parts and single features.

Substantive Words. Words that carry the meaning of a sentence: nouns, verbs, adjectives, and adverbs. They are also called content words.

Supramarginal Gyrus. A convolution of the surface of the brain that surrounds the posterior end of the sylvian fissure (*see* Fig. 9−1).

Syntax. The arrangement and relationship of words and morphemes in sentences.

Tachistoscope. An instrument allowing rapid exposure (milliseconds) of visual material.

Taxonomy. The study of classification.

Telegraphic speech. Agrammatical speech without full complement of grammatical modifiers but with the preservation of substantive words.

U-Fibers. Fibers connecting adjacent cortical regions.

Verbal Apraxia. Apraxia of speech. A pure motor but yet central disorder of speech, which is classified more in the realm of aphasia than dysarthria.

Verbal Paraphasia. Semantic paraphasias as manifested by erroneous word substitutions.

Visuographic naming. An exercise which involves writing down the names of visually presented material.

WADA Test. An intracarotid sodium amytal injection, producing temporary aphasia at the side of the language hemisphere.

Watershed Infarct. Anoxic brain damage at the borders between the territories of the main cerebral arteries.

Word Fluency. A test of naming as many items as possible within a category and within a given time. (For example, the naming of all animals within one minute.)

Index

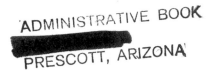